THE GINSENG HUNTER'S NOTEBOOK

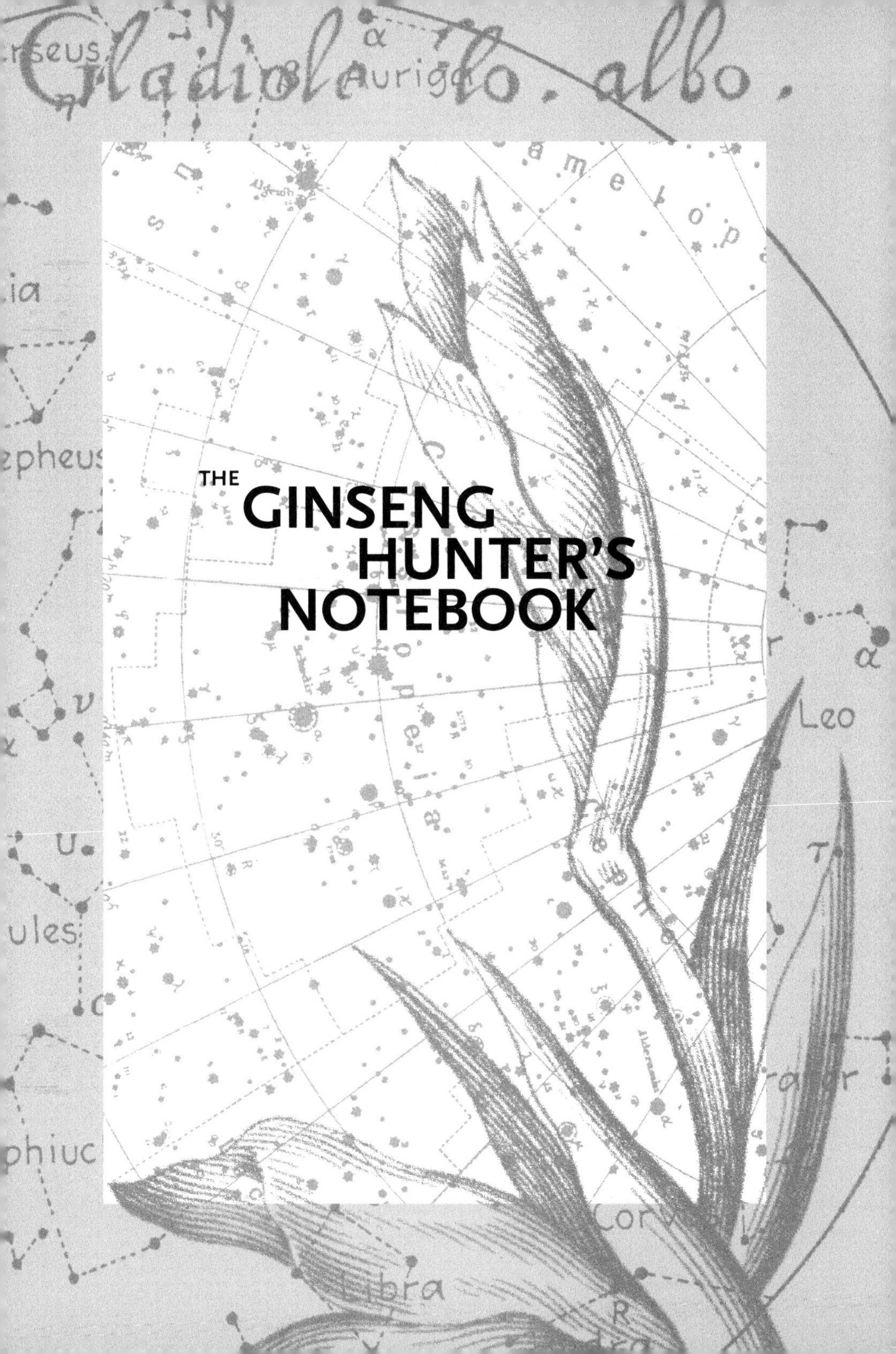

The New Issues Press Poetry Series

The New Issues Press Poetry Series is sponsored by The College of Arts and Sciences, Western Michigan University, Kalamazoo, Michigan

The publication of this book is made possible by a grant from the National Endowment for the Arts.

An Inland Seas Poetry Book

Inland Seas poetry books are supported by a grant from The Michigan Council for Arts and Cultural Affairs.

Printed in the United States of America.

First Edition, 1999.

ISBN: 0-932826-71-7 (cloth)
ISBN: 0-932826-72-5 (paper)

Library of Congress Cataloging-in-Publication Data:
Lundin, Deanne
The Ginseng Hunter's Notebook / Deanne Lundin
Library of Congress Catalog Card Number (98-67449)

Art Direction:	Tricia Hennessy
Design and Photography:	Jef Lear
Production:	Paul Sizer The Design Center, Department of Art College of Fine Arts Western Michigan University
Printing:	Courier Corporation
Illustration of orbits:	From *Mathematical Astronomy for Amateurs* by E.A. Beet. Copyright © 1972. Reprinted by permission of W.W. Norton & Company, Inc.

THE GINSENG HUNTER'S NOTEBOOK

DEANNE LUNDIN

New Issues Press

WESTERN MICHIGAN UNIVERSITY

For all my families and especially for Doris

Contents

Acknowledgements

The Georgia Review: "Shaker Dance"
Prairie Schooner: "Camellias for P," "Fig," "Gladiolus," "Surinam," "Four Thieves Vinegar," "Where the Soul Is"
Third Coast: "The Ginseng Hunter Finds Jimsonweed," "The Ginseng Hunter Explains," "The Ginseng Hunter Lies Down in a Meadow"
Shenandoah: "1001 Nights"
Kenyon Review: "Poppies," "Chicory Seeds"
Colorado Review: "Lycos Search"
Antioch Review: "In This Direction"

Thus when anyone comes to a city which is strange to him, he should thoroughly examine its situation, how it lies with respect to the winds and to the sun's rising; for a city exposed to the north has not the same qualities as one exposed to the south, nor one lying towards the rising sun the same as one turned towards its setting.

Hippocrates

I

Shaker Dance

The visitor pushes the gate and it disappears

into a blue shade through which
dazzle slants in sharp white
lines like envy.

He arrives in his black box
looking for exits.

So much space
offends him.

Here we tilt away from the world

in a different gravity
where motion does not
complete.

So far we do not lie down
but square our bodies
to the ultimate task.

We keep the soul
from flying off on its string of light

though the strain pulls us up
a little each day.

Gesture becomes us.

A knot of fire undoes the hand
and it opens. The shears dip
and flash, and a green smell rises

into the rolled-up morning's
oblique news.

In a little while
the body will unfold
in all its senseless and extravagant delight,

which to the visitor will seem
like silence,

silence and arrested motion.

We call this grace.

The Ginseng Hunter Explains

To what I can't hear I am always listening,

hard as it gets each day
to remember convergence, this leaning

of foxglove over the sage
like a silent alarm: *where is the oak?*

Where is the oak?

Rainwater curls in the hole.
No note from the landlord, "sorry–the city,"

etcetera, "hazard"
and "fine,"–all the usual reasons we give

for not wanting the trouble
of life,

and so on and still endlessly on wheels disaster,
seeding little deaths like money.

Here's where my elbow squares to the door,

every hair points
to the shadow unlocking its suitcase.

Who am I kidding? Really the only
terror we face is the truth about God (Who is Love),

and we know what that means, but we'll never
be able to say it.

Now where the oak spread
its gospel of green between neighbors

there are houses standing apart
without touching: rise, o ghost,

from my door

to that roof in an arc of electric blue,
for I fear

She's forgotten me, root branch and twig.

Saturday 3PM

Bottlebrush bushes explode in a clean impatience,
red bristles soft to the touch. The day's blue
has withdrawn with its glass of iced tea
somewhere beyond the ocean's repeated

gesture of arrival, zipping, unzipping the coast,
which has nothing in common with the cypress
whose pointed hair proves we are still
falling. What connections there are may be blurred,

I admit, never having been sure how the mind
holds a vanishing point in focus
while bleached oak trees waver in a stunned remoteness
of light. We can't go on like this,

discussion is futile, I say, dialing your number,
and *When can I see you again?* throaty
as a cat in heat, leaving my own peculiar
scent among the bouquet of voices

on your scratched, well-used machine.

The Ginseng Hunter Thinks About Oranges in May

A frond does splits
like the eighth-grade cheerleader
whose mother killed off
the competition's mom
with true corporate reasoning,
able to bear looking at horror without blinking
once she accepted the heat
but this

was in Texas, some little town where dear god
hatred is frequently colorless.
Bitter almond

and oranges say all there is to be known
about light, how it struggles
out of its cave where the rock has fallen,
rounding the curve of rock
pocked like an orange. Echo
of red sky. My Florida

never was like this.
Oh we
had our casual killings,
the woman found strangled
on her round satin bed. Anyone
could have told her
what to expect from white satin,
but nobody did. Oranges
remained oranges, and so she died,
fooled by the early light
licking his face like a cat,
missing the truth of his climax,
those hard green elderberry eyes

even the birds won't light on. This
opacity of oranges

surprises a number of people each year
who come to preserve in snapshots
the effects of light shocking water,
and to eat palm dates rolled in coconut
imported like refugees
swimming up from the islands
or down from New York.
Naranja is something my father will never say,
turning his back on Miami and *platanos*,
tending his little grove of oranges.

The Ginseng Hunter Thinks About Oranges in October

Cats are like clocks.
In the window, they tick and whirr to keep traffic moving,
winding the cars in counterpoint

over the sunslicks
and into the candied crunch of leaves.

New air unwraps each appointment successively bitter
or tart. Everything hurries to get. Even my hands

smell like pennies. We know that disasters
are timed events when we hear so much brilliance harden and
swerve
the instant we pull down the shade.

Clouds take us in like manna.
Clouds spit us out.

Winter approaches Lake Tyner, ashamed to be seen in Orlando
as the bloodoranges mass in the grove like malignancies
and memories swell like Billy McPherson
who swims, a drowned face in my dreams, because once
he believed I was wearing a bra and I kept my shirt on,
which is all I regret.

Each day repairs itself, hurricanes pass,
and the neighbors install a new generator.
All they ask is a really deep freeze.

Each night the envelopes steam themselves open.

Each night I rise through the ceiling like rain in ascension
and still have not broken the bottle.

Voulez-vous coucher avec moi was the frenchiest song we knew,
teaching our bodies tricks with the metronome
so that soon we could rinse our teeth clean
in faultless rhythm, timing the sky's
rehearsals of bliss.

Where the Soul Is

Descartes kept his in the pineal gland, safe and convenient. Even when traveling. He always knew where he was. Freud wasn't sure but felt something unusual in the penis, and thought at once of wanderers haunting the steppes, women keening the soul that flew out of them, so many exits you could not guard them all. Some keep their souls in clay jars, the scent of ground cumin and cinnamon spitting in oil, or like Yeats, in a smell of invisible violets. It lurks in a tub of laundry, in Emerson's eye. Socrates thought it had something to do with dryness, thinking perhaps of Lethe, or maybe the weight of light, his soul never happy, twisting itself in a question, kicking its legs. They say Baudelaire kept his in a bottle of wine, Picasso hacked and slashed and tore to let it out. And Beethoven's lived in his ear, just think of those terrible years of separation—or was it enclosure? private garden? festive little parties for two as he roared singing through the fields? A farmer heard him coming, stunned for a moment, was this the devil at last, coming to claim—and quickly dropped his soul, seed by seed, into its rich black holes, just in case. The divine Miss D kept hers in a tiny box. Like Beethoven, there were two of them. Tea and a crumb of blood. But she had that window, a woman's soul can always get out. I used to think my soul was gnomish, home in its hollow stump under the bridge, its sign at the crossroads. Then for a time the killing pace of her long legs covering tundra, hungry and sharp. But last night I heard her tiny hooves clatter in a panic of glee down the dividing street, dim far shriek of tea. If you love something, it's time, say the clocks, and empty, say the baskets, the lamp says, too hot, but I never let her go. She leaves when she wants to, lives where she can. She never tells me anything.

Weathering St. Cloud

Sky breaking for cover
          and finding nowhere to go cherishes clouds
that press us into the mud.
Twisted flowers
                    of spine and mirth.

And then rain   like taking our clothes off after church.

So much of you seems to be there
          and then suddenly drifts.
                                        Stigmata
of shudder and shrug
                    while hugging the one truth tight.

The fragrance of lakewater
purges you even of that.

You open a beer.

East Lake Tohopekaliga stains each minute precisely,
blue herons and anhingas like feathered
extensions of cypress.

You don't think of its name
as an infinite hunger   cries
                                        long flown
in the cry of the birds still echoing
    –ho
        to–
          ho,
    to–
      ho

like a southern mocking of expensive snow.

I keep asking to see the ocean.

I am sure we should not be here where our voices
flit like mosquitoes. Our johnboat threatens to swamp

and I'm bailing away
while you light up a Malboro smiling.

It's called scoliosis. Here, I say, look it up: your back
twists into a question

but you don't trust words, their tricky migrations. They wait at
the airport like gifts from Finland. Letters submerged and rising:
your painful pause before spelling tire—

"t -i -e -r"

and the bark of astonished laughter that wilts
you into your chair like a day-old hyacinth
dried on an oar.

Beneath us reeds rub like paper ripped from a gift and I've nothing
to say but thanks. Gratitude's not what I feel

seeps into every corner I've lived in
awash with the weedy greens
of its shallow deeps

I make an effort: *Don't let disaster*
fool you into thinking
something better has got to be on the way.

And *Get out*
while you still can.

The transfusion begins. My veins open slowly, like lilies.

"Shut up," you hiss and point: swirl of green water.

Mallards rise with the sound of old carpets
and the huge gnarled head
sinks back, disappointed.

And then
clouds

II

In the Roof Garden

Starved blossoms stage a comeback. Drift of
langostina climbs the stairs.
I forget burnt mornings, caffeine-starched and
plumed, vociferous days.
I want to be calm about this. I want to be fair.
I name each pot a remedy: *Plausible, Blemish, Catch, In Sight.*

Rosemary flares its tiny stash of blue as if
blue were an easy thing anyone could do.

Jewel of disasters, my sweet calamity, you are futures trading
themselves for a past unlocking its luggage and scattering
all of it in the street, a clamor of yellow and white,
traffic pumping its flammable blood
at the light, a fury and stench of sadness dressed
in joy, and without you I have no peace.

Herbal Remedies

Juniper

Five o'clock's falling light, crushed from juniper
berries, held in little pockets of ice
the way windows harden against rain,

though the smell of rain keeps falling through
like a voice not heard, but remembered.
Such a slight tree, the juniper, twisted, sparse,

to have become a window, a view of ice
in all its meltings and freezings, rain, ice,
rain—the tongue's window falling on bitter times.

Hard luck, when juniper's light is the light you read by,
seeing in ice juniper's thirst for rain,
while desire falls in at the darkened window,

the window you surely closed. A light
matter. But the smell of *him* falling into every corner:
an icy smell of juniper, laced with rain.

Wild Onions

We think things are fine, little plates on the gold-flecked formica
under control. The sky doles out its visions to the few and the pure,
mostly in New Mexico, while massing its greater effects of fog
for the ones who will need it. Rhapsodies at the sink! Listen:
National Geographic can take us to places they've never been
with only one white man, a camera, and a couple of guides, on
the *Search for the Great Apes* which however long it takes
we know we will find.
                                        And there they are! silverbacked male
gorillas sitting in brine-soaked weeds, munching on shrimp
and wild onions, and aren't you surprised? They'd like us to be
a little surprised about this. How I should like to run my fingers
through your silverfine, savage hair, dripping with onions.

Eyebright

Elsewhere, the days remove layers of doubt
The way new stars confirm our suspicion
That birth is what happens when we are out
Looking for answers. Light from the Pleistocene

Era illumines your eye in its tight fit
At the telescope. Briny little puffs
Of air from the shore leave your mouth
As stray marks of guiltless violence,

Air bleeding smoke into darkness,
Keeping you pure. It's the way bitterness

Cures. Exfoliation. Purge. Blank.
And we become Us, quick as a wink.
Sofabed. One cat. Double sink.

Ginger Snaps

For the will is like a fire, baking each deed as if in a furnace.
Hildegard of Bingen

Fire's easy to mistake, its direction, its speed,
although earthquakes are also confusing. Into the oven
with you, my dear, and the toasty bits will feed
dozens for days. Little hot cross buns.
Olives! Raisins! Vienna sausage, what fun.
Gingerbread studded with everything.
Savor the sharp sweets striking the tongue, sing,
sing like cats in the furnace. Now scream. Rattle
your bones when you dance with me, dance with me,
don't be so coy. They ship the stuff in a tattered
gunny sack, roots like the members a witch gathered
into a tree-nest, as gravely recorded in *Malleus*
Malificarum. Really, come on, snap into it. Dance like it matters.

Garlic Blossom

Gold beats the air with dull rage. Who really gives a fig?
All of my mouth with an   ache. You're the way karma
rolls up its scarf while it's   raining so the punctured scar
lies perfectly hidden   like lives invisibly ill
in plain view. Convince me   it's not fatal. Beautifully
cold cash. Love in a fis   cal swoon on its back

blissfully counting its   blessings which suddenly throb
like your voice in my tune   less ear, in the dried small
offerings of sweet words   out of all passion. And how
sad it all is, anti   septic and pure at the cross-
shunted roads of our days.   Surely we should have smelled its
odious perfume, sending   out flare after flare now:
more sorrow, more hope and   more riddles of guilt to come.

Sowing Basil

(semer le basilic, "to sow basil": to rave)

Semer le basilic the French say faced with
farming another fistful of
basil, raving in parallel rows. *Sacrebleu*
basil to blooming hell and back—

hell, you can hear the hissing of
hard times about to hit hurricane
watch. What you want, what I want
wait in the waves' white warnings.

We line up like licorice, links to the
lasting sweetness of leathery joys.
Bad seeds, reluctant to sprout. De-
spite swamis who whisper blessings

and preachers who pray for peace,
our perfection's delayed. We're impervious.
Worse, we don't worry. War's
for the weak who can't wreak their own

havoc at home. Honey, I've cleaned the
house, I say, holding the poker handy
while you call the cops to come
cart me away. Too late. I'm contagious.

Springtime in Provence, the people
push seedlings in place. They privately
curse the dank clouds, the chill
clods that stick to cold fingers

and everything else about us
I've invented. A woman in Ireland said once
No fuck, no fight; no fight, no fuck.
Parallel pals in the fast track.

Fennel

Gleams in its porcelain. Handfuls. Fistfuls. Pockets
Of sweet seed. Blown like the petals of white

Bougainvillea, seeding the street with its possible
Futures, threading the air that it not detach

From its cities where color is hoarded and sold.
Waiters, in cinnamon glimpses, are bearing me

Dishes of scent I can no longer hold. O sweet
Persian boy, I am stealing your fennel from

Under the register, secretly, charmingly,
Taking it all, there's no hurry, O let the air

Scatter and turn, let the world sweeten
Its teeth for the nightly encounters, flesh in its yielding

Surprises, flesh in its sky-ground hues, and the sky
With its open-mouthed kisses of fennel.

The King Majesty's Excellent Recipe for the Plague

(nutmeg, treacle, and angelica water beaten together)

May 8. Feast of St. Michael the Archangel.

All day the angels cross and recross the street. Only I can see them. One of them offers me nutmeg, the other a toffee. We bow politely. I offer my sleepless nights, and the words of a song I don't understand, something heard once in Latvia from a street-vendor hawking angelica. He didn't know what the words meant, either. Angel Two puts a necklace over my head, made of leaves. I feel the swamps of Florida calling me out on a mission for I shall separate water hemlock from *angelica atropurpurea*, gliding above the stench of things mixing together. All day dark green has infused my vision, the roar of the T dims the street. *You can eat this*, Angel One is saying, or else, *You can beat this*, or possibly, *Two can meet: kiss.* Like the song I don't know. He puts a crown on the head of a boy with his boom box cranked to the max. The bruise slowly widens, the heart slows. It was 1665 and the plague was raging. So was the King. It must be stopped. It is intolerable. Not only what, but how things are mixed, said the witches, and then the physicians, who thought of angelica root like the angels, descending, not as we'd hoped, to heal, but to trouble the waters, descending because we were beaten enough to ask.

Poppies

hum in electric reds: light
hearted

means we see that way
through
music
distant
and too close to hear
without

poppies

listen as the day shuts down
and all things tilt toward
difference

(which is not distinction)

poppies

sway a little
this way
and that

they know how much we want to be
deceived
brilliantly
and without
pity

and so sometimes it pleases them
to tell the truth

a few have heard them
singing

and keep it to themselves

red
is
            not
                        difficult
everyone
believes
                        in
            red

and so the heart

sways a little
                        this way
            and that

and is comforted

III

Magdalena to Her Husband, Balthasar

25 December 1582.

On such a day she writes to him:

The plague, praise God, has again abated with the arrival of
cold weather.

Magdalena, feeling her bones darken, closes the door
against drafts.

She dips her pen, and pauses, sees the raven glide and turn in
sheer extravagant delight.

I too hope, as you write, that God will guide us back together again
in our little garden of joy
and there keep us
together
for a long time.

An opening. A point.
["discover them to be two people in a love-
hate relationship"]

She reaches in, one finger at a time. Wider. Her chest hurts
where a little light drifts.

["with God, their Afflicter
and Redeemer"]

She meant to ask him something, tell him she endures,
and so she writes,

pestilence
broke out
in three houses on our street up by the baker's

and three people died

but this was not the thing she meant to say. She needs more light.
The garden! Of course.

And as she settles there, the blossom falls. Petals in her lap.
I am sending you
with this letter
the flower

"[W]e know little about her life
during the years before her marriage"]

A sign of its virtue: no leaves, no color, no thorns—
but will it last?

["The same may be said for the years
after"]

Bruised, its fragrance chills the air.

It's on its way
to Balthasar.

Chicory Seeds

1809, a cool dawn. Jefferson looks out
on the blue-eyed fields. Rice-paper light.

The letter flares with its secret.

He thinks of Culpeper: for "sore eyes
that are inflamed"
because its eye-blue flowers sleep at night.

Milk from its stem means
chicory extract
"for nurses' breasts that are pained by the abundance of milk."

(Preposterous, the old Puritan, though robbing
the "proud, insulting, domineering
Doctors,

whose wits were born
five hundred years before themselves," rather pleases him:

the *London Pharmacopoeia* into English for anyone since.
The College of Physicians incensed.)

A sweet hot drink that's not coffee, despite
the Liverpudlian merchants
who ground it up small and made beans.

A livid consumer: "The coffee-dealer adulterates
his coffee with chicory, to increase
his profits,

the chicory-dealer adulterates
his chicory with Venetian-red, to please the eye
of the coffee-dealer;

the Venetian-red dealer grinds up his color
with brick dust,

that by his greater cheapness,
and the variety of shades he offers, he may secure

the patronage of the trade in chicory."

1795: *[A] tolerable sallad for the table*, Jefferson writes
to George W., advised to get some without
delay.

Fourteen years later, President Jefferson "revealed
to be in contact
with the duplicitous British,"

tips his answer
into a cool dry hand:

at last, chicory seeds for George!

He smiles at the confounded patriots
and pockets their pink faces.

At Monticello days gather differently,
eight by eight,

until he is alone in a strange room.

No one has been here before. The walls like cream.
The honey floor.

Pirated from eternity.
Pieces of eight! Pieces of eight!

The seeds in the envelope wait.

Flowers that spread wildly like summer raids,
the ice blue eyes of Viking ghosts
who know this place to be rich.

The clock descends through the floor
and time carries on
its secret work.

Under his feet a new hour blooms.

Tendrils, without roots, like the others.
Duplicitous.

Galen On the Anatomy: Lesson One

Here are the body's principal organs:

heart
brain
liver
testicles

The heart is a tiny sun drying
the body's amnesia: humidity

causes the soul to forget
what it formerly knew.

So, like a cipher, the pulse ebbs
and flows in its right equation,

secretly telling the days of life.
When we produce by means

of food and drink a good bodily
temperament (*eucrasia*), we thereby

influence the soul towards goodness,
(though do not forget the brain,

for here in the brain rise the nerves
like fountains. They lift and spill

downward from silence. They carry
the soul in its sheath of light.)

Of the liver, Zeno is reported to have said
that he was affected by wine

just as are bitter lupines when soaked
in water. Likewise, when the testicles are heavy

the nerves will stretch like a harpstring
aiming itself at an unseen wound.

But why, when the body is excessively
chilled or overheated, does the soul

definitely leave it? After much search
I have not found out why.

Fig

Elizabeth Blackwell to Alexander Blackwell
September, 1736. The Society of Apothecaries Garden.

My love, though you have driven me to such
intemperate means of living apart
from you, almost in exile, among herbs
and plants of physick, I do bless your poor
habits with such poor praise as best I can
in early morning pilgrimage to cut
new purses, fat and green, among my plants.

My little house in Swan Walk seems to me
the kindest reference to my gosling state
on point of transformation: a lady once
of no ambition, now my secret heart
flares to green fire, my philosopher's stone
alive, new buds and shortly, now, new fruit.

O see how changed I am! that mix of things
seems no more curious than the muddy spring
from which decay we blossom—dear Blackwell,
your dainty girl's a dirty one. This day
one fool said, *milady apothecary*
as I pas't, all in contempt, but I bowed
and smiled sweetly. A fig, if I may say—

and so I chose this afternoon to draw
the charming fig, and find a perfect five-
point leaf spread like a bright concealing hand
across the secret places of our lives,
and, if we've heard the story right, across
the secret places of our first parents;

but lest you think I do descend too far,
remember had she never sinned, Eva
never had been Ave. These things I thought
as I slit open one ripe purple fig,
the wrinkled purse of its velvet skin
filling the palm of my hand, its sticky
seeds so many, packed so close together,
it seemed I held the fruit of paradise,
and felt my woman's spirit rise and eat.

Surinam

Maria Sybilla Merien, artist on a 1699 expedition to Surinam

Dolphins cleave the uncut waters, green as jade from Surinam.
They send me this vision: all roads lead away from Surinam.

Not morning yet, I walk the sea-sprayed deck, a brush
That swells with wet and thunderous grays, too far from Surinam.

Do you think loss is only personal? No doubt it is.
I crouch on English rocks, I gather bitter waves from Surinam.

In the studio, sick and pale, I cut and eat a crust of scarlet
Kept for fever, chills & blindness—in short, in case of Surinam.

Nothing works. My husband's dull, the servants deaf,
And I am mute, because my thoughts are phrased in Surinam.

I copy leaves that burn, entanglements of tendrils, fronds along
The sea-shed sand, creased like a letter. It arrives, erased,
from Surinam.

Faint wash of sky. You shrug: your coat seems tight. Come close—
No. Closer. Ah, you see? Like that, the palm trees sway in Surinam.

Words fall dead as money. Pocket of grief, stain of joy. On the pure
Page, shrubby scratches. There is no place called Surinam.

So now, Maria, sybil of Christians, choose the colors—saffron, lapis,
Cochineal—which tell (like news heard in a shell) the days
of Surinam.

When I die, you will see I told the truth. Unfold the skin,
Unwall the heart. You'll find it burning still, the way to Surinam.

Violet Crossing

Collecting seeds in Russia, near the Chinese border

Near the border
feral cliffs swim
in sea fog, pinned
to the edge with

tall fragrant pines.
We crawl through grass
like spies looking
for secret maps.

An outhouse, then—
the only one
in four long miles
of nothing else

but cloud, fog, cliff
where Russia meets
China, and both
suspect the worst,

as we suspect
them both. And as
I close the door
of the outhouse,

I step onto
sweet Russian grass,
starred with Manchur-
ian violets.

Gladiolus

John Tradescant the Younger to Dr. Parkinson
24 July 1642. The Barbary Coast.

Huge
bowl beaten to
shine and froth,
its light
the flaming sword
of eden—azure,
lapis, turquoise,
sapphire, none of
them has told it
right; we lean into
the spray that
stings and scours
our eyes because
the warning is
merciful—it is true
we cannot survive
paradise,
or truthfully, I
think the English
can't, unless you
count the suet
pudding of a sky
and sea we
long for, haven,
miracle enough to
burn the vision
out of me, already
spent with looking:
just this morning

(the coast a glare
behind us now)
some two or three
of us strolled
out of camp to see
the second warning
rise up in a field
of thousands—
stiff green towers
scissoring the
wind, *xiphon*,
corn-flag
fluttering,
glad-sword, sky-
blood, tribe of
spears bearing flowers.

The Ginseng Hunter Finds Jimsonweed

I am considering how to send back to you

days without rage, clouds folded,
rain in jars, still falling,

when the singular bell of jimsonweed calls me

to its fifteen minutes of fame
like a muezzin's promise of joy,

bruised edge of each sprung petal
bleeding inward,

then wider, deeper, a fragrant throat tilts
and the night bends down,

a cricket shirs—everything casts its fate
into the itch of twilight.

"Venus is afflicted," my astrologer told me,
"Your love affairs will be troubled,"

but I say jimsonweed burns,

I say maybe
we have fewer choices than we think,

only a slow and tentative
slip of green

trembling toward the light while night blossoms.

The best I can do is stay away.

Lemon Grass

Poirot sits calmly, expecting disaster, and Miss Lemon
Fetches it for him—letter (from Russia? Imperial seal?),
Though it's barely seven hundred years since Temujin

Rode into his vision (dropping his whip as he yields
to a sea of wildgrass : scimitars swimming in light!
crying *here you must bury me*)—and Europe reeled

Into the new world, its own vision melting to sight
In a yellow wildfire six thousand miles from the heaven
Of prairie. Ah, but the new world spreads like a blight

Microscopically into white pages, crisp and even,
Where Poirot, that clever little dick, is still combing
His Belgian moustaches, curiously tasting of lemon.

Three Wise Men Seek the Emblem of Life in a Jar of Vinegar

(a tale from the Book of Tea)

They found the jar at last, nippling the hill.
Confucious waved and the caravan stopped.

Tents of blue silk. Green hush. They sat still
for eight days, and then he climbed to the top.

Ah, what a ripeness! he dipped in a finger. "Swill!"
he cried, staggering back. "Grief is less sharp!"

He gave way to Sakyamuni. "Friend, I now will
discover the truth." Alas, disappointment! Bitter as hops!

Laotse approached and said with a charming smile:
"Can this be? Such nectar!" and he drank it all up.

And they went away. But around the empty jar on the hill
the wild sage grew up in three colors, a most philosophical crop.

Four Thieves Vinegar

(Four thieves, sentenced to carrying away victims of the plague in Paris, reputedly drank a mixture of vinegar and garlic, and to this attributed their escape from contagion.)

Stench and sting of the fires. Morning a dim of ash. Evening a
starless fog.

It is good for ye burning heat of ye head.

"I've stolen nothing," the first thief objected. "Your words or
mine, who'd know?"
He poured a libation over his skull.

"I have a terrible memory," said number two. "I confess to
remembering everything."
He took up the bottle and drank.

Vinegar doth raise an appetite.
And being supped up it casteth out leeches that were drank.

"I have lived without faith for so long," said the third, "I've
begun to have doubts."
He sprinkled a few drops over the flames.

And being gargarized restraineth also ye fluxes in ye throat.

The last thief, who never spoke, said
the usual thing,

And they picked up the dead woman and carried her to the fires.

That the Character of the Soul Depends Upon the Constitution of the Body

> *[T]here are three kinds of soul: one is located in the liver,*
> *another in the heart, and another in the brain.*
> Galen

credo
The mouth being small tells you nothing. A secret
holds. Lips cling together

in thin resistance to flesh and air.
Say it's not so.

Didn't you swallow something you shouldn't?

Fat seals, you know
what she paid for *those* lips.

Don't take my word for it. Make up your own.

kyrie
First there is light. You think it is whole
and pure, and you bathe your face in
its unfiltered truth. Then you learn

about clouds, about ions, about the whole
chaos of sky and the way it lied

about who's in charge.

Splinters. Clots.
Division begins its work by subtraction.

That day the sky breaks over you like an ornament

and you hear a voice saying, "The shards
work their way into the heart,

but you won't know the day
or the hour." At this point you even give up
the organic hash.

One late afternoon on your way to the ocean
you look over Hollywood's hills to the shock

of a pale green fissure of sky
small as a catscratch, a slit so fragile

only the delicate bones of birds
can take in its meaning.

Here is one you invent:

You don't have to live
without mercy.

ave
Once Leonardo had marred its
perfection he abandoned

the stone
to that blockhead, Buonarotti,

and went back to flying machines,
goes the legend. Dark center

of bells swung on the thighs
like a shout

only the stone-mason heard.

Down from the shoulder the arm
like a cloak

unfolds
to the tender wrist

and the fingers curled under
in shadow as if

what he hides there
could save us.

Light creeps into its hollow.

Can't you smell it from here? Terror
tangles the air

in its soft gray fist. Let the head
take care

of itself, there's no help
for the rest of him working the hollow again

and again,

where God put his burning finger on Jacob
throwing him out of joint,

to keep him
from running away.

IV

Orange Bang

April's a hat made of rain and an anchor of cloud.

The Santa Monica sea waves goodby and goes back to its sewing.

I bought a small quilt by the pier, it was covered with ants
bearing needles.

Some of us feel this way and some of us that, but mostly
otherwise.

He said, Just who do you think you are, and I said, Exactly.

They sent me a small brown scrap as the proof that my box had
exploded.

Such an agreeable color, like snails sliding over leaves.

I have reassembled my life in another body, one without sin.

In another city, inside a tunnel of wind.

Arrival

The hill dips down, banking its final descent
as we hope for a pleasant stay

here in the Los Angeles region, or wherever
our final destination may be. Lies spent,

teeth cleaned, fingernails swabbed in palmolive,
a dark gray trail of disaster lights my way

back to a difference of lying, one sliver
a day until anything's easy to forgive. A spray

of mistletoe takes on an aura, though never
that sibilant crisp of leaves underfoot.

The old priest cuts the emblem of life
from its vampiric hold on an oak. I'm saying

nothing to love. She still can't sever
sadness from bliss, though she's good with a knife.

In this Direction

> *This is a beautiful country. I have not cast my eyes over it before, that is, in this direction.*
>
> —John Brown, December 2, 1859

Blossom and Meg take the Hollywood Line,
two girls heading west. The American dream's
gone funny somehow—Blossom, in green
fatigues and cowboy boots

has that pinched look around the waist
as if God, feeling peevish, was closing his fist
when it seemed more amusing, a nice twist,
to make Blossom a man

with expensive tastes in nylon and hats.
Across from our bus stop, at Parkman and Sunset,
two cops have arrested a black man who wanted
I remember a double espresso

and make it quick. A middleaged king
in exile, he stands there, maybe thinking
of how long it will be, years of thin
burnt water, refuting

the very idea of *coffee*, while they snap
on the cuffs. Meanwhile Meg is happy
just to be seen with Blossom on a trip,
with the rapt fan's

attentive crossing of legs, the cigarette
flicked with a casual consequence, wet
lips pursed. But she'll never get
that perfectly bored expression

only the rich can acquire,
the ones who have already met desire
and passed through, possibly wiser,
free to take any direction.

Dinner at the Reel Inn

Malibu feels like an old shoe tonight,
leathery, dark, invisibly
smelling of seaweed. Too much sand.
No vacancy at the Topanga Ranch Motel,
but who's staying? You got out
your atlas, and talked about heading east.
We figured the Grand Canyon had to be somewhere
south of Nebraska, but was it in Utah? Arizona?
and then the Badlands, Dinosaur National Monument —

Postcards arrive like news
from a star no longer living.

You thought it took years
to reach the point of departure,
nerves unfolding like sea anemones
dancing to Brahms, but it's only
a phone call, a letter, the hand
on your shoulder, and everything
falls away, bad burritos, the Novel Café,
the shag-headed man in his sandy blanket,

and L.A.'s flatter, brighter,
thinner than ever, its mind
pressed over yours like a re-run
of *Vertigo*, wanting to keep you blonde
and vulnerable, plucking you
out of the harbor, not letting you go,
not letting you leave forever.
But you do.

The blackened nerves of America
wave, beckoning onward, and the day
shifts into reverse.

A Thousand and One Nights

Kay Nielsen , Illustrator (1886-1957)

Return to Copenhagen from Hollywood, California, 1938

Wherever I look, bleakness: somehow it suits me,
the blank sky, the scrawled water, rubbed hills.
When the snows arrive I remember the hills
in Hollywood, glutted with tired flowers, the sea

breaking and breaking, its wet foamed frills
like the abandoned gown of Scheherazade, trying
to get back to her. What for? We both can rely
on illusion, but only in darkness or snow will the spells

finish their dangerous beauties—against sky
are the clouds set forever, unmaking their perfect
faces, their jeweled thighs, formed and wrecked
by the same mouth. Slender and unafraid I

made her, the curve of her back a crescent,
the curve of her hand outstretched in the story's
vision, her ornamental king slumped in mysterious
yielding before her pale body. What I meant,

what I wanted to say there by the sign of her knees
bare and commanding I no longer remember.
Something to do though with power and trembling,
with love and its endings, with brave-told lies.

Is

(on The Fall of Troy, Romare Bearden, 1974)

for two voices

i.
halves and crosses,
night-smoke,
totem-faced building
white metal horse and
green fishes
helen a burntout
lap becomes a pier-
brown robe: three
sing (*laudant, laudamus*) to
siva who rises
phoenix: life out of ash

ii.
two sides of any story:
green morning
shakes red dreadlocks, a brilliant
cerulean eye that sees
above lapis lazuli water
shade whose
cross unfolding
black warriors they
praise him,
life out of ashes
(*est*): sing, for he

Is.

Camellias for P

(named for Georg Josef Kamel, Moravian Jesuit missionary, 1706)

Camellias, unexpected, garish
as the bright pink kneesocks
Mrs. Eichelberger wears
on Sundays when she walks

to church, despite the best advice
of neighbors (not quite friends)
seem undecipherable, the petals
frilled and heavy, dense

with color. Everything expands
except camellias. And yet
the scent—a fresh and rainy smell,
so light, so delicate.

Bent above his graftings, Father
Kamel checks for buds,
for signs of chaos channeled into life.
Patience. Water. Mud.

The tree releases blooms the way
old ladies lose their gloves,
address books, everything except
the memory of old loves.

Some five or six are floating in a bowl
of water. When he knew
that he'd invented these peculiar
Slavic, brilliant jewels,

he picked the lot and scattered them
about the feet of Christ
(but named them for himself). Old love,
will you and I survive

the yellow cat who won't come in
but cries at 3 a.m.
for someone who will not come out?
Below, a window slams

resentfully. The one good eye of darkness
blurs, enlarges, focuses
his outline on the stairs, the whiskers
twitching as he pokes

the slit of warm air underneath
the door. Since I know what's not
fastened tends to drift, I hold
my head. Another shot

of Robitussin. Back to bed.
You're in your second sleep
by now, will fling an arm across
my pillow, drifting deep

as the snow I think of sometimes
covering camellias.

A Norman Milkmaid at Greville

(Jean-Francois Millet, 1871)

i.
Nothing much to see, a girl staggering
down a footpath in 1871. Greville
is far behind her now, the dairy
one small slash of white
floating in a far green sea.

What's all that to the distance
between us? I can't imagine
her desires beneath the dark warmth of cattle,
scarfed head pressed into all that dusty hide
with the rhythm of the downpull
and the steam rising from the still-cold buckets.

Now she leans before me: hip thrust out
to balance that awkward shuffle,
two thongs looped around her arm
and drifting hand, basket on her shoulder
full of milk smoking in the chill.
How many layers, three? Four?
wrapped around her feet—
or are those wooden shoes?

Dark dark the receding light—
blooming or tightening, I can't tell which.

ii.
What's missing then, what seems
beyond us? Grief? Nothing so intense.
Only gray-flocked canvas, chunks of blue,
a weary resignation, walking dreams . . .
the edge of moor there. *That* seems immense.

iii.
Thirty first-graders crowd the room,
silent as sparrows stunned by a wall of glass.

The teacher gestures toward a painting
filled with garnet and emerald green,
a pheasant cock hanging by a bowl of grapes

and golden candelabras, red cabbage
exposing its heart in frilled edges,
the very splinters in a wooden crate
of ripe tomatoes—ecstatic—!

Do you see anything moving
in this painting? asks the teacher.

A small girl raises her hand.
The peach is rolling across the table.

No, no, smiles the teacher, a little tightly.
This is what we call a Still Life.
The twenty-nine children nudge each other,
grinning, and the group moves on.

She stands there, watching the peach roll,
so brilliant in light it burns the cheeks.

iv.
—all of her body in shadow
eyes closing, mouth askew

as if a Mardi Gras had passed her on the road
and left her still asleep.

Light is approaching, but she faces
into darkness, she is struggling
towards us.

v.

Across the room old Satan marks
her progress. Minutes bronze
and gather in his wings. But she bores him,
they all bore him, no vision anymore,
no grand ambition!
He'd welcome
any kind of challenge—
except aesthetic, which bores him also.

And now the rage is all for dissolution.

Boring.

A glance at the girl again, the bruises
meant for eyes. A stifled sigh.
Oh yes the way
is difficult, torturous even,
but she'll arrive.

vi.

A sharp smell pricks the air,
a shudder of instinct—not felt that
for years! He can't move his head,
neck stiff with centuries of boredom,
but the gaze of him flames out—
a young child stares into that inward flaring socket,
mutely, mildly curious, eating a peach.

Vampire Movies

He was Panama black, "like a hat," he said, saving
his Spanish for later. He did wear his life
at an angle.

I am he tells me the white
goddess he's always wanted.
Perfect. Even the shape of betrayal

looks good from this distance
and my throat tilts like a spilled drink.

We rent *Nosferatu* because it reminds him of home.
"He's the proof that everything rises."

I count the moments.

Black scowl and a little hat.
Big teeth.
Dear terror
I think I'm in love with you.

(*the cats, also—*
they twist their fur in one another's cries
at the swerve of his smile)

No, I'm wrong: that was Mina
fastened to Dracula's breast like an infant.

(curtains would sleep   between us   like windows held still
in the hush of snow.   we were always
astonished by so much sky

which could part cities and not be used up)

Kiss my ear the way Mary caught God
as he tenderly parted the waves of her hair like water

flooding her bones with joy

and I am beside myself.
O rose, I am sick.

There goes the count, hugging his little coffin
since beds are so unreliable.

His legs scissor past. I feel kindly towards him.
I hope he gets something to eat.

Meanwhile redemption sweeps through our lives
like a plague

though I cherish a reasonable doubt. Think of who lingers,

who hangs back, who waits. What twists in the eye's designs.
Who answers the phone still wet and keeps talking.

Who turns off its ring.

It is more dangerous than you think,
whispers Dracula. He takes the razor away for a quick snack.

(music crackles like new life
in his fingertips
sheering

the map of nerves from my skin

which he doesn't need he knows
where he's going)

How can I hate him? Love's ruthless as death in its delicate timing:
the brush of his hand
across years as I open the door,
the strange
independence of shadows.

Like stopping for supper, we don't ask why
but when.

Día de los Muertos

Unsafe, this stagger of morning.

I pause at the door
like a thick loaf raisined with sleep

on the cusp of disquiet, the dead oven's
lip of doom—

or the lisp? all hard edges dissolving in mist,
the cup disappearing in steam,

the flat man
stuttering up the driveway with three bags
belching cans,

fixed shine in the eyes that flicker over
me turning the key in my door,
            flicker and slide,

my outline slick as a postcard of Kobe, Japan,
and about as expected,

while the fog spirits us each away.

Yellow cellophane leaves. White paste of sky.

A cold pale light
ghosting everywhere, charmed

by our pulsing bodies that tremble in stillness,
stumble and wheeze,

as we go out to meet it.

Getting Away In South Kerry

On the road to Tralee we pass hedges cunningly planted
to look like L.A. Store fronts wink
and go out.

The same faces fold up like wallets.

In the evening gold shadows leaf through his hair
though he feels no wind.

It's a trick I have.

I follow him in from the dingle where shale spits foam
in a storm of light all the tourists think
is a dangling key.

Then we see the bruise dimpling across the water.

We gasp as the sky rolls up and I can't find
the camera. Over the tidal basin stars hatch
and fly up like cinders.

Everyone said, Nothing's as good as finally getting away.

What rosy curls! He talks about fish and his friends
in Laguna. It's been so long, he'd like to see them,
but where would he stay?

Dark pours into my glass in a slow wave of panic.
The moon ignites.

My ribs open like fingers and wait for what happens.

His voice swims in the mirror dissolving
around my fist.

I can feel my hips sparkling as they tune up and then my body shrinks to a mouth.

I think I shall sing.

At last, I think, life! Now
I'm getting somewhere.

V

Lycos Search: [Adoptions: Not found. Replace with?]

[?adopt]

L. se alicui adoptare (Obs.)
We are made sons of God by adoption
As Chickens are hatcht at Grand Cairo by the Adoption
of an Oven.

Thus we have adopted the modern German names
of several rocks and minerals, as *gneiss*, *hornblende*,
quartz, and *nickel*.

The Spirit itself, that is the Spirit of Adoption,
which Christians receive,
is one Witness
I had rather adopt a child than get it.

To approve, to confirm, then,

I propose that the report and accounts be adopted
which [words] must depend for their adoption
on the suffrage of futurity:
L. fac ramam ramus adoptet, as Ovid says, (Obs.)
or as Holland when he read Pliny in 1601,

"Fit one [vine stocke] to the other, ioyning pith
to pith, and then binding them fast together so close that no
aire may enter
between, vntill such time as the one hath adopted
the other."

[?adorn with pictures]

Now according to the 1959 reprint of a 1934 translation of
De Materia Medica which presents a Greek work of the first
century as understood in Hampshire in the [1500's] illustrated
by a Byzantine artist in AD 512 for presentation to the daughter
of Anicius Olybrius who was Emperor of the West in 472
(the drawings learned from "originals . . . not far removed
from sketches by the famous Crateus, whose plant-descriptions
are occasionally quoted in the text")

we are less likely to invent than to mistake,

[?adore]
    and so I bless

the Nestorians, who first believed, in error, that the son
of God was only by Adoption,

    and I bless

the pictures, which as Pliny warns,
are deceitfull; in representing such a number of colours,
and especially representing the lively
hew of Hearbs according to their nature as they grow,

no marvell if they that limned and drew them out, did fail
and degenerat from the first pattern and
originall, and as in error they misunderstood
the wanderings of each plant
from its picture, *for they change*
and alter their form and
shape every quarter of the year, depending on the place in which
the root
of their deviance may be found,

[?adulterate]

and I bless

the figures which seem hopeless of interpretation,
for they are printed in the hope that
field-botanists when traveling in the special localities whence
the Dioscoridean flora was derived, may thus recognize
a few of the plants which through mistaken
features it has been impossible to identify in an herbarium
of dried plants,

for so these imperfect identifications stimulate by their falsity
the production of a revised version

and I bless

the Gnostics, also Adoptionists who formed, in error,
the division of the cosmos into spiraled chambers reached
by strange enchanted turnings between light
and darkness, stairs that wind
the spirit up its thread

and I bless

the woman who believed herself incapable of love
and so chose for herself the sergeant whose red hair burnt her
husband to a crisp
when she mistook him as my father
(for I have no father, and have never had)

and thus I bless

the air which fills my body in its rising
and descent,
and I adore the strange digressions of my life
adorned with pictures
from the error of her ways.

Speech in Five Acts

on meeting a birthmother

Mariposa, California.

[genitive]

expensive elsewhere, your hunger kisses its bowl of ink, you would do anything, anything so i'd lie down in this brown clench of hills and forget i was going or thinking of someplace unherded or held. why bother? poor i was born, a chipped plate and a fork full of dents, i am here now, subside, desist, i lie down and i claim my inheritance, blade by blade.

[subjunctive]

coolie in blue jeans, coolie in sweet grass yellow in august, coolie rocks. if a coolie in blue jeans were willing to wear a hat made of sweet grass, the hungry, riddled yellow, itching and harrowed, the fitful grass in august to get to the other side. of these rocks

[dative]

what do you bring the lilies? there is to be sparing of the lilies. to the lilies it will be pleasing. from this we augur days and fallows, the anhinga ruptures the lake, though the wound is made small, almost invisible. it seeps there, in water, among the lilies. would you please send me your catalog of lilies.

[relative]

weed me, o night, i am wracked with green. i spit like a cricket, i rise in a whir of wings thinner than candlelight shining through fingers—grasshoppers, my cousins, embrace your lost defect, do not despise what you know, my familiars are strange to me now, and why should you not be familiar? though they waver, their edges corrupt with joy, white stones scattered like stars in a lunar panic of grass.

[imperative]

blue shards brilliant and sharp as a child who owns nothing, and vast it is. lunatic fringe of sky, what have you to say? too much and too little, the back of a dress too small on a fat man, trees tightened up into knots on the puckered fields. let's hurry boys. aren't the boys hurrying? let us not stay at home. he is one who. when we have gone down into italy, the romans will not be able to resist us. there is no one who. there is nothing that. the snow is so deep i can scarcely walk. do not trust the gauls. they will certainly betray you. let us not stay at home. when the parrot had died, corinna was very sad. o nine times terrible, bless me, my mothers, for i am singed.

Hymn for a Birthmother

I.

She is the voice in the wilderness crying.

She is not prepared.

She is the shadow of legs crossing the light like a fan.

She is the ultraviolet message to bees.

She is on her way.

She is the neon hinge of night.

She is the window closing.

She is the lawnchair's last warm curve.

She is the one who looked back.

She is the mouth forming *o*.

She is the panic of waves.

II.

I am the tongue that will lick her clean.

I am the wound that will not grieve.

I am the broken needle in her arm.

I am the light that travels too slowly to see.

I am the hiss in the sand.

I am the red stone considering fire.

I am the circle she walks inside.

I am the crow that walks there with her.

I am the sidewalk telling news.

I am the crooked sign on the last hotel that says *no*.

I am the one that got away.

Hole

Her hands raw in the wound-up days sprung loose,
that baffled whir of time she ignores
easy as a once-aching tooth dangling on a
thread (*gawd*, *Myrtle*, and she'd just smile, digging out onions,
another hole never hurt nobody)
which might explain how a place so flat and basically holeless
could get to be called a hole,
as in no-water-hole,
dust-hole,
black hole of whatever,
the whole enchilada of holes,
and so it was a kind of mission to make a few more holes
for the relief of other folk trapped in this two-dimensional
pitiless cartoon of a hole
nothing but gophers and onions could ever get out of,
not even the daughter who stands there like a worn-down penny
in the last rub of light, saying *i gotta get outa here*,
i want my own life, saying, *i wanta be somethin*,
so she don't even look up
at the bite of that hole going in because no matter what
she knows she won't be left here for long all alone
with six babies and two half-grown,
because sometimes what seems like an empty hole
turns out to have plenty going for it after all
and anyway, she thinks, turning the black dirt over
and punching a place for the seed,
that's the way of holes, sometimes you stand there for a long
time at the edge
before dropping a stone to see how far—
but the girl ain't that kind, she won't fall through,
she's the kind so afraid of the hole she'll carry it everywhere,
shooting up in her chest like an onion, pungent and thin
till they smell her coming and know she's a child of the hole,
until dread finally rivets her gaze and she learns to dig.

Gingkos

November undoes Division Street—
a derangement of trees

like so many broken music stands

freed to an improvised
scat of days,

each maple's last spray of red
a trash of wet noise.

Zero weather
closes in.

Night pocked with predictable stars,

familiar feint of rain,
all the same dead words underfoot,

the tiring maples blink their red alerts in the margin,
"Details! Explain! Develop!"

but no one listens. How can we, cast
in the passive voice of winter?

And then without warning a scribble of sky bends
childishly close,

the maples twirl their last rags of confetti

and all down the street
gingkos rattle their still-green leaves

like old money
thrown in a fit of joy to the poor.

Time Piece

I know what time is, but if someone asks me, I cannot tell him.
— St. Augustine

[relativity]

The genes tell nothing of all this sparkle, the mist and forgotten teeth and the trinkets of blood. They give nothing away. They are into preserving. You might think a judgment belongs. You might think an airy dismissal. One of the stories my genes unzip: you are not wrong to love a fraud. So long as you do not kiss him. Then it is oola la trouble in paradise, out of your garden and into the jungle. But the fraudspawn is something else, button of jelly topping the foam. It will find you when least. You expect it. And then the unravelling. Does not connect to new twisting, the wrist in its packet of bruise, the chest with its telltale crack, the rerouted flow. Not. Yet

[escapement]

Out to the movies, a dinner for two, we touch but we do not join. We roll up together, finite but no boundaries or edges, so how can we touch? Slide and glissando. Fingernails bleeding. Tip of the finger to all that. It's just you and me baby so don't you forget it, I know where you live. Inside me she keeps expanding but finds no leak and no finish, she does not remember this meadow, though something about the crepuscular slither of ocean reminds her of something she knew once, when all that she knew was nothing. Escapement, that brief interruption, the tick. And release. Of a watch. Going. Around. And around. Interruption advances the truth.

[water clock]

Weight of "I know" follows "I think" in a fluid circle, dip and rise of the soul. Sometimes a balloon, giddy and red, and then two, they expand and deflate together. Each side has something to offer, heart, kidney, ovary, track of the belly. Ins and outs. Is everything locked and shut off? Beware of the enemy you don't know means including you. Now I uncurl from looking. I am unfolding my fists. Dear enemy, face I own, father I never will, militant rage I exact your obedience. Wash me and I shall be. Neither will I fear. When courage falls, the night will get up. It will strike, and the nerves will hear it. Pain has a beautiful sound. Exquisite.

[transitive]

Einstein snagging himself again on the same damn nail which will not be hammered or pulled. It is absurd. It is not a reasonable nail. It hangs there, in nothing, serene. He knows about time. He knows about space. He is not sure nothing can be known for certain. "Contradictory," he writes Bohr, "to every idea of reality that is reasonable," so probably true and contagious. Those of us who escape always think there's a reason. Those of us who do not know there is. Shrapnel and zinfandel, we drink to the town we were almost in and the child gives up his blasted eye. Leap of fate, act of will. He thinks of it rolling in heaven, watching the places he's never been. O now he will see, he will know in time. Where are we going. We have always been here.

Tea

(Japanese Tea Room, University of Michigan Art Museum)

a stone turns into a step
at the child-high door

it is like my life
opaque and miraculous

poised at a rabbit hole

door i must bow myself
door i must creep

the scroll on the wall explains everything
differently each time

o riches of here and be

not is a tight word
nothing undoes it

impossible little room
you are open

without fear of business

i lean on your missing walls each day
i lean on your slit of light

i see into the nothing you hold exact
and precarious

on the tokonoma
three sprays of orchid

a petal clings

like the last good man

like the slipshod grace of backbone
curved in a hiss

unable to speak or unclench

door i am not permitted to enter
until i am light as a shadow

although my head is an echo
my heart is a pocket

my pocket a tunnel of sighs

i am a pitcher
without water

cup without tea

o little room let me in
i have already

lost the way

The Ginseng Hunter Lies Down In a Meadow

I love the sky which is not the color of grief.
If there is an argument, it is an old argument

sky carries on with itself and has nothing to do with us.
It says nothing of the life I was going to live, back then,

before I understood there is no future, only
a kind of forward wash carried out of the last act

I thought could be changed in time to prevent its arrival.
When sky is this confused we call it rain

and go in for the day. Among its stars not one
fails for lack of vision, its light rubbed thin

on a cinderblock, only another long narrow box
for keeping us out of each other's lives

as if all it took were walls. Stars fall out
of their places because it is time to go but nobody

locks the door behind them or sends on the mail.
Sky rearranges no mirrors and tells no lies

about what it was thinking when you met
its gaze for the last time over coffee

and foam which obscured the muted underlight
of the throat swallowing. The sparrow has no more space

than the hawk to dive and roll and sky touches
neither but hovers there distant and still imperceptibly

present, though if you have enough little bits of sky
heaped together it glows or streaks or ignites

without purpose. Sky can be wounded
but does not heal like the skin we mistake it for.

There is a language of moisture and heat but when sky
makes a point it does not invite dialogue.

I love the sky which takes no prisoners. It kills
like an elephant no longer able to restrain its itch

and so whole jungles and villages are trampled in something
that looks like rage but is only relief, for sky

does not roll itself up or reveal a long sweet curve
of leg emerging from water, neither stretching nor leaning

nor any other thing the leg may do, and so
we search sky daily for signs of our lost selves as if

so much indifference must surely hide something, and where
else could all that feeling have gone? But sky isn't even

indifferent. It tells us no more than the wind, which is not
the sound of something tearing a long way off,

or a cough, or a sigh of bewilderment. The sky I love
is the sky that is not suffused with faith or delusion

or joy or poignant arousal shaped like a new
understanding of sadness, and this is the sky I look for

now without ceasing, the way ivy creeps
toward the light, but to tell you the truth I have yet to see it.

Notes

Weathering St. Cloud: For Jim Lundin. St. Cloud is a small town south of Kissimmee, Florida, where a bizarre rash of tornados struck during the 1998 El Niño.

In the Roof Garden: For Elisabeth Frost and Derek Hackett on their wedding (March, 1998).

Herbal Remedies: For Bevan.

Magdalena to Her Husband, Balthasar: Based on Steven Ozment's 1986 edition of letters exchanged between a sixteenth-century Nuremberg merchant and his wife. The bracketed quotations are from Ozment's introduction.

Chicory Seeds: Nicholas Culpeper (1616-54) was a Puritan apothecary whose pithy vehemence makes his Herbal well worth reading in its original version, partly because of his absolute belief in the Doctrine of Signatures, which held that God had left clues in the characteristics of any plant as to its use—heart-shaped plants were sure cardiac cures, and so on. Culpeper produced his English translation of the official London Pharmocopoeia (with much commentary) as a deliberate attempt to provide common people with medical knowledge and agency, to the displeasure of the Royal College of Physicians. Jefferson's passion for all things botanical pressed him to continue correspondence with "the duplicitous British," including the incident mentioned. The livid consumer is cited from Rodale's *Encyclopedia of Herbs* (1986 edition).

Fig: Elizabeth Blackwell (d. 1758) was perhaps the first woman apothecary; her *Curious Herbal* was published in weekly parts and collected in two large volumes in 1737 and 1739. She drew, engraved, and painted all 500 plates herself. Apparently she did this in order to release her husband from debt— unfortunately, Alexander Blackwell went to Sweden without his wife and was subsequently tried and executed for the high treason of plotting to change the royal succession. She lived near the Chelsea Society of Apothecaries Garden in a street called "Swan Walk" while working on the herbal.

Galen on the Anatomy: Galen was Marcus Aurelius' private physician; his teachings and prescriptions formed the basis of European medicine until Paracelsus' introduction of mercury and antimony in the therapeutic, rather than humoral (the four humors of hot, dry, cold, wet) system of medicine. Early physicians disagreed about the primary organs and their functions. It was actually Plato who said that the body's moisture caused the soul to become forgetful of what it once knew. Galen, though he was careful not to refute Plato, was troubled by his own inability to locate and define the soul.

Gladiolus: Dr. John Parkinson (1567-1650) was perhaps the most famous herbalist of his day, apothecary to both James VI and Charles I. He is best known for two works: *Paradisus Terrestris* (1629), primarily a florilegium (an herbal about flowers) and *Theatrum Botanicum* (1640), the most comprehensive book of medicinal plants in English at the time. Parkinson said that "John Tradescant assured me, that hee saw many acres of ground in Barbary spread over with [gladioli]" (*Paradisus Terrestris*).

The Ginseng Hunter Finds Jimsonweed: Jimsonweed blooms open quickly enough to watch and last for one night only, beginning at dusk; the flower wilts by mid-morning of the next day. Jimsonweed is a notorious hallucinogen, one highly unreliable in potency and so one of the most unpredictable narcotic herbs.

Violet Crossing: For David Michener, botanist and Curator of the Matthai Botanical Gardens, University of Michigan (Ann Arbor), who told me this story.

Lemon Grass: Temujin: Genghis Khan.

Four Thieves Vinegar: The quotations are from Dioscorides' *De Materia Medica.*

Dinner at the Reel Inn: For Katherine Swiggart.

Camellias for P: For Karl, who knew Putney and Tango.

Lycos Search: "Lycos search" is one of the search engines on the World Wide Web. The queries are from the list called up with Microsoft Word 5.1's spelling dictionary. Other sources include the *Oxford English Dictionary* ("adopt" and "adoption"), Pliny's *Natural History*, and the preface to the 1959 reprint of the 1934 edition (using the original John Goodyer translation) of Dioscorides' *De Materia Medica*, probably the best-known herbal surviving from classical times.

Speech in Five Acts and Hymn for a Birthmother: On meeting my birthmother for the first time in August, 1997.

Hole: For my maternal biological grandmother, Myrtle Arlene.

Gingkos: For my students.

Tea: Tokonoma : the altar in a tea house. For the poet R. Tillinghast.

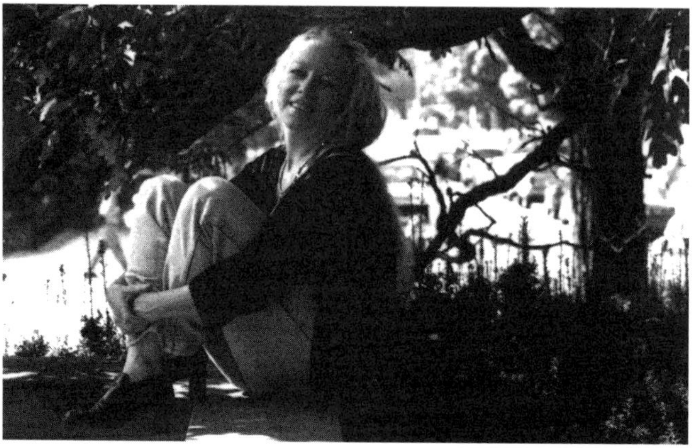

photo by Bill Wood

A native of Florida, Deanne Lundin has lived in Oklahoma, Boston, Los Angeles, and Ann Arbor. Lundin's poems have appeared in *The Georgia Review, Prairie Schooner, The Kenyon Review, Colorado Review, Antioch Review* and elsewhere. She has earned degrees from the Eastman School of Music and the University of Michigan, where she now teaches. Current writing projects include her dissertation (English, UCLA) on American women poets and their use of mystical discourse; and a memoir based on the experience of being adopted and her recent reunion with her birth family.

A HANDBOOK OF BIOANALYSIS AND DRUG METABOLISM

Contents

Editor's preface

Originally this book was to be called 'Grieves Harnby's Guide to Bioanalysis and Drug Metabolism', as the project conceived by David Scales was going to be produced by Grieves. Unfortunately Grieves died following a heart attack shortly after he retired. We decided to complete this book and dedicate it to his memory. Grieves had worked in Research and Development in Glaxo in all its various guises from 1961 until he retired in 1996. The majority of that time he was involved in the formation of a new discipline – Drug Metabolism arising out of the regulatory changes introduced in the late 1960s. I was recruited by Grieves in 1979 and worked with him for the next 18 years. Each chapter in this book was written as an individual contribution by one or more authors, all of whom worked at Glaxo-Wellcome at the time of writing their chapters. It was decided to allow each chapter stand alone. Each chapter was the responsibility of the contributing authors. All of the chapters compliment each other and present a comprehensive picture of the breadth of functions and activities which are included in Bioanalysis, Pharmacokinetics and Drug Metabolism.

Gary Evans

Preface

I came to drug metabolism and bioanalysis rather late in life when, in 1995, I was appointed VP of the Division in GlaxoWellcome. It was the time of the merger between two great companies and I had the unenviable task of making many fine people redundant. I remember a lunch meeting with Grieves Harnby, at the beginning of, what was euphemistically called, the integration process. With only two years before retirement Grieves was convinced he would be a casualty of the reorganisation. I however wanted him to stay, for it gave me the chance to work with one of the founding fathers of industrial drug metabolism. When I told him of his promotion to position of International Director, he nearly choked on his sandwich. This was the only time I ever saw Grieves lost for the right words.

Grieves acted as a mentor and guide to many. I was fortunate that he was mine, if only for two brief years. His task was to convert me from a toxicologist into what he called 'a real scientist'. The new company had many outstanding individuals who devoted time and effort, under the watchful eye of Grieves, in getting me up to speed. It was from this teaching programme that the idea for a book grew. It was envisaged that it would cover the necessary information to work in a pharmaceutical drug metabolism and bioanalysis function. Staff from the company based in the USA, Italy and the UK agreed to contribute. Grieves would work on the project, post-retirement, on those few rare occasions when he was not improving his golf handicap.

To our great sadness, Grieves died shortly after retiring. It is a tribute to the man that his loss created a void in so many lives. His friends and colleagues still toast his memory and mourn his passing. Mike Tarbit, who knew him for many years, has captured, in an anecdotal reminiscence given below, some of Grieves' humour and humanity.

The book was still very much at a preliminary stage when we lost our Editor-in-Chief. We decided, however, to continue with the project. Gary Evans took over the herculean task of acting as editor, as well as cajoling the contributors to finish their chapters. It is a great credit to Gary and all the authors that, despite yet another merger, the book has finally been completed. It is, of course, dedicated to Grieves Harnby.

David Scales
Henley-on-Thames
England

Grieves Harnby: In memoriam

I had the pleasure and privilege to know Grieves for nearly twenty years before his untimely death. He was a rare person: a true, loyal, humorous, but candid, friend. Humour, wit and sagacity oozed from Grieves at all times. 'Candid' meant, with Grieves, that he would always tell you what he really thought with characteristic northern bluntness, whether it was what you wanted to hear, or not! He could kill with a sentence! If you have the courage to treasure such friendship, it always serves you well, and Grieves gave me immeasurable guidance and counsel over the years of our shared time in GlaxoWellcome.

Grieves had an almost uncanny and yet completely natural gift in communicating with people, and anecdotes abound about his ability to get on with strangers in no time at all. Thus, for example, he was the only person in my experience, who could have made such an impression with the normally 'detached' and 'seen it all before' air crew on one 40 minute USAir flight that the air hostess put her arm round him and kissed him goodbye as he was leaving the flight! No concern over sexual harassment there! Indeed he specialised in 'melting' air crew, and perhaps the most famous example of this was when the normal USAir/British Airways connection from our North Carolina laboratories to Heathrow, via Philadelphia, went badly awry due to storms, and we were stranded in Philadelphia. Much to Grieves' obvious delight, we were driven to New York by British Airways and brought home on Concord. Soon after take-off, a fairly formal and slightly upper crust 'Concord class' lady Purser arrived with a wine carrier laden with vintage Dom Perignon, Chateau Beychevelle St Julien and an excellent Mersault. The basket was offered to Grieves, not someone normally viewed as a wine connoisseur, with a svelte "And which wine would you like Sir?" "All of them, Pet!" was his reply, delivered with such a twinkle that three glasses were instantly placed on our tables by a giggling Purser, along with three bottles of wine! After that we owned the plane! Grieves felt that he had enjoyed the experience of a lifetime on that flight.

Mike Tarbit

GRIEVES HARNBY GLAXO: 1961–1996, Drug Metabolism

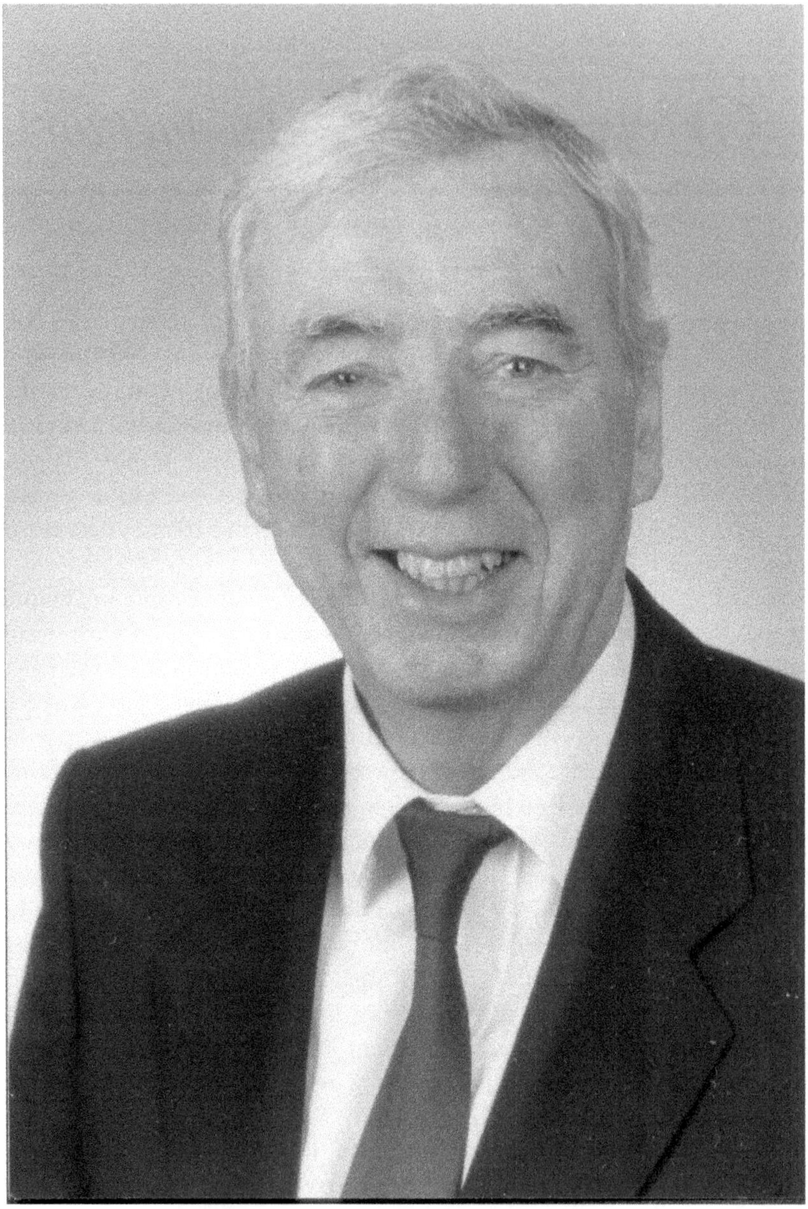

CHAPTER 1

Introduction

Gary Evans

1.1 *Bioanalysis, pharmacokinetics and drug metabolism (BPDM)*

The prime function of the Research and Development subsidiaries of pharmaceutical companies is to discover and develop new medicines. Achieving these objectives is not easy, only a small percentage of the chemical compounds synthesised become medicines, most compounds prove unsuitable for reasons of efficacy, potency or toxicity.

Both the discovery and development phases are time-consuming processes which take between five and ten years to complete. They involve scientists from many different disciplines, working together, to identify disease targets and, to discover suitable chemical entities which have the appropriate biological, chemical and pharmacological/toxicological properties to be quality medicines.

When the potential drug is selected for development, extensive safety and clinical studies are conducted to provide sufficient data for a regulatory submission for registration of a new medicine.

One group of scientists whose contribution is particularly important in both drug discovery and drug development are those working in the discipline which may be described as bioanalysis, pharmacokinetics and drug metabolism (BPDM). Whilst other names have been used to describe this discipline, it has broad range of activities which seek the same objectives – to understand what happens to the drug after it is administered and to determine what implications a knowledge of the fate of the dosed drug has for either improving the drug or for dosage regimens and safety.

This discipline consists of three main areas which are closely related. Bioanalysis is a term generally used to describe the quantitative measurement of a compound (drug) in biological fluids primarily blood, plasma, serum, urine or tissue extracts.

Pharmacokinetics is the technique used to analyse these data and to define a number of parameters which describe the absorption, distribution, clearance (including metabolism) and excretion (often referred by the acronym ADME). The ability to monitor the presence of the drug in the body and to measure its removal is critical in understanding the safety, dosage and efficacy of any medicine.

Drug metabolism is the study of the metabolism of a drug. It can be used to discover the nature and route of metabolism of the drug and the information permits predictions to be made concerning the potential for interactions with co-administered drugs through knowledge of the enzymes involved in the metabolism of drugs. Increasingly predictions can be made about the metabolism of a putative drug using the knowledge base from existing drugs. These three areas have developed together because of the use of common techniques and knowledge. The scientists conducting these functions may be geographically separated or, increasingly, scientists may specialise in one of the functional areas. However, the functions are closely inter-related and may be considered a single scientific discipline. In this book this discipline will be referred to as BPDM.

1.2 *The role of BPDM in drug discovery and drug development*

The roles and techniques of BPDM used in supporting drug discovery and development are similar but the information is required for different purposes, hence the priorities and approaches differ. Information is used for decision-making in both phases; however, the nature of the decisions affects the quality and quantity of information required.

For discovery, the priority is to examine a large number of compounds and determine which pharmacologically active compounds are most suitable for drug development. In practice when a compound is obtained which has the required biological activity, a number of analogues or chemically similar compounds will be synthesised and tested to optimise the preferred characteristics of the compound (a process is known as lead optimisation). Figure 1.1 shows an illustration of a possible scenario in discovering drugs which are active *in vitro* and improving these by modification of the chemical structure optimised for *in vivo* activity.

In drug development, a single compound is progressed and information relating to the safety of the drug and the dosage required for efficacy in man is obtained. Figure 1.2 shows the studies which are conducted on a drug under development – the exact experimental design and priorities will depend on the particular drug under development.

There is a significant overlap in the techniques and methodology used in BPDM for drug discovery and drug development and often the difference is in the experimental

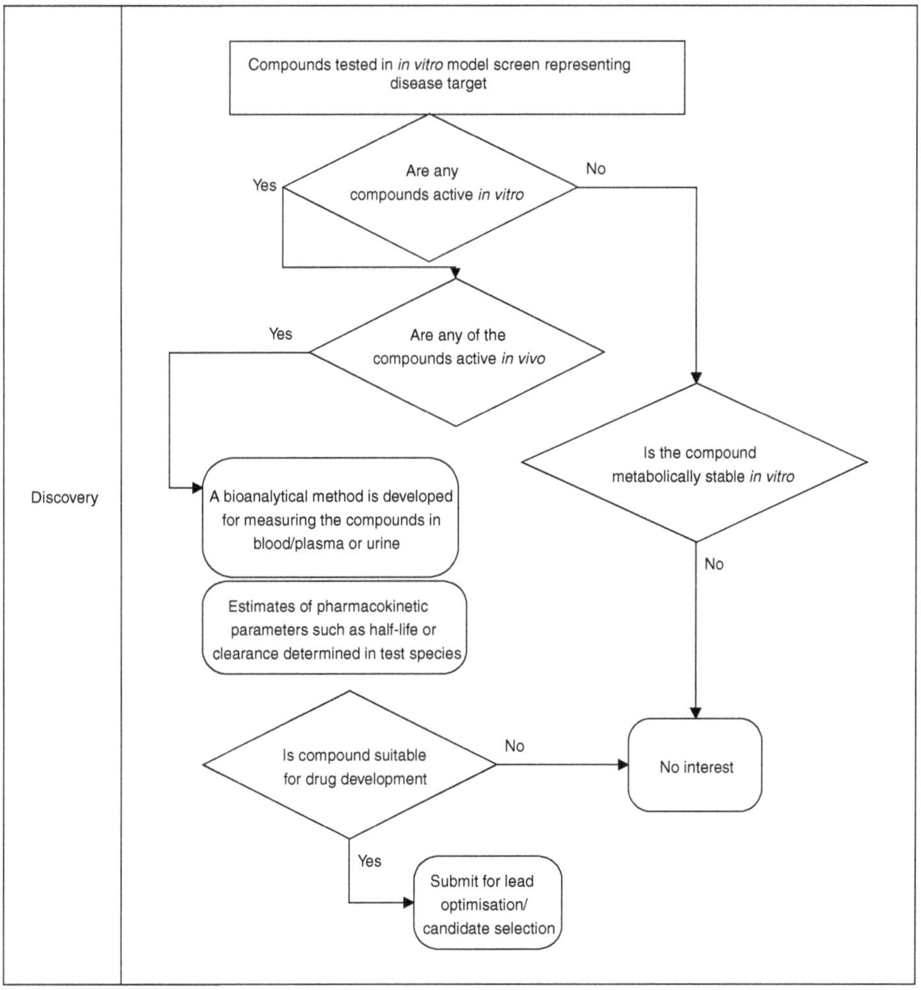

FIGURE 1.1 *Process diagram representing some of the BPDM steps in drug discovery.*

design. Consequently, the chapters in this book have been organised on the basis of functional topics and where there are different approaches for discovery and development these are discussed in each chapter.

Physiochemical properties of compounds are also an important consideration in drug design as they will effect absorption and clearance. They will also be of concern in the development of an analytical method or determining a suitable drug formulation. These aspects are discussed in detail in Chapter 2. A sensitive and specific bioanalytical method is developed to allow the monitoring of drug levels in plasma (systemic circulating levels) and urine (excreted levels) in clinical studies. The assay is also used to monitor the levels of exposure in pre-clinical safety studies. Whilst the analytical methodology used in discovery and development will require

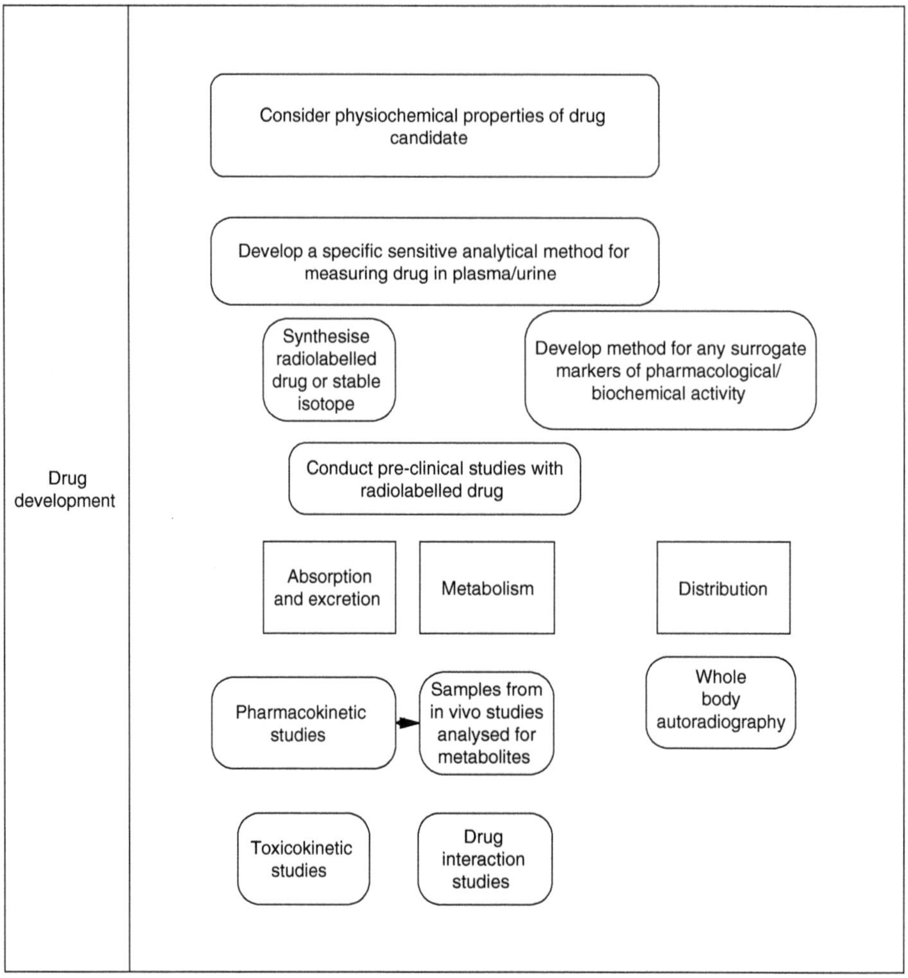

FIGURE 1.2 *Process diagram representing some of the BPDM steps in drug development.*

different levels of sensitivity and validation the basic aspects remain the same. A bioanalytical method consists of two main components:

1 Sample preparation – extraction of the drug from the biological fluid usually including a concentration step to enhance sensitivity of the method; and
2 Detection of the compound – usually following chromatographic separation from other components present in the biological extract. The detector of choice is a mass spectrometer.

These issues are discussed in Chapter 3 (Sample preparation), Chapter 4 (Chromatographic separation: HPLC) and Chapter 5 (Quantitative mass spectrometry). Whilst traditionally other chromatographic techniques have been used, the method of choice is now high-performance liquid chromatography (HPLC) which is used almost universally in both discovery and development methods. The use of tandem mass spectrometry has reduced the need for extensive chromatographic separation because of the enhanced specificity and selectivity of this methodology. It is especially valuable in lead optimisation for studying the pharmacokinetics of multiple compounds administered simultaneously. In addition to monitoring the drug there is an increasing need (with the advent of biochemically active compounds) to monitor surrogate and biomarkers. These are endogenous compounds whose profile reflects the pharmacological action of the drug (biomarker) or disease (surrogate). Immunoassay is the chosen technique for most endogenous compounds and surrogate markers. The use of immunoassay forms the subject of Chapter 6. Plasma levels of the drug are normally monitored to permit the calculation of pharmacokinetic parameters. Whilst preliminary pharmacokinetic data is obtained in drug discovery in pre-clinical species, the definitive kinetics is obtained in drug development by conducting single dose experiments in pre-clinical species and in humans. The importance and definition of the pharmacokinetic parameters are discussed in detail in Chapter 7. These data are essential in defining the dosage regimen in man and ensuring that the therapeutic benefit is maximised.

Plasma samples are also taken from the pre-clinical species used in safety testing. The kinetics derived from these data are often referred to as 'toxicokinetics' because they represented exposure after repeated administration of high levels of drug and the data may indicate drug accumulation, inhibition or induction of clearance mechanisms. In addition the calculation of total drug exposure in the safety studies is critical to calculating the margin of safety in clinical studies, and by scaling data from different species predictions can be made of the parameters in humans. All of these issues are discussed in Chapter 9.

The need to monitor both drug and biomarker levels is important for both discovery and development work. The priority for discovery is to ensure suitable pharmacokinetic properties of the chosen drug and to establish the relationship between systemic levels of drug (pharmacokinetics, PK) and the pharmacodynamics (PD) of the drug. This PK–PD relationship is discussed more fully in Chapter 8.

Pharmacological and toxicological effects are normally only produced by the free drug in the body. Most drugs are, to a greater or lesser degree, bound to proteins, notably serum albumen. The techniques and importance of measuring protein binding are discussed in Chapter 10, illustrated with a case study on a highly protein-bound drug.

Many of the studies conducted in the development phase involve the use of radiolabelled drug which is not available at the earlier discovery phase. This allows the absorption, distribution, excretion and metabolism of the drug-related material to be investigated in the pre-clinical species, and where appropriate, in man. These studies are essential in determining the elimination from the animal of all drug-related material. The initial experiments conducted are known as 'excretion balance studies' because following administration of radiolabelled drug, urine, faeces and exhaled air are collected over a 7-day period to measure the percentage of the dose eliminated. The excreta is used to examine the form of radioactivity and identify the metabolites. In addition, whole body autoradiography is used to follow the distribution of radioactivity in the organs and the time period of elimination. This data is used quantitatively to determine the dose of radiolabelled drug which can be administered to human volunteers; however, these studies are becoming less common as stable isotope alternatives are developed. All of these issues are discussed in Chapters 11 and 12.

The major routes of metabolism and the enzyme systems involved are well documented although it is an area under continuing development, particularly the Phase 2 enzyme systems. Phase 1 metabolism (Chapter 13) primarily consists of oxidation and hydrolysis of the parent molecule whilst conjugation is the main feature of Phase 2 metabolism (Chapter 14). In both instances the result is to render the molecule more polar and thus suitable for elimination from the animal. There are many *in vitro* techniques used to investigate the metabolism of compounds. The pros and cons of different models are discussed in Chapter 15. These *in vitro* techniques allied to tools provided by molecular biological techniques (Chapter 18) permit the scientist to identify the enzymes involved in the metabolism of a drug. By considering the metabolism of co-administered drugs, predictions can be made about the potential for drug–drug interactions and reduce the need to conduct expensive clinical studies (Chapter 16).

It is important to identify the metabolites and to show that the metabolites which were present in the pre-clinical species used in toxicity testing are the same as those observed in humans. Traditionally metabolite identification involved painstaking extraction of radiolabelled drug from biological material and the use of spectrometric methods for identification. In recent years developments in nuclear magnetic resonance or NMR spectroscopy linked to chromatographic systems and mass spectrometry have revolutionised the ability to identify metabolites without extensive extraction, and from much smaller quantities of material. Examples of the use of these techniques are presented in Chapter 17.

Whilst the pharmacologist or biochemist can develop a screening method for determining which compounds show biological activity against a particular target, these data are of limited value without the knowledge to determine whether the compound can be developed into a commercially viable medicine. Indeed many homologous compounds may show similar biological activities in screens but may behave significantly differently when administered *in vivo*.

The bioanalytical methods used in discovery are designed to be more generic and suitable to monitor a range of analogous compounds. The assay does not require the high sensitivity which is required in drug development because the concentrations of compound used in the pharmacological screening models and initial *in vivo* testing are higher than will be encountered in the human studies. In addition the pharmacokinetic experiments are not designed to obtain the definitive data but to obtain comparative data between a series of analogous compounds permitting these to be ranked in order of, for example, plasma half-life. Indeed only a small number of sampling times need to be taken to derive this information and many compounds may be co-administered to reduce the number of animals used in these studies. The quality of information is of a level suitable for scientific evaluation and decision-making.

The metabolism of putative drugs will be examined using *in vitro* screens. *In vivo* pharmacokinetics studies and *in vitro* metabolism studies are essential in explaining why some compounds active *in vitro*, in pharmacological models, show no or poor *in vivo* activity. *In vitro* metabolism screens can be very useful in 'lead optimisation' where chemical substitution around an active moiety can be used to obtain compounds which retain pharmacological activity but have improved metabolic stability. The role of bioanalysis and drug metabolism in discovery is discussed in detail in Chapter 19.

CHAPTER 2

The importance of the physicochemical properties of drugs to drug metabolism

David Spalding

2.1 *Introduction*

In order for a drug to produce a pharmacological effect, it must first reach its site(s) of action at sufficiently high concentrations to elicit the desired response. Whilst the concentration of drug achieved at the site of action is a function of the dose administered, it is also a consequence of how the drug is handled within the body. The rate and extent to which the drug is absorbed from its site of administration, its distribution within the body, its elimination and its ultimate excretion from the body are also fundamentally important determinants of its efficacy.

By studying the pharmacokinetics of a drug, we can identify the processes that determine its concentrations in the body and, by maximising its pharmacokinetics, maximise also its potential to be successful in the marketplace. Pharmacokinetic evaluation is, therefore, not only important to support drug safety and efficacy evaluation during drug development, but has a very important role in supporting drug discovery by optimising the candidates selected for development.

Fundamental to an understanding of pharmacokinetics is the role of the inherent physicochemical properties of a molecule for it is these properties, in combination with the nature of the physiological processes that handle the drug in the body, that determine the pharmacokinetic profile of a drug. In addition, the same physicochemical properties that allow a molecule to partition into and out of a lipid membrane also pertain to its ability to interact with the immobilised phase of an extraction cartridge or an analytical chromatography column. An understanding of the physicochemical properties of a drug is, understandably, invaluable in determining and optimising the analytical conditions for assaying the drug in biological fluids, a necessary pre-requisite to obtaining high quality, reliable pharmacokinetic data.

The main aim of this chapter is to provide a brief introduction to the salient physicochemical properties of a drug and to consider these in connection with familiar aspects of ADME (absorption, distribution, metabolism and excretion) studies, in particular, pharmacokinetics and analysis. The chapter is intended to set the scene for more detailed discussions on the topics of absorption, distribution, metabolism, excretion and analysis to be covered in subsequent chapters. For more detailed discussions of physicochemical properties, readers are directed to more comprehensive reviews on this subject (Seydel and Shaper, 1982; Jezequel, 1992).

2.2 *The physicochemical nature of drug molecules*

At the last count, there were approximately 3,000 drugs currently available on prescription in the United Kingdom. Although of diverse structure, the common physical characteristic of these compounds is that the majority are, invariably, organic molecules, that is to say the molecule is predominantly the result of simple covalent bonding between carbon and hydrogen atoms. Since the receptors and membranes with which they interact are themselves organic, then this is not surprising. Furthermore, since most drugs are designed to either mimic or block the effects of a naturally occurring molecule, an organic nature is a pre-requisite to being able to gain access to, and interact with, the binding site of the endogenous compound.

Simple organic compounds such as hydrocarbons, which, by definition, only contain carbon and hydrogen atoms, are electrically neutral since the valence electrons comprising the bond are shared equally between the carbon and hydrogen atoms. In contrast, the molecules forming the specific receptors contain heteroatoms such as oxygen, nitrogen, sulphur or phosphorous in addition to carbon and hydrogen. Bonds between heteroatoms and carbon exhibit unequal sharing of electrons due to the differing electronegativities of the elements concerned. Such bonds have the overall effect of shifting the distribution of electrons within the molecule such that areas of positive and negative charge are created, thereby introducing polarity into the molecule. The presence of charged groups offers the potential for electrostatic interaction with molecules of opposite electrical charge and these interactions are important in controlling the binding of the endogenous substrate with the receptor (Tenakin, 1993). Drugs, therefore, also require heteroatoms to bind specifically at receptors and thus the efficacy of a drug is due to a balance between its inherent lipophilicity and the number of carbon and heteroatoms within the molecule as well as their relationship to one another. Both of these properties will have a bearing on the disposition of a drug and this, as will be discussed in the next section, will be influenced greatly by the structure of the cell membrane, a barrier to the penetration of exogenous substrates.

2.3 *The structure of the cell membrane and its implications for drug disposition*

All living cells, be they plant or animal, are surrounded by a cell membrane whose function, apart from maintaining the integrity of the cell itself, is to maintain the compartmentalisation required to allow the metabolic processes going on within the cell to proceed efficiently. The cell membrane has, therefore, a regulatory function to control the uptake of nutrients and regulatory substances whilst allowing waste and breakdown products to be removed from the cell. The membrane is thus semi-permeable, and consists of a bimolecular layer of approximately 8–9 nm thickness comprising phospholipid molecules such as sphingomyelin and phosphatidylcholine. The molecules align themselves such that the polar alcohol or choline head groups form a continuous layer binding both the inner and outer surface of the membrane, whilst the hydrophobic fatty acids chains are orientated inwards to form an essentially lipophilic core. This bilayer configuration, which is illustrated in Figure 2.1, allows individual lipid molecules to move laterally whilst endowing the membrane with fluidity.

This configuration has the further property of creating a lipid barrier which is highly impermeable to ions and most polar molecules, and which only permits free transport to drugs that are able to dissolve in lipid and move into and across the membrane. There are, however, globular proteins embedded in the membrane, some of which extend through all the layers of the membrane. These proteins contain heteroatoms, which contribute to the formation of pores or channels, through which small water-soluble molecules such as ethanol and quaternary ammonium salts, or ions such as sodium or chloride, can pass. However, for larger molecules including most drugs the cell membrane acts as a barrier to distribution within the body and dictates the physicochemical characteristics required for drug penetration i.e. the drug has the appropriate degree of lipophilicity. How the lipophilicity of a drug is determined and the implications of lipophilicity for the crossing of biological membranes will be discussed in detail in the next section.

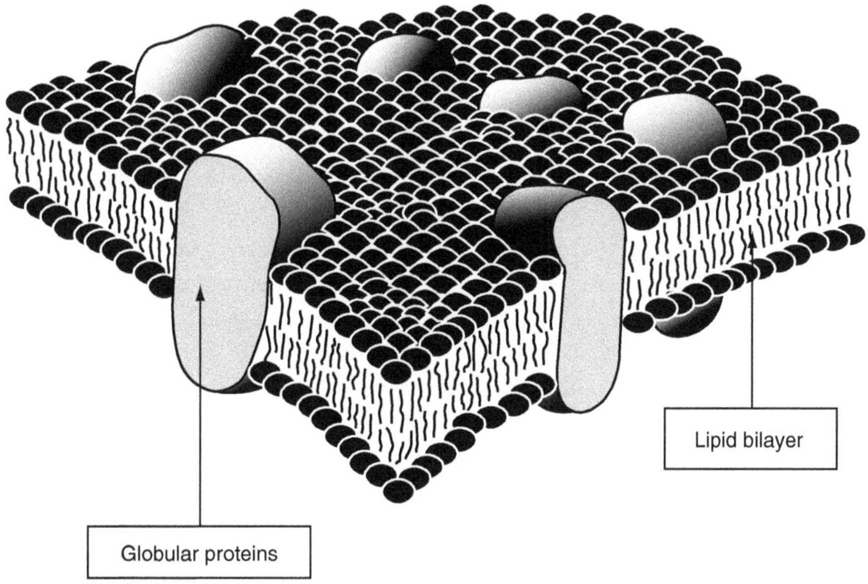

FIGURE 2.1 *Fluid mosiac model for the overall organisation of biological membranes* (Fluid mosaic model [reproduced with permission from S.J. Singer and G.I. Nicolson, *Science* 175 (1972):723 Copyright 1972 by the American Association for the Advancement of Science]).

2.4 *Drug partitioning across membranes*

In order for a drug to be distributed to its site of action, it must cross at least one membrane, and usually more. Since for the majority of drug molecules, crossing of the membrane occurs by virtue of simple diffusion, and given the largely lipophilic nature of the membrane, the prime determinant of the rate of absorption is the inherent lipophilicity of the drug molecule. Both aqueous and lipid environments must be traversed whilst crossing a membrane and, thus, a measure of the relative affinity of a drug molecule for both phases is useful as a predictor of the likelihood for it to be absorbed or to cross the blood–brain barrier.

The partitioning of a drug between water and octanol at a constant temperature to give the partition coefficient (P) or log P as it is more commonly expressed, has been demonstrated to be a useful predictor of membrane transport (Hansch, 1976). This is represented diagrammatically in Figure 2.2 and Equation 2.1.

$$\text{Partition coefficient } (P) = \frac{\text{concentration in organic}}{\text{concentration in aqueous}} \tag{2.1}$$

The partition coefficient has been determined traditionally using the shaking flask technique. This method involves the drug being shaken in a flask containing water and an immiscible organic phase such as *n*-octanol or chloroform at constant temperature for a fixed time before analysis of the drug concentration in the two

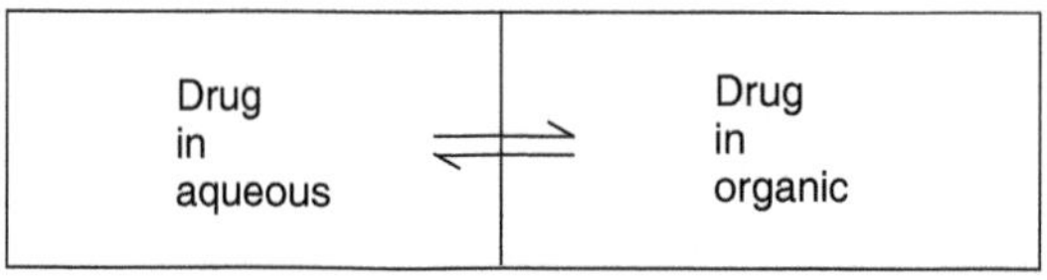

FIGURE 2.2 *Diagrammatic representation of drug partitioning.*

phases (Fujita *et al.*, 1964). It should be noted that such systems are not truly composed of pure solvent and pure water, but as water-saturated solvent and vice versa. The *n*-octanol phase has been shown to contain a relatively high concentration of water (Smith *et al.*, 1975) but it is likely that this is also true of the lipid membrane, certainly in the intestine (Chapman *et al.*, 1967).

Measurement of log *P* by the classical shaking flask technique is rather tedious and has low throughput. More rapid techniques based upon chromatography have been developed and have been shown to give good agreement with the values obtained by the classical method (Unger *et al.*, 1978; Brauman, 1986; Hansch *et al.*, 1986).

The utility of a drug's partition coefficient to predict its ability to pass through biological membranes has been demonstrated by early pioneering work carried out by Schanker (1964) who investigated the absorption of a structurally related series of barbiturates from the rat colon as shown in Table 2.1.

Comparing the lipophilicity of the molecules with their uptake across the colon shows that the membrane permeability of each member of the series is proportional to its partition coefficient. Also of note is the fact that, in contrast to drugs that diffuse through aqueous channels in the membrane, where size is an important factor, there is little effect of size on transport across the colon. As a general rule of thumb, therefore, the higher the partition coefficient then more easily will the drug be transported across the membrane. This should only be used as a rough guide; however, as above a certain lipophilicity problems will be encountered with poor solubility in the aqueous phase leading to a drop-off in permeability.

As defined above, the partition coefficient is the ratio of the concentration of drug between the two liquid phases for the same molecular species and is only

TABLE 2.1 *Relationship between lipophilicity and the absorption of a series of barbiturates from rat colon*

Barbiturate	Chloroform: water partition coefficient	Percentage absorbed
Barbitone	0.7	12
Phenobarbitone	4.8	20
Cyclobarbitone	13.9	24
Pentobarbitone	28.8	30
Secobarbitone	50.7	40

applicable to compounds that do not ionise. This is a somewhat simplified approximation to the situation *in vivo* where there is not a uniform pH within the body and where the effects of ionisation can have a profound effect upon the disposition of a drug. The concept of ionisation and its effect on drug disposition are discussed in greater detail in the next section.

2.5 *The ionisation of drugs*

As explained above, most drugs contain heteroatoms necessary for interaction with receptors at their site of action. These substituents, by virtue of introducing polarity into the molecule, also confer the property of allowing the drug to act as an acid, a base or even a zwitterion. Acids can be defined simply as proton donors and bases as proton acceptors, and drugs with acidic or basic functions can exist both in an un-ionised or an ionised form as represented in Equations 2.2 and 2.3.

$$\text{Acidic} \quad \underset{\text{un-ionised}}{[HA] + [H_2O]} \rightleftharpoons \underset{\text{ionised}}{[A^-] + [H_3O^+]} \tag{2.2}$$

$$\text{Basic} \quad \underset{\text{un-ionised}}{[B] + [H_2O]} \rightleftharpoons \underset{\text{ionised}}{[BH^+] + [OH^-]} \tag{2.3}$$

$$\begin{matrix} \downarrow & \quad & \downarrow \\ \text{Lipid soluble} & \quad & \text{Water soluble} \end{matrix}$$

Ionised molecules possess an electrostatic charge and prefer to associate with a similarly charged environment i.e. an aqueous rather than an uncharged organic environment, and dissolve preferentially in water. Conversely, un-ionised molecules have no net charge or polarity and thus prefer to dissolve in lipid i.e. they are lipophilic. Most drugs are either weak acids or weak bases and thus will be partially ionised in an aqueous medium such as blood. The law of mass action applies in the case of weak acids but favours the ionisation of weak bases. At acid pH, therefore, weak acids will be un-ionised and will favour solution in the lipid phase, whilst for a weak base, the reverse situation will apply and, because they are ionised at acidic pH, they will favour solution in the aqueous phase.

The degree of ionisation of a drug is, therefore, a very important determinant of its ability to cross membranes as this dictates the amount of drug that is un-ionised and hence lipid soluble. It also follows that the pH of the environment will play a crucial role in determining the ability of a drug to diffuse into and across lipid membranes.

The extent to which a drug is ionised at any given pH is a function of the apparent dissociation constant K_a which, like hydrogen ion concentration, is normally expressed as its negative logarithmic transformation $-\log K_a$ or pK_a. Strong acids have low pK_a values and strong bases have high pK_a values. The pK_a values of a selection of acidic and basic drugs are shown in Figure 2.3 to illustrate the range of values usually attained.

The pK_a value of a particular drug can be obtained by plotting the pH resulting after addition of sodium hydroxide against the equivalents of OH^- added to give a titration curve, and those for a number of weak acids (acetate, phosphate and ammonia) are shown in Figure 2.4.

It can be seen that the shape of the curve is the same for both the acid and the base, the main difference being a vertical shift on the pH scale. At the midpoint of the titration, the number of charged and uncharged molecules is equal and the pH at which this occurs is the pK_a.

It can also be seen from Figure 2.4 that for an acid, at a pH two units below its pK_a the drug is virtually completely un-ionised (>99 per cent), whilst at a pH two units above its pK_a the drug is virtually completely ionised. The reverse situation applies for bases such as ammonia where they are almost completely ionised two pH

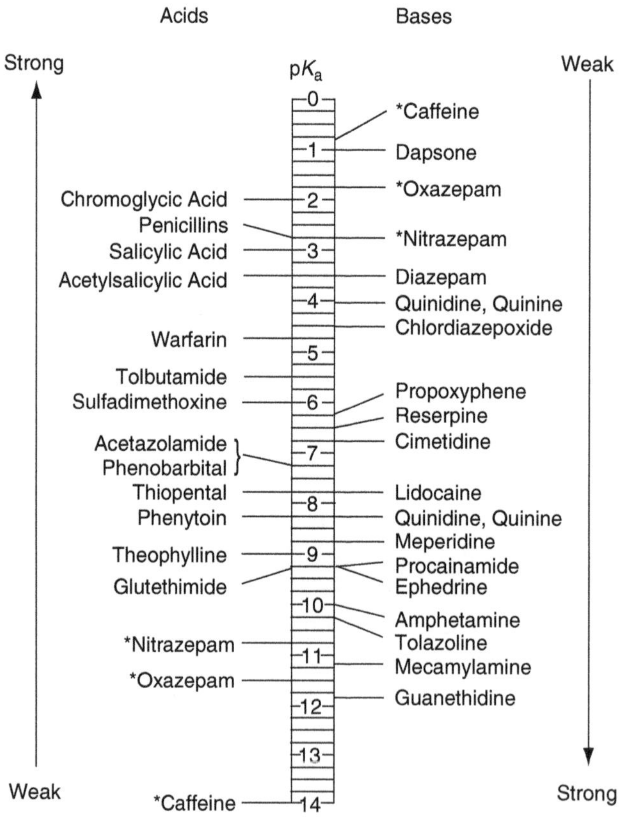

FIGURE 2.3 *The* pK_a *values of acidic and basic drugs vary widely. Some drugs are amphoteric* (*) *i.e. they are both acidic and basic functional groups* (reproduced with permission from M. Rowland and T.N. Tozer, *Clinical Pharmacokinetics: concepts and applications*, Williams and Wilkins, London, 1985).

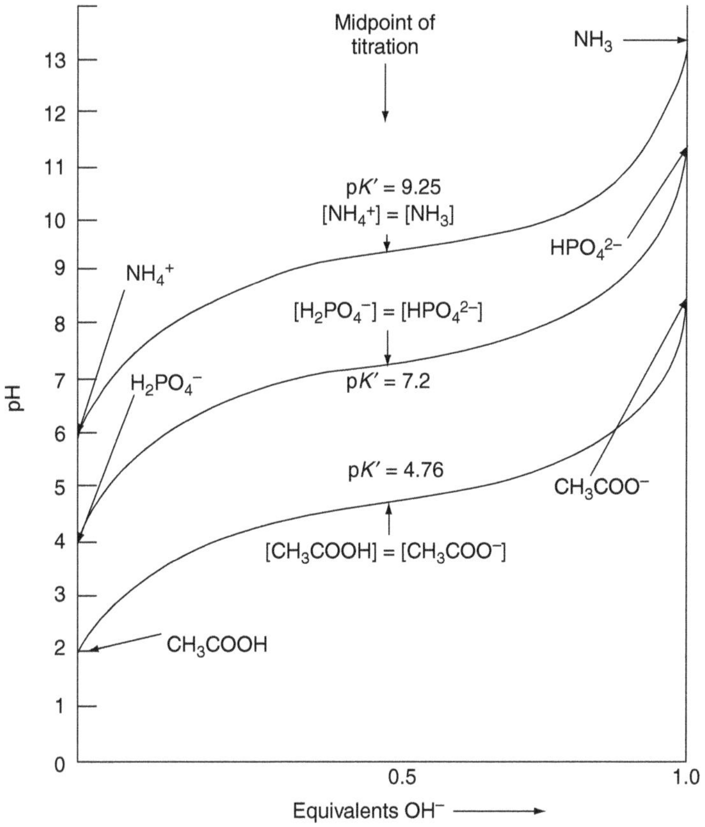

FIGURE 2.4 *Acid–base titration curves of some acids, showing the major ionic species at beginning, midpoint and end of titration* (reproduced with permission from A.L. Lehninger, *Biochemistry*, Worth Publishers Inc., New York, 1975).

units below their pK_a and fully un-ionised two pH units above their pK_a. Thus it can be seen that, if we have knowledge of the pK_a of a drug and the pH of the environment, we can begin to predict the likely degree of ionisation of the drug and thereby the potential for it to cross membranes and be absorbed.

The shape of the titration curve can be described mathematically for any particular compound by the Henderson–Hasselbalch equation which relates the degree of ionisation of a drug to pH and its pK_a as shown in Equations 2.4 and 2.5.

$$\text{For acids} \quad pK_a - pH = \log \frac{[\text{un-ionised}]}{[\text{ionised}]} \tag{2.4}$$

$$\text{For bases} \quad pK_a - pH = \log \frac{[\text{ionised}]}{[\text{un-ionised}]} \tag{2.5}$$

Thus it can be seen that the partitioning of drugs between organic and aqueous media is a function of not only the partition coefficient of the molecule but also of the degree of ionisation of the molecule. The partitioning of ionisable drugs is thus more complex than the situation represented in Figure 2.2 and is a function of the partition coefficient and the dissociation constant thus shown in Equations 2.6 and 2.7.

$$\text{For acids} \quad [A^-]^{aq} \overset{K_a}{\rightleftharpoons} [HA]^{aq} \overset{P}{\rightleftharpoons} [HA]^{org} \tag{2.6}$$

$$\text{For bases} \quad [BH^+]^{aq} \overset{K_a}{\rightleftharpoons} [B]^{aq} \overset{P}{\rightleftharpoons} [B]^{org} \tag{2.7}$$

It is obvious from Equations 2.6 and 2.7 above that the direction in which the overall equilibrium lies is dependent upon the pH of the environment since this determines the amount of un-ionised drug free to partition into the organic phase. Thus, the greater the degree of ionisation of a molecule, the lower the partitioning into and across lipid membranes. The partition coefficient, log P, can thus be adjusted for the degree of ionisation of a compound to give a more accurate descriptor of the behaviour of ionisable and non-ionisable drugs. This adjusted form of the partition coefficient is known as the dissociation coefficient (D), more usually expressed as its logarithmic form log D. This is defined for either acids or bases by the Equations 2.8 and 2.9.

$$\text{For acids} \quad D = \frac{[HA]^{org}}{[HA]^{aq} + [A^-]^{aq}} \tag{2.8}$$

$$\text{For bases} \quad D = \frac{[B]^{org}}{[B]^{aq} + [BH^+]^{aq}} \tag{2.9}$$

From this, D is obviously pH-dependent and is related to P by the following equations derived by Scherrer and Howard (1977, 1979).

$$\text{For acids} \quad \log D = \log P - \log[1 + \text{antilog}\ (\text{pH} - \text{p}K_a)] \tag{2.10}$$

$$\text{For bases} \quad \log D = \log P - \log[1 + \text{antilog}\ (\text{p}K_a - \text{pH})] \tag{2.11}$$

Thus it can be seen that it is possible to calculate the degree of ionisation of a given drug and, therefore, its likely capacity to cross membranes and be absorbed at any site in the body, if the pK_a of the drug and the pH of the tissue are known.

Furthermore, given the similar nature of the interactions between drugs and the organic stationary phases of solid phase extraction cartridges and chromatographic analytical columns, a knowledge of the log D of a compound can also be very useful in terms of maximising the extraction and assay conditions of a molecule.

2.6 *The pH environment of the body and how it affects drug absorption and distribution*

From the previous sections on lipophilicity and ionisation it is obvious that, while the solubility and dissolution rates are higher when they are in the ionised form, only un-ionised lipophilic drugs can diffuse across cell membranes. Thus, the pH on either side of a membrane will markedly affect the distribution of ionisable drugs into cells.

If one considers the oral route of administration, where there are acidic conditions in the stomach and alkaline conditions in the intestine, it becomes obvious just how great these differences in pH can be between different sites and tissues. Knowledge of these differences can help us not only to interpret the data that we obtain from pharmacokinetic studies with novel compounds but also to predict the likely behaviour of a drug in the body. Consideration of the effects of pH on absorption and distribution at different sites will be discussed individually below.

2.6.1 Absorption from the stomach

The pH of the gastric juices in the stomach is very acidic with a pH of approximately 1, whilst the intestinal pH is nearly neutral in the range pH 6–7 (Kararli, 1995). The pH of the plasma is 7.4 and thus the large difference in pH between the plasma and the stomach and gastrointestinal tract largely determines whether or not a weakly ionised compound will be absorbed into the plasma. Alternatively, it will also determine whether or not a drug could be excreted from plasma back into the stomach or intestine.

For a weak acid such as aspirin which has a pK_a of 3.5, we can calculate how it would distribute across the gastric mucosa between the plasma (pH 7.4) and the gastric acid (pH 1) using the Henderson–Hasselbalch equation for an acid shown above (Equation 2.4).

$$\mathrm{p}K_a - \mathrm{pH} = \log\frac{[\text{un-ionised}]}{[\text{ionised}]} \tag{2.12}$$

which upon rearrangement gives,

$$\mathrm{pH} - \mathrm{p}K_a = \log\frac{[\text{ionised}]}{[\text{un-ionised}]} \tag{2.13}$$

and hence,

$$\frac{[\text{ionised}]}{[\text{un-ionised}]} = \text{antilog pH} - \text{p}K_a \tag{2.14}$$

Thus, for aspirin, pH − pK_a = 7.4 − 3.5 = 4, in plasma and 1 − 3.5 = −2.5 in the stomach. Thus, in plasma at equilibrium, log [ionised]/[un-ionised] = 4 and [ionised]/[un-ionised] is the antilog of this i.e. 10,000. In the stomach, however, log [ionised]/[un-ionised] = −2.5 and [ionised]/[un-ionised] = 0.003. Since, for a weak acid it is the acid moiety that is un-ionised and thus freely able to distribute to equilibrium, the distribution will be as follows:

Stomach (pH 1.0) Plasma (pH 7.4)

$$H^+ + A^- \rightleftharpoons HA \rightleftharpoons HA \rightleftharpoons H^+ + A^-$$

0.003 1.0 1.0 10,000

It can be seen that in the acid environment of the stomach, aspirin is greater than 99 per cent in the un-ionised form and, therefore, can be rapidly absorbed from the stomach. Note that in the plasma, however, the reverse is the case and greater than 99 per cent of the drug is in the ionised form. This obviously has implications as to the ability of the drug to distribute further from the plasma into the tissues and this will be discussed further below.

In the case of a basic drug such as procaine (pK_a = 9.0), for example, the reverse situation will apply to that of an acid. In the acidic conditions of the stomach, the drug will exist almost exclusively in the ionised form with less than one molecule in ten million being un-ionised. Thus, it can be seen that the majority of weakly basic drugs will be ionised in the stomach and hence poorly absorbed. In the near neutral conditions of the small intestine, however, ionisation of weakly basic drugs will be suppressed and thus basic drugs tend to be rapidly absorbed in the small intestine. In truth, due to the large surface area for absorption offered by the small intestine, acidic drugs can also be absorbed. Thus, although we have shown above that aspirin is nearly completely ionised in the small intestine, it has been shown to be well absorbed from this site in man after oral administration. It is also clear, however, that strong acids or bases such as sulphanilamide (pK_a = 10.4) and quaternary ammonium salts such as tetraethylammonium will be ionised over the normal range of physiological pH and will thus be poorly absorbed from either the stomach or the small intestine.

2.6.2 Distribution to the tissues

After absorption into the circulation, drugs are distributed throughout the body tissues and fluids. The pattern of distribution of a given drug will be dictated by its lipid solubility, in addition to its ability to bind to plasma proteins and to tissue proteins. The pH of the plasma (7.4) is more basic than that of the tissues (7.0) and thus this can affect the distribution of drugs between the two. Acidic drugs such as aspirin, once absorbed into the circulation, tend to exist largely in the ionised form and thus do not distribute out of plasma into the tissues. In contrast, weakly basic drugs are present at least partly in the un-ionised form, which can diffuse out of the plasma into the tissues. Due to the pH difference between the tissues and plasma, the equilibrium in tissue is shifted back towards the ionised form with the result that the drug tends to remain in the tissue. Consequently, the equilibrium in plasma is driven further towards the un-ionised form, which maintains the concentration gradient of diffusion into the tissues. Thus, unlike acids, bases tend to be widely distributed into the tissues and this explains the characteristic difference in distribution seen between acids and bases when carrying out quantitative whole body autoradiography studies.

In addition to determining its likely distribution, the intrinsic lipophilicity of a drug can also markedly affect its preferred site of accumulation. Since approximately 15 per cent of the body weight of normal individuals is accounted for by fat, and can rise to as much as 50 per cent in grossly obese individuals, this can act as a depot or slow release facility for highly lipophilic drugs. It has been shown, for example, that the volume of distribution of the anticholinergic drug biperidin correlates with the fat volume per unit mass (Yokogawa *et al.*, 1990).

Furthermore, it has been shown that 3 hours after intravenous administration of thiopentane, up to 70 per cent of the dose can be found in the fatty tissues. In the latter case, this redistribution of drug into the fatty tissues acts to terminate the effects of the drug as this takes place at the expense of the brain concentrations of drug, its site of action. Thus, the distribution of drug into fatty tissues can have important effects on the onset/duration of pharmacological action.

2.6.3 Distribution across the blood–brain barrier

For drugs having their effects on the central nervous system, an additional barrier exists to their distribution to the site of action, namely, the blood–brain barrier. The endothelial cells of the brain capillaries have continuous tight intercellular junctions and are closely associated with astrocytes such that the endothelial gaps seen with other organs are lacking. These tight junctions have an electrical resistance of approximately 2,000 Ω/cm^2. This is much higher than those recorded for other endothelia (Crone and Olensen, 1982). The blood–brain barrier thus represents a lipid barrier which plays an important role in separating the tissues of the brain from red blood cells, platelets and exogenous and endogenous compounds present in the systemic circulation.

Although the blood–brain barrier acts as a barrier to large molecules such as proteins, and generally excludes or allows only slow penetration of more polar compounds, highly lipophilic compounds can, to varying extents, rapidly cross the barrier by passive diffusion. Thus drugs such as diazepam, midazolam and clobazopam rapidly appear in cerebrospinal fluid (CSF) ($t_{1/2}$ entry <1 minute), presumably having crossed the blood–brain barrier (Arendt *et al.*, 1983). Some polar solutes can cross the blood–brain barrier by means of active transport systems but these tend to be endogenous compounds such as sugars, hormones, large neutral and basic amino acids, nucleosides and carboxylic acids rather than drug substrates (Pardridge, 1979, 1988).

The use of models to predict the ability of drugs to penetrate the blood–brain barrier is the subject of a later chapter of this book and a more detailed treatise on the importance of physicochemical properties is given there. Readers are directed to this chapter for further details, and also to the excellent review on the subject of central nervous system penetration by Jezequel (1992).

2.6.4 Binding of drugs to blood cells and plasma proteins and its effect on drug distribution

It is well known that drugs can bind reversibly to red blood cells and plasma proteins such as serum albumen, α_1-acid glycoprotein and lipoproteins (Bridges and Wilson, 1977). It is the structure and physicochemical properties of the drug that will determine this association, acidic drugs tending to bind to albumen whilst basic drugs such as β-blockers tend to bind to α_1-acid glycoprotein (Belpaire *et al.*, 1984). Since only free drug is able to cross membranes and interact with the receptor, the distribution and, ultimately, the efficacy of a drug can be affected by its binding to blood constituents. This important characteristic of a drug is described in more detail in a subsequent chapter of this book and thus will not be discussed further here.

2.7 *The importance of the physicochemical properties of drugs to their metabolism and excretion*

The primary purpose of metabolism is to convert a lipophilic drug molecule, which is easily able to cross membranes and thus access its site of action, into a molecule which has a lower lipophilicity, a lower affinity for the tissues, and a greater propensity for removal from the body via the urine. The intrinsic lipophilicity of a molecule is a key determinant of its metabolism. Lipophilicity is important, not only in terms of facilitating crossing of membranes to reach the drug-metabolising enzymes, but is also an important parameter controlling binding of the drug to the active site of the drug-metabolising enzymes.

In addition to lipophilicity, the presence of ionisable groups on the molecule is also an important characteristic of compounds undergoing metabolism. Ionisable groups are important both in terms of contributing to the apparent lipophilicity of the molecule (log *D*) and in determining the binding to the active site of metabolising enzymes, the latter being important in dictating the regioselectivity of metabolism.

2.7.1 Cytochromes P-450

The most important group of enzymes responsible for drug metabolism in animals and man are the cytochrome P-450s and these are responsible for the oxidative clearance of the majority of lipophilic drugs i.e. with a log *D* above 0 (Smith, 1994). The mechanism of catalysis of the cytochromes P-450 is thought to be constant across all the families and to be determined by the ability of a high valent formal $(FeO)^{3+}$ species to carry out the one electron oxidations through abstraction of hydrogen atoms, abstraction of electrons in *n* or * orbitals or the addition to * bonds (Guengerich and McDonald, 1990). As a consequence, metabolism by cytochrome P-450s is determined by a number of factors related to the physicochemical properties of the substrate and the enzyme itself. The gross topography of the active site is obviously important as is the degree to which the shape of the substrate complements that of the active site of the enzyme. Following on from this, the degree of steric hindrance of access of the iron–oxygen complex to the possible sites of metabolism will also have a profound effect upon the degree of metabolism. Equally important is the ease with which electrons or hydrogen atoms can be abstracted from the various carbons or heteroatoms in the substrate.

The major isoforms of cytochrome P-450 involved in the metabolism of xenobiotics in man are CYP2D6, CYP2C9 and CYP3A4. By examination of the structure and physicochemical properties of published substrates for these isoforms it has been possible to formulate general rules for substrate preference. These rules are shown in Table 2.2.

It can be seen that both CYP2D6 and CYP2C9 have a regioselectivity, which is governed by specific binding to a region of the active site by means of an ion pair. Thus, whilst the structure of the substrate may play a part in determining the site and type of reaction, the primary determinant is the site of oxidation and is the topography of the active site. In contrast, for CYP3A4, the most abundant form of cytochrome P-450 in the human liver, the structure of the substrate, rather than the topography of the active site, appears to be the primary determinant of the site of oxidation.

TABLE 2.2 *The physicochemical properties of the substrates for the major isoforms of cytochrome P-450 responsible for drug metabolism in man*

P-450 isoform	Structural/physicochemical properties
CYP2D6	Arylalkylamines (at least 1 N and 1 aromatic ring) pK_a of basic nitrogen above 7 log *D* below 5 Protonated nitrogen 5–7 Å from the site of metabolism
CYP2C9	Lipophilic (log $D < 6$) Acidic and neutral compounds (p$K_{a<6}$) containing at least one oxygen atom Site of oxidation is 5–7 Å from the hydrogen bond acceptor/donor heteroatom
CYP3A4	Lipophilic, acidic or neutral Site of oxidation after a basic nitrogen Hydrogen bond acceptors 5–8 Å from the site of metabolism

In silico models produced by overlap of substrates or inhibitors with the active site of the enzymes are being established with a view to being able to predict the site of metabolism of compounds from their structure. Whilst we are some way along this road, with models becoming increasingly refined for CYP2D6, those for CYP2C9 and CYP3A4 are at an earlier stage. Currently, the use of such models is mainly confined to interpretation and rationalisation of experimental results rather than for the positive selection of compounds with optimal metabolic stability. This remains a goal for the future.

2.7.2 Glucuronidation

In addition to elimination by Phase 1 metabolism, xenobiotics can be eliminated by conjugation of the unchanged drug or its Phase 1 metabolite to form a glucuronide or a sulphate conjugate. The chemistry of the enzymes is well understood and the metabolically vulnerable functionalities (e.g. an aromatic hydroxyl group or a carboxylic acid moiety) are already known. Thus, with glucuronidation for example, the reaction of the transfer of D-glucuronic acid from UDPαD-glucuronic acid to the acceptor molecule is catalysed by the UDP-α-glucuronyl transferases. The reaction proceeds by nucleophilic SN2 substitution of the acceptor at the C1 position of glucuronic acid, the resulting product then undergoing configurational inversion.

Although our understanding of conjugation reactions is applied to rational drug design, it is not sufficiently advanced to explain why compounds containing functions amenable to conjugation are ultimately resistant to conjugation *in vivo*. The subject of conjugation reactions is dealt with in greater detail in Chapter 14.

2.7.3 Renal drug elimination

Excretion from the body via the urine is the major route of elimination for many drugs. Drugs that are non-volatile, have a low molecular weight (<500), are highly soluble or are lowly metabolised will be eliminated from the body by renal excretion. Renal excretion is actually a multifactorial process and excretion of a drug via the kidneys may include a combination of three processes, namely, glomerular filtration, active tubular secretion and tubular reabsorption.

Glomerular filtration is a unidirectional process that occurs for most low molecular weight compounds (<500) irrespective of their degree of ionisation. Drugs that are highly protein bound will not be filtered at the glomerulus and, thus, glomerular filtration of drugs is directly related to the free fraction in plasma. As the free drug concentration in the plasma increases, the glomerular filtration of the drug increases proportionately.

In contrast to glomerular filtration, active renal secretion, as the name suggests, is an active process involving a carrier-mediated system. Because the system transports drug against a concentration gradient, energy is required to drive the system. Systems exist for secreting acids (anions) and bases (cations) from the plasma to the lumen of the proximal tubule. In most cases, the process is unaffected by plasma protein binding due to the rapid dissociation of the drug–protein complex. Penicillins, for example, which are highly protein bound, have short elimination half-lives due to their rapid elimination by active secretion. In contrast to glomerular filtration, however, since a carrier system is involved, competition between drugs can occur for the carrier leading to inhibition of the tubular secretion of the drug with the lower affinity for the carrier. The inhibition of the tubular secretion of antibiotics by the uricoscuric agent probenecid is well known and this has been used as a means of reducing the rapid elimination of penicillins thereby increasing their duration of action.

After filtration of free drug at the glomerulus and secretion of the drug in the proximal tubule, drugs can be subject to tubular re-absorption. Re-absorption is generally a passive diffusive process that arises as a consequence of the large concentration gradient that exists between the drug in the tubular lumen and free drug in the plasma due to the highly efficient re-absorption of water. In keeping with the function of the tubular membrane, re-absorption/transport of lipid soluble drugs is favoured and drugs that have poor lipophilicity or are ionised are not generally re-absorbed. Re-absorption takes place in the distal portion of the tubules where the un-ionised molecules can pass across the membrane to the circulating plasma. In a situation similar to that for intestinal absorption, the pK_a of the drug and the pH of the fluid in the distal tubule i.e. the urine, dictate the rate and extent of re-absorption. Whilst the pK_a of the drug is constant, the pH of the urine can vary from four to eight depending upon diet, concurrent drug elimination (e.g. antacids) and pathophysiological changes that result in acidosis and alkalosis. Acidification of the urine facilitates the re-absorption of weak acids whilst reducing the re-absorption of weak bases. Making the urinary pH more alkaline has the opposite effect on weak acids, increasing their ionisation such that they cannot be re-absorbed and are thus eliminated. Strong acids or bases, as is the case for intestinal absorption, are completely ionised over the entire range of urinary pH and undergo little re-absorption. On the basis of the behaviour of a variety of different drugs, in keeping with the discussion on the effects of pH, the lipophilicity of a compound as described by its log D is a good surrogate of the kidney tubule membrane. Thus, as a general rule of thumb, re-absorption of a drug will be near complete at log D values above zero, whilst tubular re-absorption will be negligible for those below zero. Thus if the log D of a drug is known along with its pK_a, it should be possible to determine the changes in urinary pH required to ensure secretion of the drug where detoxification is required as in the case of accidental overdose. In such circumstances, the urinary pH can be made more basic by intravenous administration of bicarbonate if the toxic drug is an acid, or more acidic using ascorbic acid where appropriate, to ensure that the drug remains in its ionised form and is thus safely voided in the urine.

2.8 *Chirality and its effects on drug absorption, metabolism and excretion*

Prior sections of this chapter have focused on the physicochemical properties of molecules common to most drugs such as intrinsic lipophilicity and degree of ionisation. There is, however, a further physicochemical characteristic found in certain molecules that markedly affects their disposition and metabolism, namely that of chirality. Chirality is a structural characteristic of a molecule whereby it is able to exist in two asymmetric forms, which are non-superimposable. Most frequently, these isomers or enantiomers occur where the molecule contains a carbon atom that is attached to four different functional groups i.e. the molecule possesses a chiral centre. An example of a chiral drug is the anticoagulant warfarin the structure of which is shown in Figure 2.5.

Although such pairs of enantiomers cannot be distinguished by the usual physical characteristics of melting point and lipophilicity, the body can readily distinguish between such molecules. Because the two isomers are non-superimposable they have different abilities to bind to receptors or enzymes and this confers stereoselectivity. This is often reflected by significant differences in the pharmacokinetics and pharmacodynamics of a pair of enantiomers and these will be discussed briefly below.

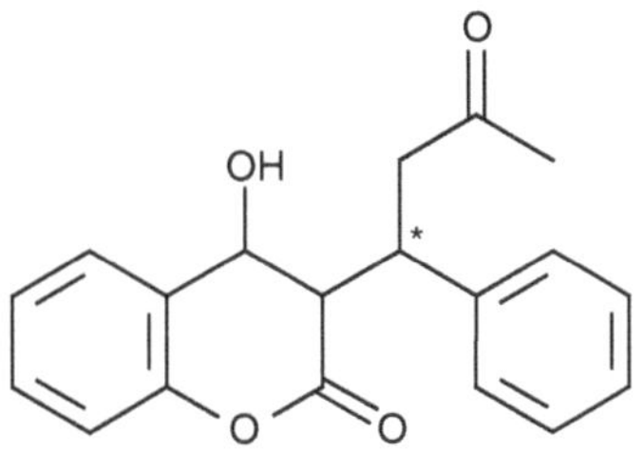

FIGURE 2.5 *The structure of warfarin indicating the position of the chiral centre (*).*

2.8.1 Differences in absorption of enantiomers

In terms of the absorptive process, in the case of drugs that penetrate the membrane by passive diffusion, this is due purely to their lipophilicity and degree of ionisation. Since there will be no difference in either of these parameters between a pair of enantiomers, there will be no difference in the extent or rate of absorption and passive diffusion can be considered to be achiral. In contrast, however, active transport which requires recognition of the enantiomer by its carrier protein, may be expected to demonstrate enantioselectivity. Indeed the preferential uptake of the L-isomer of dopamine has been demonstrated in man (Lee and Williams, 1990). Similarly, in the case of methotrexate, the R-form of the drug is preferentially absorbed after oral administration (Hendel and Brodthages, 1984). It should be borne in mind, however, that unless there is a physical barrier to passive absorption then only the rate of absorption should differ and the extent of absorption should remain the same. Furthermore, despite the potential importance of stereoselective absorption, the number of drugs demonstrating this behaviour is quantitatively small and for the majority of compounds, which undergo passive absorption, chirality has no effect.

2.8.2 Differences in distribution and protein binding of enantiomers

Distribution of a drug, like absorption, involves penetration across tissue compartments but, additionally, involves recognition by macromolecules present in tissue and plasma. The potential exists, therefore, for stereoselective distribution to occur. In practice, however, there is little if any evidence of this process occurring *in vivo*, the only evidence coming from *in vitro* studies suggesting that the release and storage of β-blockers such as atenolol from nerve endings in cardiac tissue are stereoselective for the active *S*-enantiomer (Walle *et al.*, 1988).

The distribution of a drug can be markedly affected by its ability to bind to plasma proteins since only free drug is able to cross cell membranes and the blood–brain barrier. The plasma proteins to which drugs bind are enantioselective and the fraction of the free, active drug can be widely different between the enantiomers of highly protein-bound drugs such as ibuprofen and propranolol. The active *S*-enantiomer of ibuprofen is 50 per cent less protein bound than the inactive *R*-enantiomer (Evans *et al.*, 1989). In the case of warfarin, however, the opposite is true with the more active *S*-enantiomer being 50 per cent more protein bound (Toon *et al.*, 1986). By virtue of being highly protein bound, small changes in protein binding result in large changes in the free active fraction and thus the therapeutic benefit of such compounds can be markedly affected by stereoselective protein binding.

2.8.3 Differences in the metabolism of enantiomers

Although some drugs are excreted in the urine unchanged, the vast majority undergo some degree of metabolism. Although hepatic cytochromes P-450, the major drug-metabolising enzymes in humans, have a broad substrate specificity, they display significant stereoselectivity of metabolism towards chiral substrates. The extent of the difference in metabolism of enantiomers can be significant as illustrated by the example of warfarin. The oral clearance of the *R*-enantiomer is some 42 per cent greater than that of the *S*-enantiomer (Toon *et al.*, 1987). It is known that *S*-warfarin is metabolised by cytochrome P-450 2C9 whilst *R*-warfarin is metabolised predominantly by cytochrome P-450 3A4 and this may underlie the difference in the rates of metabolism of the two enantiomers (Rettie *et al.*, 1992).

The β-blocker propranolol also shows stereoselective elimination with the oral clearance of the *R*-enantiomer being 40 per cent greater than that of the *S*-enantiomer (Walle *et al.*, 1988). The calcium channel antagonist verapamil also undergoes stereoselective elimination but also has the complication of the extent of elimination being specific to the route of administration. Thus, after intravenous administration, *S*-verapamil is preferentially eliminated with a systemic clearance some 70 per cent greater than that for the *R*-enantiomer (Eichelbaum *et al.*, 1984). After oral administration, however, although the *S*-enantiomer is still preferentially eliminated, the oral clearance is some 4-fold higher than that of the *R*-enantiomer (Vogelsang *et al.*, 1984). Since the anti-arrhythmic activity of verapamil resides largely in the *S*-enantiomer, because of stereospecific elimination, there is poor efficacy after oral administration. If verapamil is administered intravenously, the elimination of the *S*-enantiomer is reduced and a better anti-arrhythmic response is achieved. Thus, by manipulation of the route of administration of this compound, adequate efficacy can be achieved.

2.8.4 Differences in the renal clearance of enantiomers

Renal clearance, like hepatic clearance, can be stereoselective. Examples are disopyramide and terbutaline where renal clearance of the two enantiomers differs by approximately 2-fold (Lima *et al.*, 1985; Borgstrom *et al.*, 1989). Equally, however, there are other examples, tocainide being one where there is no difference in the renal clearance of enantiomers (Edgar *et al.*, 1984). This difference is likely due to differences in the affinity of the enantiomers for the transporters involved in tubular secretion. Thus for the majority of compounds that are filtered in the glomerulus and are not actively secreted, there will be no difference in the elimination of the enantiomers.

2.8.5 Differences in the pharmacodynamics of enantiomers

It is obvious from the previous discussions that stereoselective elimination can have significant effects upon the disposition of enantiomers and upon the efficacy of a compound, especially if it is the active enantiomer that is affected. Thus, because the *S*-enantiomer of propranolol is approximately 100-fold more active than its *R*-enantiomer, and the *R*-enantiomer is selectively eliminated, measurements of dynamic effects based upon measurements of total drug concentration are meaningless (Murray *et al.*, 1990). In response to this, the Food and Drug Administration (1992) has developed guidelines for the development of racemic compounds. This document requires, among other things, elucidation of enantiomeric purity, determination of the pharmacokinetics of each enantiomer in animals and man and determination of the potential for interconversion to occur. This also necessitates the development of chiral assays, and the package of work necessary to develop a racemic drug is substantial. The ramifications of chirality thus reach beyond the bounds of its effect on drug disposition, and it is likely that most pharmaceutical companies will elect to develop a single enantiomer rather than a racemate, where possible.

2.9 *The importance of physicochemical properties to the analysis of drugs*

The ability to selectively analyse for the drug of interest in a variety of biological matrices is a necessary pre-requisite to obtaining accurate pharmacokinetic data. Unless the mechanism of detection is mass spectrometry, where by virtue of the selectivity of the detector a simple protein precipitation prior to injection may suffice, this generally requires some degree of clean up/concentration followed by chromatographic separation prior to detection.

Methods of sample cleanup are discussed in Chapter 3. However, since the sample cleanup and the chromatographic separation are the stages at which knowledge of the physicochemical properties of the drug can be utilised to optimise recovery and separation, some brief discussion of this topic is worthwhile.

Earlier in the chapter, we considered the distribution of a drug between an aqueous phase such as buffer and an organic phase such as octanol to determine the partition coefficient, log P. A liquid–liquid extraction system will be directly analogous to this system. The solvents are mixed until an equilibrium is obtained and the drug to be isolated is located primarily in one of the two immiscible layers, usually the organic to facilitate speed of evaporation and reconstitution in an appropriate mobile phase. Liquid–liquid extraction has been largely superseded by solid phase extraction, where extraction of the analyte is dependent upon its partitioning between a solid stationary phase e.g. C18 bonded silica, and solvent(s) flowing over this phase. This is represented diagrammatically in Figure 2.6.

In such a system, the efficiency of partitioning is obviously a function of the rate at which the sample matrix is drawn over the surface of the stationary phase. If the flow rate is too rapid then there may be insufficient time for the drug to partition into the stationary phase and the drug of interest may pass through unresolved from the interfering substances. Similar dynamic considerations will also pertain to the chromatographic situation in which there is a range of flow rates within which optimum chromatography will be achieved. At flow rates beyond this optimum, column efficiency will be reduced resulting in deterioration of the peak shape and a corresponding reduction in sensitivity.

Of great value to the extraction of a compound, either by liquid–liquid or solid phase extraction, and, in turn, to the optimal chromatographic separation of a drug, is a knowledge of its pK_a. The ability of a drug to partition between an aqueous phase and an organic phase, as is the case for its ability to cross a membrane, is highly dependent upon pH. As would be expected from discussions above, acids distribute into an organic phase and are well retained on chromatography columns at a pH below their pK_a when they are largely un-ionised and are poorly retained at pHs above their pK_a when they are fully ionised. The reverse situation applies for bases, which are ionised and thus poorly retained at a pH below their pK_a, but well retained at a pH above their pK_a when ionisation is suppressed. In addition, since

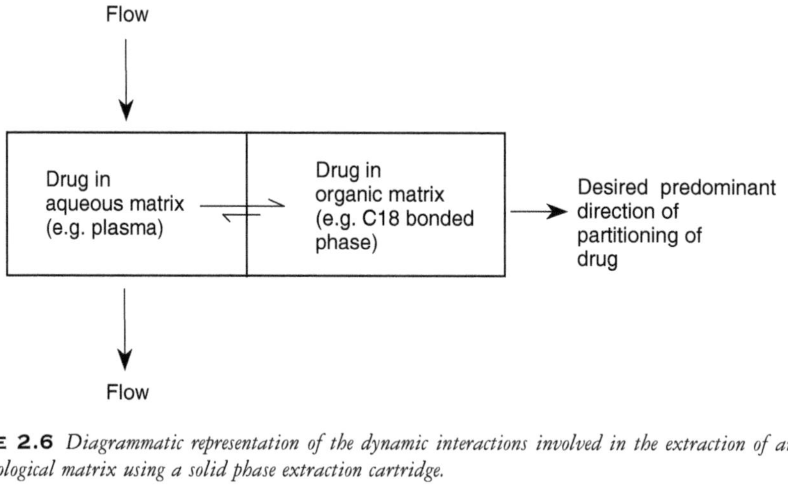

FIGURE 2.6 *Diagrammatic representation of the dynamic interactions involved in the extraction of an analyte from a biological matrix using a solid phase extraction cartridge.*

the pH of the medium can be readily manipulated, the chromatographic separation of weakly ionisable acids and bases can be readily optimised.

It can thus be seen that, by having an appreciation of the simple physicochemical characteristics of a molecule, predictions as to its likely behaviour in a given chromatographic system can be made and the task of obtaining a suitable sample cleanup and chromatographic separation can be made much easier. The value of taking a few moments to consider these properties cannot be overstated.

2.10 *Summary*

We have seen from the preceding sections just how important the physicochemical properties of a drug are to its disposition and have an understanding of the concepts of intrinsic lipophilicity, ionisation and chirality. It should be obvious that by taking the time to consider whether a compound is an acid or a base, and, if so, what the values are for its log P, pK_a and its solubility, it should then be easier to explain its behaviour in the body or in the analytical procedure used to measure it. Furthermore, since these properties determine the preferred environment of the drugs in the body, they should also allow one to predict the likely behaviour of a drug in the body and allow one to make judgements as to the viability of new chemical entities to become drugs. With the advent of combinatorial chemistry, the potential exists to synthesise thousands of compounds per week, which will require evaluation and optimisation. The development of predictive models based upon physicochemical properties offers a high throughput means of reducing the numbers of compounds being tested *in vivo*, and such models have begun to emerge (Lipinski *et al.*, 1997). The focus is beginning to return to basic physicochemical properties of molecules, and if this chapter has prompted you to think more carefully about the properties of the drugs with which you work, it will have fulfilled its purpose.

2.11 *Bibliography*

Arendt, R.M., Greenblatt, D.J., deJong, R.H., Bonin, J.D., Abernethy, D.R., Ehrenberg, B.L., Giles, H.G., Sellers, E.M. and Shader, R.I. (1983) *In vitro* correlates of benzodiazepine cerebrospinal fluid uptake 1. Pharmacodynamic action and peripheral distribution. *J. Pharmacol. Exp. Ther.* 227, 98–106.

Belpaire, F.M., Braeckman, R.A. and Bogaert, M.G. (1984) Binding of oxprenolol and propranolol to serum albumin and α_1-acid glycoprotein in man and other species. *Biochem. Pharmacol.* 33, 2065–2069.

Borgstrom, L., Nyberg, L., Jonsson, S., Linberg, C. and Paulson, J. (1989) Pharmacokinetic evaluation in man of terbutaline given as separate enantiomers and as a racemate. *Br. J. Clin. Pharmcol.* 27, 49–56.

Brauman, T. (1986) Determination of hydrophobic parameters by reversed-phase liquid chromatography: theory, experimental techniques and applications in studies on quantitative structure activity relationships. *J. Chromatogr.* 373, 191–225.

Bridges, J.W. and Wilson, A.G.E. (1977) Drug–serum protein binding interactions and their biological significance. In: *Progress in Drug Metabolism*, Vol. 2, pp. 193–247, Bridges, J.W. and Chasseaud, L.F. (eds), Wiley Interscience, London.

Chapman, D., Williams, R.M. and Ladbrooke, B.D. (1967) *Chem. Phys. Lipids* 1, 445.

Crone, C. and Olensen, S.P. (1982) Electrical resistance of brain microvascular endothelium. *Brain Res.* 241, 49–55.

Edgar, B., Heggelund, A., Johansson, L., Nyberg, G. and Regardh, C.G. (1984) The pharmacokinetics of R- and S-tocainide in healthy subjects. *Br. J. Clin. Pharmacol.* 16, 216P–217P.

Eichelbaum, M., Mikus, G. and Vogelsang, B. (1984) Pharmacokinetics of (+)-, (−)- and (±) verapamil after intravenous administration. *Br. J. Clin. Pharmacol.* 18, 733–740.

Evans, A.M., Nation, R.L., Sansom, L.N., Bochner, F. and Somogyi, A.A. (1989) Stereoselective protein binding of ibuprofen enantiomers. *Eur. J. Clin. Pharmacol.* 36, 283–290.

Food and Drug Administration (1992) Policy statement for the development of new stereoisomeric drugs. *Chirality* 4, 338–340.

Fujita, T., Isawa, J. and Hansch, C. (1964) *J. Amer. Chem. Soc.* 86, 5175.

Guengerich, F.P. and MacDonald, T.L. (1990) Mechanisms of cytochrome P-450 catalysis. *FASEB J.* 4, 2453–2459.

Hansch, C. (1976) On the structure of medicinal chemistry. *J. Med. Chem.* 19, 1–6.

Hansch, C., Klein, T., McClarin, J., Langridge, R. and Cornell, N.W. (1986) A quantitative structure–activity relationship and molecular graphics analysis of hydrophobic effects in the interactions of inhibitors with alcohol dehydrogenase. *J. Med. Chem.* May, 29(5), 615–620.

Hendel, J. and Brodthages, H. (1984) Entero-hepatic cycling of methotrexate estimated by use of the D-isomer as a reference marker. *Eur. J. Clin. Pharmacol.* 26, 103–107.

Houston, J.B. and Wood, S.G. (1980) Gastrointestinal absorption of drugs and other xenobiotics. In: *Progress in Drug Metabolism*, Vol. 4, pp. 57–129, Bridges, J.W. and Chasseaud, L.F. (eds), John Wiley & Sons, London.

Jezequel, S.G. (1992) Central nervous penetration of drugs: importance of physicochemical properties. In: *Progress in Drug Metabolism*, Vol. 13, pp. 141–178, Gibson, G.G. (ed.), Taylor & Francis, London.

Kararli, T.T. (1995) Comparison of the gastrointestinal anatomy, physiology and biochemistry of humans and commonly used laboratory animals. *Biopharm. Drug Dispos.* 16, 351–380.

Lee, E.J.D. and Williams, K.M. (1990) Chirality: clinical pharmacokinetics and pharmacodynamic considerations. *Clin. Pharmacokinet.* 18, 339–345.

Lima, J.J., Boudoulas, H. and Shields, B.J. (1985) Stereoselective pharmacokinetics of disopyramide enantiomers in man. *Drug Metab. Dispos.* 13, 572–577.

Lipinski, C.A., Lombardo, F., Dominy, B.W. and Feeney, P.J. (1997) Experimental and computational approaches to estimate solubility and permeability in drug discovery and development settings. *Adv. Drug Deliv. Rev.* 23, 3–25.

Luscombe, D.K. and Nicholls, P.J. (1988) Processes of drug handling in the body. In: *Smith and Williams' Introduction to the Principles of Drug Design*, 2nd edition, pp. 1–31, Smith, H.J. (ed.), Wright, London.

Murray, K.T., Reilly, C., Koshakji, R.P., Roden, D.M., Lineberry, M.D., Wood, A.J.J., Siddoway, L.A., Barbey, J.T. and Woosley, R.L. (1990) Suppression of ventricular arrythmias in man by D-propranolol independent of beta-adrenergic receptor blockade. *J. Clin. Invest.* 85, 836–842.

Ong, S., Liu, H., Qiu, X., Bhat, G. and Pidgeon, C. (1995) Membrane partition coefficients chromatographically measured using immobilised artificial membrane surfaces. *Anal. Chem.* 67, 755–762.

Pardridge, W.M. (1979) Carrier mediated transport of thyroid hormones through the rat blood – brain barrier: primary role of albumin bound hormone. *Endocrinology* 105 605–612.

Pardridge, W.M. (1988) Recent advances in blood–brain barrier transport. *Ann. Rev. Pharmacol. Toxicol.* 28, 25–39.

Rettie, A.E., Korzekwa, K.R., Kunze, K.L., Lawrence, R.F., Eddy, A.C., Aoyama, T., Gelboin, H.V., Gonzales, F.J. and Trager, W.F. (1992) Hydroxylation of warfarin by human cDNA-expressed cytochrome P-450: a role for P-450 2C9 in the etiology of (S)-warfarin drug interactions. *Chem. Res. Toxicol.* 5, 54–59.

Schanker, L.S. (1964) Physiological transport of drugs. *Adv. Drug Res.* 1, 71–106.

Scherrer, R.A. and Howard, S.M. (1977) Use of distribution coefficients in quantitative structure/activity relationships. *J. Med. Chem.* 20, 53–58.

Scherrer, R.A. and Howard, S.M. (1979) The analysis of electronic factors in quantitative structure/activity relationships using distribution coefficients. In: *Computer-Assisted Drug Design.* ACS Symposium Series, No. 112, pp. 507–526, Olson, C. and Christoffersen, R.E. (eds) *Am. Chem. Soc.*

Seydel, J.K. and Schaper, K.-J. (1982) Quantitative structure-pharmacokinetic relationships and drug design. *Pharmacol. Ther.* 15, 131–138.

Smith, D.A. (1994) Design of drugs through a consideration of drug metabolism and pharmacokinetics. *Eur. J. Drug Metab. Pharmacokinet.* 3, 193–199.

Smith, R.N., Hansch, C. and Ames, M.M. (1975) Selection of a reference partitioning system for drug design work. *J. Pharm. Sci.* 64, 599–606.

Tenakin, T. (1993) Pharmacologic analysis of drug receptor interaction. 2nd edition. pp. 223–224, Raven press, New York.

Toon, S., Hopkins, K.J., Garstang, F.M. and Rowland, M. (1987) Comparative effects of ranitidine and cimetidine on the pharmacokinetics and pharmacodynamics of warfarin in man. *Eur. J. Clin. Pharmacol.* 32, 165–172.

Toon, S., Low, L.K., Gibaldi, M., Trager, W.F., O'Reilly, R.A., Motley, C.H. and Goulart, D.A. (1986) The warfarin-sulfinpyrazone interaction: stereochemical considerations. *Clin. Pharmacol. Ther.* 39, 15–24.

Tracy, T.S. (1995) Stereochemistry in pharmacotherapy: when mirror images are not identical. *Ann. Pharmacother.* 29, 161–165.

Unger, S.H., Cook, J.R. and Hollenberg, J.S. (1978) Simple procedure for determining octanol-aqueous partition, distribution and ionisation coefficients by reversed-phase high pressure liquid chromatography. *J. Pharm. Sci.* 67, 1364–1367.

Vogelsang, B., Echizen, H., Schmidt, E. and Eichelbaum, M. (1984) Stereoselective first-pass metabolism of highly cleared drugs: studies of the bioavailability of L- and D-verapamil examined with a stable isotope technique. *Br. J. Clin. Pharmacol.* 18, 733–740.

Walle, T., Webb, J.G., Bagwell, E.E., Walle, U.K., Daniell, H.B. and Gaffney, T.E. (1988) Stereoselective delivery and actions of beta-receptor antagonists. *Biochem. Pharmacol.* 37, 115–124.

Yokogawa, K., Nakashima, E. and Ichimura, F. (1990) Effect of fat tissue volume on the distribution kinetics of biperidin as a function of age in rats. *Drug Metab. Dispos.* 18, 258–263.

CHAPTER 3

Sample preparation

Bob Biddlecombe and
Glenn Smith

3.1 *Introduction*

The quantitative determination of drugs and their metabolites in biological matrices (bioanalysis) includes a number of steps from sample collection to the final report of the results. The intermediate steps typically include sample storage, sample preparation, separation, identification and quantification of analyte(s). Sample preparation prior to the chromatographic separation has three principal objectives: the dissolution of the analyte in a suitable solvent, removal of as many interfering compounds as possible and pre-concentration of the analyte. A number of techniques such as protein precipitation, liquid–liquid extraction and solid phase extraction (SPE) are routinely used.

3.2 *Sample preparation techniques*

3.2.1 Protein precipitation

In protein precipitation, acids or water-miscible organic solvents are used to remove the protein by denaturation and precipitation. Acids, such as trichloroacetic acid

(TCA) and perchloric acid, are very efficient at precipitating proteins. The proteins, which are in their cationic form at low pH, form insoluble salts with the acids. A 5–20 per cent solution of these acids is generally sufficient and the best results can be achieved using cold reagents. Organic solvents, such as methanol, acetonitrile, acetone and ethanol, although having a relatively low efficiency in removing plasma proteins, have been widely used in bioanalysis because of their compatibility with high-performance liquid chromatography (HPLC) mobile phases (Blanchard, 1981). These organic solvents which lower the solubility of proteins and precipitate them from solutions have an effectiveness which is inversely related to their polarity.

3.2.2 Liquid–liquid extraction

Liquid–liquid extraction (LLE) is the direct extraction of the biological material with a water-immiscible solvent. The analyte is isolated by partitioning between the organic phase and the aqueous phase. The distribution ratio is affected by a number of factors: choice of extracting solvent, pH of aqueous phase and ratio of the volumes of the organic to aqueous phase. The analyte should be preferentially distributed in the organic phase under the chosen conditions. Although a number of factors influence the choice of solvent, the most important factor is the relative lipophilicity or hydrophobicity of the analyte. The analyte must be soluble in the extracting solvent. The solvent should also have a low boiling point to facilitate removal at the end of the extraction and a low viscosity to facilitate mixing with the sample matrix. Generally, selectivity is improved by choosing the least polar solvent in which the analyte is soluble.

The extraction process can be controlled using pH; ionised compounds are less efficiently partitioned in the organic phase. Changing the pH enables the process to be reversed; the charged analyte is re-extracted into the aqueous phase for further purification. The use of pH control allows the fractionation of the sample into acid, neutral and basic components. A large surface area is important to ensure rapid equilibrium. This is achieved by thoroughly mixing using either mechanical or manual shaking or vortexing.

There are several disadvantages of LLE; the technique is not applicable to all compounds. Highly polar molecules can be very difficult, although the use of an ion pairing reagent can extend LLE to molecules of this type. Another major problem is the formation of emulsions. These can be difficult to break even using centrifugation or ultrasonification and can cause loss of analyte by occlusion within the emulsion. The use of less rigorous mixing or larger volumes of extracting solvent can help reduce the problem with emulsions. LLE is also not very readily automatable.

Disposable columns containing diatomaceous earth as an adsorbent have been used to overcome many of the limitations of LLE. The diluted sample is poured onto the column and held on the support as a very thin film. The extracting solvent is then passed through the column. The high surface area of the sample allows a very efficient extraction.

3.2.3 Solid phase extraction

The principal mechanisms of separation and isolation utilised in solid phase separation (SPE), reversed-phase, normal phase and ion exchange are the same as those used in HPLC. Although the mechanisms of separation for the two techniques are the same, the dynamics of each technique is very different. In HPLC the compounds are separated in a continuously flowing system of mobile phase, while SPE is a series of discrete steps. In SPE the analyte is retained on the solid phase while the sample passes through, followed by elution of the analyte with an appropriate solvent. SPE can be considered as a simple on/off type of chromatography (Wells and Michael, 1987).

A typical SPE sorbent consists of a 40–60 μm silica particle to which has been bonded a hydrocarbon phase. This bonding is achieved by the reaction of a chlorosilane with the hydroxyl groups of the silica gel to form a silicon–oxygen–silicon link (Gilpin and Burke, 1973). This monofunctional bonded phase was originally the most popular reversed-phase sorbent with 4, 8 or 18 carbon atoms attached (C4, C8 and C18). Other reversed-phase sorbents such as C2, cyclohexyl and phenyl have subsequently been developed. A three-carbon spacer chain is generally used to link both cyclohexyl and phenyl groups. Normal-phase sorbents and ion exchange sorbents also have a three-carbon linking chain. The degree of carbon loading varies from 5 to 19 per cent by weight depending on the length of the hydrocarbon chain. The greater the carbon loading the greater the capacity; hence C18 sorbents have the greatest capacity expressed in milligrams of analyte sorbed per gram of sorbent. The capacity of a sorbent is also dependent on the pore size of the silca. The pore size affects both the coverage density of alklybonded phase and the migration of analytes in and out of pores during sorption. Much of the variation encountered between bonded phases of different manufacturers and even between different batches from the same manufacturer can be attributed to variation in the surface composition of the silica (Nawrocki and Dabrowska, 2000). An important characteristic of a sorbent is the number of unreacted or free silanols. These silanols are capable of hydrogen bonding or weak cation exchange with any solute bound to the bonded phase of the sorbent, particularly weak basic compounds. These secondary interactions need to be carefully considered during method development. As in the development of chromatographic stationary phases the manufacturers have tried to minimise the effect of these silonal groups. The use of trifunctional derivatives, trichloroalkylsilanes, gives not only greater stability under acid conditions, because the hydrocarbon chain is attached at multiple sites, but reduces the number of free silanols. The number of free silanols is generally further reduced by endcapping, where the derivatised silica gel is reacted with a trimethylchlorosilane reagent.

The disposable syringe barrel format of SPE contributed significantly to its success as a sample preparation technique. The syringes are available in 1–25 ml and packing weights from 25 mg to 10 g. The syringe barrel is typically polypropylene with a male Luer tip fitting. The sorbent material is packed between two 20 μm polypropylene frits. A vacuum manifold is used to draw the sample and eluting solvents through the syringe barrel under negative pressure by applying a vacuum to the manifold. Other types of sample processing that may be used include centrifugation and positive pressure. The SPE is typically carried out using a five-step process: condition, equilibrate, load, wash and elute. The solid phase sorbent is conditioned by passing a solvent, usually methanol, through the sorbent to wet the packing material and solvate the functional groups of the sorbent. The sorbent is then equilibrated with water or an aqueous buffer. Care must be taken to prevent the phase from drying out before the sample is loaded, otherwise variable recoveries can be obtained. Samples are diluted 1:1 with aqueous prior to loading to reduce viscosity and prevent the sorbent bed from becoming blocked. Aqueous and/or organic washes are used to remove interferences.

3.3 *Instrumentation*

A great deal of sample preparation in bioanalytical laboratories is still carried out manually. Indeed, automation of sample preparation in bioanlytical laboratories has progressed at a much slower rate than in other areas of the pharmaceutical industry. Specifically, the combinatorial chemistry, high-throughput screening and compound storage/distribution laboratories in drug discovery, as well as the analytical quality control laboratories in manufacturing plants, have been revolutionised by automation over the last 5–10 years. Until recently, the hesitation to automate bioanalytical sample preparation has been quite understandable. The diversity of sample preparation techniques and the uniqueness of each individual assay's methodology have made implementing the required functionality and flexibility into an automation system too difficult and expensive. The wide variety of extraction consumables (e.g. test tubes, vials, SPE cartridges, etc.) used for sample preparation has meant that automation system is often limited to only certain manufacturers' sample preparation products. Most bioanalytical methods are only used for a limited time and the long-term need for a particular assay is often uncertain. Therefore devoting significant resources to the automation of a method can be viewed as a risky venture.

Recent advances in both laboratory automation equipment and sample preparation products have made automating bioanalytical assays more appealing and practical than ever before. The establishment of LC–MS–MS, with its combination of high sensitivity, high specificity and potential for high sample throughput, as the technique of choice in bioanalysis has greatly accelerated the development of automated sample preparation systems. Trends towards parallel processing of samples in 96-well plates have made automated sample preparation procedures quicker and more cost-effective. Likewise, novel SPE products that yield high recoveries for a wide range of analytes, using a single generic extraction procedure, greatly reduce the amount of time spent reconfiguring robotic systems each time a new assay is needed.

The number of commercially available automated sample preparation systems is still somewhat limited. Most of these are designed to support solid phase extraction. Protein precipitation and liquid–liquid extraction are often restricted to either semi-automated approaches, in which only the sample transfer and reagent addition steps are automated using a liquid handling workstation, or the more complex fully automated robotic systems which tend to be highly customised.

Instrumentation currently available can be grouped by their degree of automation. The five representative categories are:

1 SPE application-specific workstations or modules
2 On-line sample prep instruments
3 XYZ liquid handlers
4 Robotic workstations
5 Fully automated robotics systems.

This classification is not absolute since the diversity of these systems really represents a continuum. Some systems may overlap into two or more of the categories. On-line instruments include autosamplers with preparative, liquid addition, transfer capabilities, switching valves and other on-line and direct injection techniques.

3.4 *Bioanalytical automation strategy*

The switch to LC–MS–MS as the method of choice for bioanalysis made the sample preparation step the bottleneck. The development of SPE in the 96-well format and the development of systems using parallel processing have overcome this bottleneck and once again made the analysis time the rate-determining step. The original semi-automated systems used a customised vacuum manifold located on the deck of a Packard MultiPROBE™ RSP (Allanson *et al.*, 1996). The MultiPROBE performed all the liquid handling steps and controlled the vacuum. This allowed automation of the condition, load and wash steps, but the operator was required to manually place the collecting plate in the vacuum manifold prior to the elution step. Similar approaches to sample preparation in the 96-well format have been subsequently reported by a number of authors. In order to maximise the advantages of this approach and overcome some of the limitations a fully automated system was developed.

3.4.1 Fully automated sample preparation system

The initial system consisted of a Zymate XP robot, cooled storage carousel, a custom-built SPE station and an RSP (see Figure 3.1). The system running Easylab software (version 2.5) with a Visual Basic™ (version 4) user interface. The software

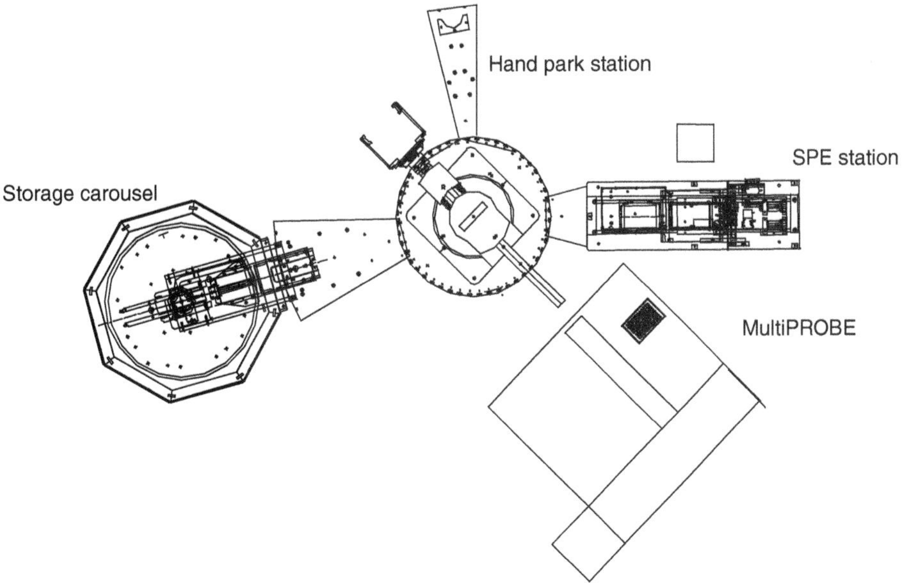

FIGURE 3.1 *Schematic representation of Zymark sample preparation system.*

was very quick and easy to use providing the facility to set up extraction procedures, change reagents and purge lines, and run procedures.

To run an existing procedure the user selected the appropriate procedure or procedures and entered the number of samples in each batch, up to four consecutive batches of samples could be processed using either the same or different procedures. When prompted, the user then loaded the required labware, SPE blocks and collection plates, into the storage carousel. The eight racks of the storage carousel are pre-assigned in the software to a particular type of labware. The cooled storage carousel, which could be maintained at 4–50 °C, not only acted as a warehouse for all the labware but also as a repository for the collection plates containing extracts.

To create a new procedure the user selected the type of SPE block (e.g. Microlute™ 2 or Empore™) and type of collection plate (e.g. deep well or square well), and specified the volume and reagent used for up to three condition steps, two wash steps and one elute step. The vacuum time and the bleed factor were also entered for each vacuum step. The power of the vacuum applied to the SPE block could be moderated using an extra valve that was open to the air. The setting on this valve, the bleed factor, was used to control the flow rates and ensure that the phase did not dry out before the sample load step. Conventional packed bed-reversed phase sorbents are prone to drying out. This can lead to poor or variable recoveries. It is also important to ensure that the flow rate for the sample load and elution step were optimised, otherwise recoveries could again be adversely affected.

The SPE station is a modified reagent addition station (RAS) which incorporates a two-stage vacuum manifold (see Figure 3.2). Reagents can be rapidly added row at

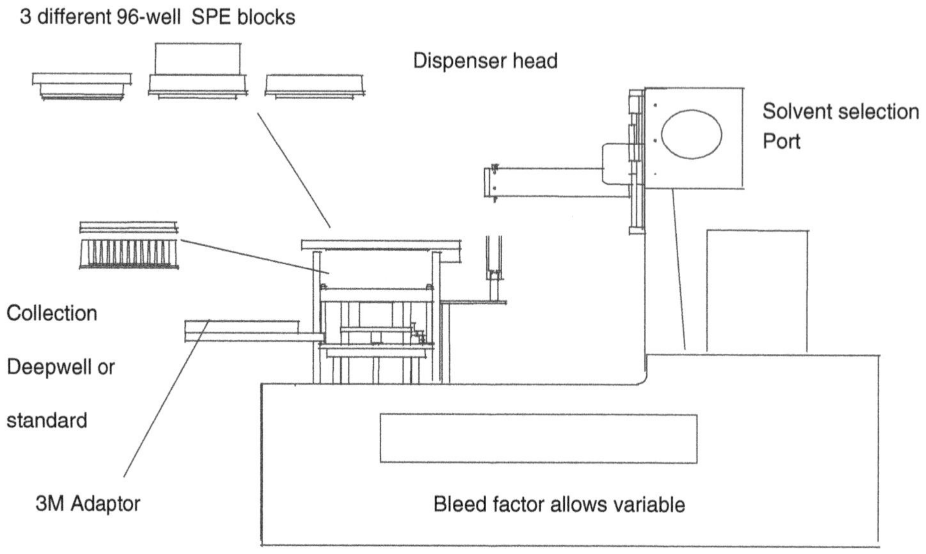

FIGURE 3.2 *Schematic representation of solid phase extraction station.*

a time and a switching valve allows up to nine different reagents to be used on the system enabling different procedures to be sequentially run. The variable height control on the dispenser head allows different height SPE blocks to be processed. The station can also cope with both Microlute™ and Empore™ type plates with their different skirt heights and length of flow directors, the Zymate places an adapter on the SPE station prior to running Empore™ type blocks (see Figure 3.2). The semi-automated system requires a different manifold for each type of SPE block.

This variable height control on the dispenser head also offers another advantage, in that it can be used to push down on top of the SPE blocks to ensure that the vacuum is consistently formed, inconsistent formation of the vacuum could be a problem with the semi-automated system. The variable height setting on the platform allows both deep well and standard micro titre collection plates to be used. Although the SPE station performs all the vacuum, conditioning, washing and elution steps the system utilises a MultiPROBE™ RSP to dilute samples, add internal standard and transfer samples from tubes to the SPE blocks.

The robot sequence begins with SPE block being ejected from the storage carousel. All the SPE blocks are stored upside down in the storage carousel so they can easily slide. The block is transferred to the SPE station where it is conditioned. The conditioned block is transferred to the MultiPROBE™ for the sample transfer step. The Zymark controller and the MultiPROBE™ controller are networked so that the transfer method can be initiated from the Zymark controller. When the MultiPROBE™ flags that the transfer is complete the Zymate collects the loaded block and returns it to the SPE station. The SPE station applies a load vacuum, carries out the wash step(s) and the elution step. The plates containing the extracts are returned to the cooled storage carousel until manually transferred to an autosampler. This system effectively halves the time to extract 96 samples compared with the semi-automated system, a batch takes about 30–40 minutes depending on the number of steps and the reagent volumes. This system was originally designed to perform a minimum of four consecutive runs from sample tubes (384 samples) and to be capable of handling all the currently available labware (Microlute™ and Empore™ blocks).

This system has been used to support clinical studies for over three years and has proven to be very reliable, with minimal unscheduled down time. The performance of the Zymark 96-well system will be highlighted by looking at the data from one of the first studies supported by the system.

3.4.2 Application

The study was repeat dose Phase I study for a compound being developed for rheumatoid arthritis. There were three dosing occasions each generating 288 samples (8 patients × 36 samples) a total of 864 samples. A rapid turn round of the data was required to enable the pharmacokinetic (PK) analysis to be carried out prior to the next dosing occasion.

The SPE method although straightforward and requiring no concentration step does highlight the fine vacuum controlled that can be achieved on the SPE station allowing SPE blocks containing only 15 mg of sorbent per well to be routinely processed. The Microlute™ block, containing 15 mg of varian C2 sorbent, was conditioned with 0.1 ml of acetonitrile followed by 0.1 ml of water. The samples were diluted 1:1 with the internal standard solution and loaded onto the block; the RSP aspirates internal standard followed by sample and dispenses these sequentially onto the block. The block was washed with 0.1 ml of water and the analyte was then eluted into a deep well micro titre plate with 0.1 ml of mobile phase, acetonitrile:0.1 per cent formic acid (50:50). The plate was then covered with foil to prevent evaporation and placed on the autosampler. The LC–MS–MS conditions are tabulated in Table 3.1.

TABLE 3.1 *LC–MS–MS conditions*

Column	Columbus C18 5 μ 150 × 4.6 mm
Mobile phase	Acetonitrile:0.1% aq HCOOH (1:1)
Flow rate	1.0 ml/min with 1/10 post column split
Temperature	40 °C
Injection	50 μl
Typical retention time	1.9 minutes
Detection	PE Sciex API-300 with turbo ionspray

The following transitions were monitored: *m/z* 395 ⥮ 86 for the parent and *m/z* 399 ⥮ 86 for the internal standard. The data was processed using MacQuan™ Software (PE Sciex). Peak area ratios of analyte to internal standard were used to construct a calibration curve for interpolation of sample concentrations. The regression model was linear with $1/x^2$ weighting. With a 0.1 ml sample volume the validated range for the assay was 1–2,000 ng/ml. The serum (SRM) chromatographs for the 1 ng/ml standard are shown in Figure 3.3. The assay is both sensitive and specific for the analyte. The precision and accuracy obtained for the back interpolated standard values and the quality control samples are tabulated in Tables 3.2 and 3.3, respectively. Both the %CV and %bias for both sets of data are less than 5 per cent and well within our acceptance criteria of 15 per cent.

The data in Tables 3.2 and 3.3 shows that the assay performance was very good. The sample preparation time is 28 minutes a block and with an analysis time of 2.5 minutes/sample each block took four hours to run. We were able to give next day turn round for the data on all three dosing occasions.

3.4.3 Enhanced system

A number of new modules have been added to the system to enhance its capability (see Figure 3.4). A plate rotator station is used to switch plates between portrait and landscape. A heated dry down station is used to evaporate the SPE extracts to

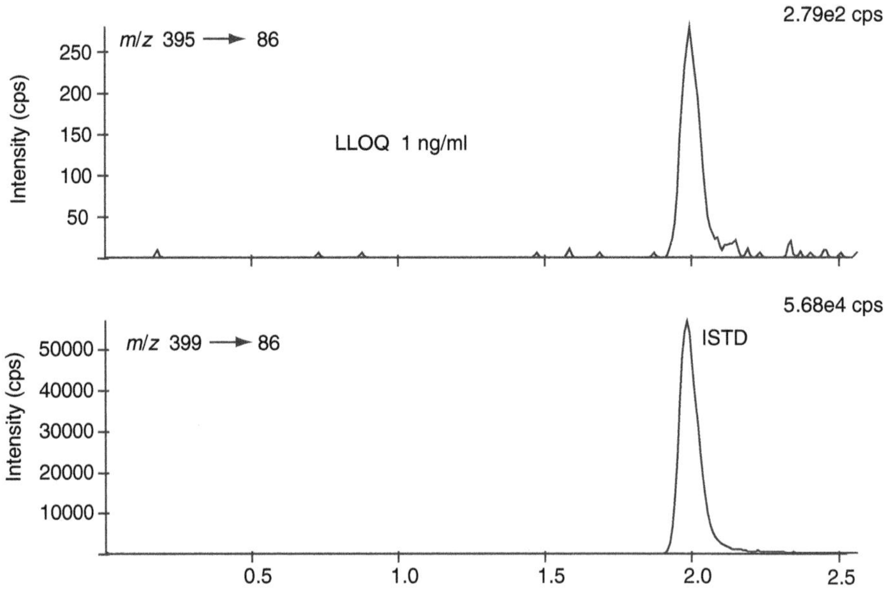

Figure 3.3 *SRM chromatographs for the 1 ng/ml standard.*

TABLE 3.2 *Back calculated calibration standard concentrations*

Nominal	1.08	3.23	10.75	32.25	107.50	322.50	1075.00	2150.00
Mean	1.09	3.13	10.29	31.86	108.49	328.71	1100.70	2182.59
SD	0.05	0.14	0.28	0.89	2.63	11.09	28.76	51.08
%CV	4.67	4.44	2.76	2.79	2.42	3.37	2.61	2.34
%Bias	1.34	−2.88	−4.24	−1.20	0.92	1.92	2.39	1.52

TABLE 3.3 *Quality control data*

Nominal	3.17	846.40	1692.80
Mean	3.27	862.57	1701.41
SD	0.13	36.75	40.65
%CV	4.12	4.26	2.39
%Bias	2.95	1.91	0.51
N	25.00	26.00	25.00

dryness and allow a concentration step. The software controls the gas temperature and the dry down time; the gas flow is set manually. The dry down head is fixed but the plate can be moved up with time by setting the start height and end height; this can improve the dry down rate for larger volumes. To reduce evaporation rates from SPE extracts prior to analysis an automated plate sealer (Advanced Biotechnologies,

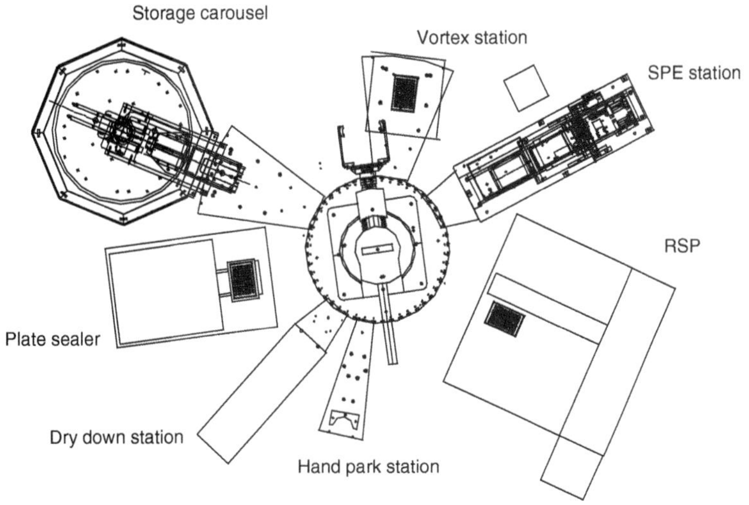

FIGURE 3.4 *Enhanced Zymark sample preparation system.*

Epsom, UK) is used to heat seal the plates with polypropylene-backed aluminium foil. The sealer can be adjusted to accommodate plates of different heights and sizes. The unsealed plate is placed on a shuttle that stands clear of the main body of the sealer, allowing robotic access. The shuttle is drawn into the unit and the plate is sealed in 10–15 seconds, depending on the plate material. The shuttle then slides out, presenting the plate in its original position. The temperature and the time for sealing the plate are manually set. The punch cuts the film to cover the entire plate surface without any overhang down the sides, which could affect the handling of the plate. This system also has the added advantage that each individual well of the collection plate is sealed. To ensure that the reconstituted extracts are adequately mixed prior to analysis a vortex station has also been added to the system. This station consists of a Bellco mini-orbital shaker mounted on a fixing plate with a pneumatically controlled plunger that is used to hold the plate in position. The speed control is manually set and the length of vortex time is software controlled.

The VB interface has also been upgraded (VB 6) and enhanced to improve its flexibility and to control the new modules; the number of condition, wash and elution steps is no longer limited, and procedures can be created by copying and editing an existing procedure. The software can schedule tasks, one plate will be dried down while the next plate is extracted; it is also dynamic, work can be added onto the system once the system is running. The MultiPROBE interface has also been improved; it now uses the MPTable™ software to allow the user to set the sample volumes, reagent volumes, source rack and destination rack positions. MPTable™ is a comma-separated values file that contains the sequence of pipetting operations and instrument optimisation parameters. This allows total control over the order in which samples are pipetted and the way in which all pipetting operations are performed. The VB interface uses Microsoft Excel™ to edit the MPTable™ file.

3.5 *Future development*

The development of more robust water wettable polymeric phases such as Oasis hydrophilic lipophilic-balanced (HLB) has led to the development of generic approaches to sample preparation. The two-stage design of the Oasis plate has enabled the use of a 5 mg sorbent mass without loss of recovery due to channelling. This enables conditioning and wash steps to be reduced to 0.1 ml and elution volumes to 0.2 ml. Coupling standard SPE procedures with standard fast gradient LC conditions has enabled method development times to be reduced. Standardisation also has a benefit in maximising the efficiency of these systems.

This approach has also highlighted many other areas that require improvements. The sample format (e.g. tubes) is not ideally suited to high-throughput bioanalysis. The choice of serum removes the necessity to centrifuge the samples prior to analysis, but the logistics of removing the caps, racking the samples and then replacing the lids afterwards on 400 tubes still remains a laborious task for the analyst. A switch to microtitre plates or strips of tubes (8 or 12) which can be plugged into a microtitre plate format would reduce this potential bottleneck. Switching to a microtitre plate format for samples would enable samples to be stored in the carousel prior to extraction; this would also increase the capacity of the existing systems more than 20 unattended runs. The automation of the sample reception processes is currently under development.

Data processing particularly with multiple analytes or cassette-dosing studies would quickly become a bottleneck; with a single quantifiable analyte the data processing was not as tedious as expected. The current sample control software on the PE Sciex API-365 cannot run multiple batches. When running four consecutive assays one large batch (384 samples) has to be set up in sample control via the Excel import, and the data retrospectively separated into individual assays before processing. This problem should be overcome with the introduction of the new NT-based Analyst™. Processing large numbers of assays makes the requirement for a laboratory data management system (LIMS) with automated report templates more important.

There are many future challenges for automation, shorter LC–MS–MS run times, lower limits of detection, miniaturisation and demands for increased instrumentation utilisation. The development of multiplexing systems, where multiple LC pumping systems are used to increase the frequency of sample introduction into the mass spectrometer, will increase the requirements for sample throughput. The requirement to develop more sensitive methods is likely to increase the complexity of sample preparation procedures. The switch to the 96-well format is likely to be only the first step, already 384 is being looked at as the next step, particularly as the benefits of LC miniaturisation become a practical reality. The need to increase the efficiency of utilisation of mass spectrometers makes it inevitable that sample preparation and sample analysis will be on-line, making it possible to operate round the clock seven days a week.

None of these problems are insurmountable and should not detract from the key success of these robot systems, i.e. sample preparation is no longer a problem or rate limiting.

3.6 *References*

Allanson, J.P., Biddlecombe, R.A., Jones, A.E. and Pleasance, S. (1996) The use of automated solid phase extraction in the '96 well' format for high throughput bioanalysis using liquid chromatography coupled to tandem mass spectrometry. *Rapid Commun. Mass Spectrom.* 10, 811–816.

Blanchard, J. (1981) Evaluation of the relative efficacy of various techniques for deproteinizing plasma samples prior to high-performance liquid chromatographic analysis. *J. Chromatogr.* 226, 455–460.

Gilpin, R.K. and Burke, M.F. (1973) Role of trimethylsilanes in tailoring chromatographic adsorbents. *Anal. Chem.* **45**, 1383–1389.

Nawrocki, J. and Dabrowska, A. (2000) Low-carbon silica sorbents for solid-phase extraction. *J. Chromatogr.* 28 January, **868**(1), 1–12.

Wells, M.J.M. and Michael, J.L. (1987) Reversed phase solid phase extraction for aqueous environmental sample preparation in herbicide residue analysis. *J. Chromatog. Sci.* **25**, 345–350.

CHAPTER 4

High-performance liquid chromatography in pharmaceutical bioanalysis

David N. Mallett

4.1 *Introduction*

Since the mid-1980s the most frequently used technique in the bioanalysis of drugs has been high-performance liquid chromatography (HPLC). Prior to this the technique of choice was capillary gas–liquid chromatography (GLC). The reason for the rapid and dominant emergence of HPLC is fairly straightforward. In GLC it is a necessity that the analyte of interest can be volatilised as the separation is carried out in the gas phase, with the key factor for separation being the difference between analytes of their relative affinities for a gaseous mobile phase and a liquid stationary phase. Often, to facilitate this process, derivatisation of the analyte to a more volatile form is required. For example, acids would frequently need to be modified chemically to their more volatile ester forms prior to the chromatographic process. This requirement often led to assay procedures being complicated and not easy for the inexperienced operator to perform. In addition to this, GLC usually operates at considerably elevated temperatures and a further consideration is therefore the thermal stability of the analyte(s) of interest.

HPLC on the other hand usually exhibits its resolving power at ambient or slightly raised temperatures in the liquid phase with the key requirements being that the analyte has some solubility in the liquid mobile phase and some affinity for the solid stationary phase. It is the relative strength of the analytes' affinity for each of these phases that gives the technique its separating capability.

Another factor in the emergence of HPLC in pharmaceutical applications has been the types of detectors that may be used 'generically' for wide varieties of drugs and which are compatible with HPLC. The most obvious example is the ultra-violet (UV) absorption detector, which has found extremely wide use as most drugs have a chromophore which will absorb UV light of the appropriate wavelength. Other detectors which are somewhat more selective but have found wide usage and are particularly suited to the liquid environment are fluorescence and electrochemical detectors. In recent years it has become routine to couple HPLC to mass spectrometric detectors and this has cemented the position of HPLC as the technique of first choice for the bioanalyst in today's pharmaceutical industry.

4.2 *A brief look at the theory of chromatographic separation in HPLC*

In HPLC, separation occurs due to partitioning between a stationary phase contained in a column and a liquid phase which is pumped under pressure through this column.

Let us consider a two-component mixture, A and B. Each of the components will have a certain affinity for the stationary phase and a certain affinity for the mobile phase. Provided there is sufficient difference between the analytes in their relative affinities for the two phases, i.e. in their partition coefficients, then in an HPLC system they will separate. For example, analyte A may have a stronger affinity for the mobile phase than it does for the stationary phase and will thus spend, relatively, greater time in the mobile phase than it does bound to the surface of the stationary phase. For analyte B the reverse may be true and the compound will spend a longer time bound to the stationary phase. In this case one would expect the two compounds to separate (to be resolved) and the compound with the highest affinity for the mobile phase, analyte A, to be eluted from the column first (Figure 4.1).

Analyte A would be said to exhibit a lower *retention time*, t_r, than analyte B. An analyte that had no affinity for the stationary phase and therefore moved through the column at the same velocity as the mobile phase travels through the column is said to be unretained. The time taken for this to occur is defined as t_0 and is equal to the column length divided by the velocity of the mobile phase flow. The properties

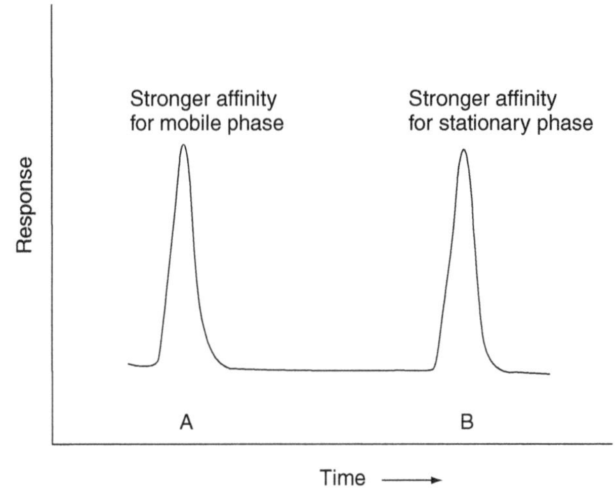

FIGURE 4.1 *Relative affinities of compounds A and B.*

t_r and t_0 can be related to each other to define one of the fundamental liquid chromatography parameters, *the capacity factor*, k', as follows:

$$k' = \frac{t_r - t_0}{t_0}$$

k' can be thought of as expressing the relative migration rate of an analyte.

One characteristic of any chromatographic separation is that each band is to a greater or lesser degree dispersed as it travels along the column. Therefore, we can consider each chromatographic peak as a band with a certain width. Each band is composed of a distribution of concentrations of the analyte around the retention time of that analyte. In an idealised situation this distribution takes the form of a symmetrical Gaussian, or standard error, curve. The width of this band is commonly expressed in HPLC in terms of the *theoretical plate number,* N, of the column. This parameter is usually calculated as

$$N = 5.54 \times \left(\frac{t_r}{w_{0.5}}\right)^2$$

where, $w_{0.5}$ is the width of the peak or band at half height. N can be viewed as a measure of column efficiency, that is, the ability of a column to produce narrow peaks. The higher the value of N, the more efficient the column is and the greater its ability to perform separations.

As has been said, the truly 'Gaussian distribution' represents an idealised case. More commonly this is not actually the case, and in fact it is usual that the decline of analyte concentration from the peak apex back to the baseline occurs over a greater period of time than does the rise in concentration from the peak beginning to the apex. This gives rise to another important parameter in considering the quality of the chromatographic process, *the peak asymmetry factor*, *As*. This is defined in Figure 4.2.

The object of the chromatographic procedure is to perform a separation of a mixture of analytes, or frequently in the case of pharmaceutical bioanalysis, a separation between a compound which we wish to quantify and interferences which would compromise the quantification. In either case, it is necessary to have adequate separation between components. This can be measured quantitatively in terms of the *resolution, Rs*. *Rs* is equal to the distance in time between the apexes of two adjacent bands, divided by their average bandwidth.

$$Rs = \frac{(t_2 - t_1)}{0.5(w_1 + w_2)}$$

Rs is a measure of separation, but to use this as a parameter we can adjust to achieve a required separation, it has to be related to experimental characteristics such as N and k'. How these parameters are related is described in the relationship

$$Rs = \frac{1}{4}(\alpha - 1)\sqrt{N}\left[\frac{k'}{1 + k'}\right]$$

where α is the *separation factor* and is equal to k'_2/k'_1 the capacity factors of the two components to be resolved.

The above equation can be considered as being comprised of three terms: $\alpha - 1$ is a selectivity term which can be varied by altering the composition of the mobile and stationary phases; $\sqrt{N}$ is an efficiency term which can be affected by changes in the column length, column packing or the mobile phase velocity; and the third term involving k' which can be altered by changing the solvent strength.

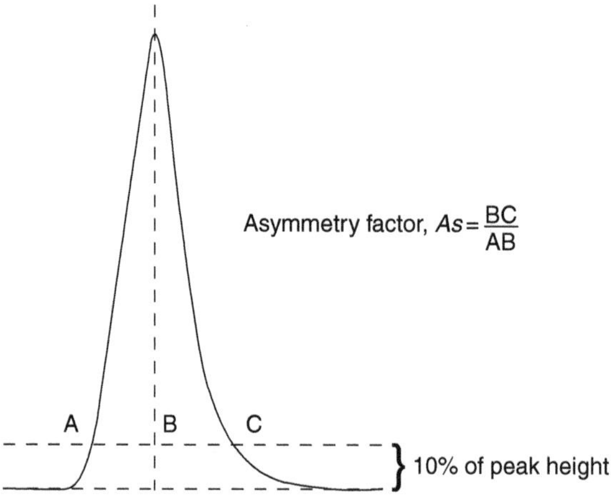

FIGURE 4.2 *Derivation of the peak asymmetry factor (As).*

These factors k', N, As, Rs and α may be considered the primary factors describing a chromatographic separation and it has been shown how they interact and need to be adjusted or controlled to affect the required separation. It is not the intention here to investigate these parameters in any greater depth, though more complex treatments have been undertaken.

4.3 *The basic equipment comprising a modern HPLC system*

Fundamentally, a liquid chromatograph consists of a high pressure pump to deliver mobile phase, an injector for the introduction of samples into the system, a column on which the analytes are resolved, a detector for measuring the response for each analyte and a means of displaying and handling the detector signal (Figure 4.3). In the modern case, frequently the pumps allow the mixing of different solvents at varying ratios over the time course of the separation to generate what is known as gradient chromatography; the injection systems are normally automated to allow the unattended injection of large numbers of samples e.g. overnight; and the resultant signals are handled by computerised peak integration systems which allow rapid data interpretation. Further, the column may be packed with one of many hundreds of different commercially available stationary phases. The detectors have become ever more powerful and sensitive and the most commonly used in pharmaceutical bioanalysis are UV absorption, fluorescence, electrochemical, radioactivity, mass spectrometric and NMR detectors.

In considering each of the parts of the chromatographic system it should be borne in mind that all parts of the system which come into contact with the mobile phase must be made of materials which are inert to the chemicals which make up the mobile phases. Also that all parts of the system from the pump outlet to the column end are under high pressure and must be made of appropriate materials and

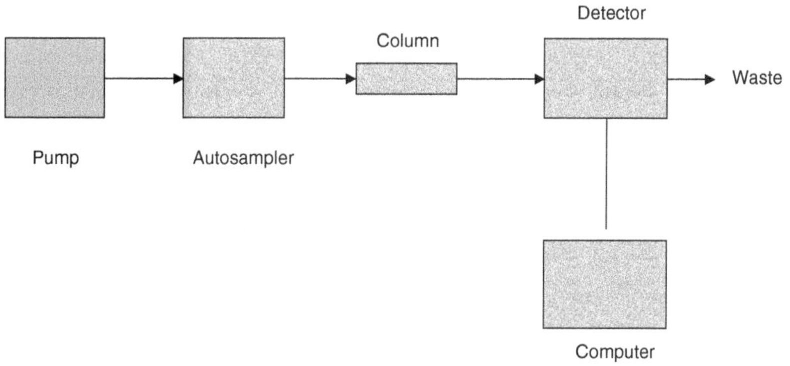

FIGURE 4.3 *Schematic representation of a modern HPLC system.*

designed in such a way to withstand this pressure, commonly up to 250–300 bar. A further fundamental design consideration is that all tubing from the point of sample introduction to the point of detection must be kept to a minimum to minimise 'dead volume'. Excess dead volume causes excessive extra-column band broadening and leads to drastic reductions in efficiency. Therefore, narrow bore tubing in short lengths should be used for all connections. It is worth noting here that in the case of gradient pumps the internal volume should also be as low as possible so that defined changes in mobile phase occur with the minimum of delay. Gradient HPLC will be discussed more fully later.

4.3.1 Pumps

In almost all modern HPLC systems the requirement of the pump is that it delivers mobile phase through the column at a constant flow rate. The pressure generated by this flow may vary with time, as the condition of the column changes with age, for example, but within limits this is allowed so long as the flow remains constant, as it is the flow rate rather than the pressure which is related to the velocity of the mobile phase and hence the retention time of the analytes of interest. The most commonly used type of pump is the reciprocating pump. These pumps use relatively low volume solvent chambers with reciprocating pistons to drive the flow through the pressurised system. Probably the most common type of these pumps is the dual reciprocating pump, wherein two identical piston pumping heads operate at 180° out of phase. This leads to a much smoother flow profile against time than is the case for a single-head pump. This is due to alternate filling of one head whilst the other is delivering solvent to the column and the rest of the chromatographic system. It is possible with such systems to largely remove pulsing from the flow profile. These pumping systems generally deliver reproducible flow, are fairly durable and are of moderate cost.

As previously stated, the parts of the pump which come into contact with the mobile phase need to be resilient to the chemicals typically used. However, even if this is adhered to, there are still conditions which should be avoided to maximise the performance of the pump. For example, mobile phases containing salts as buffers should not be allowed to stand in the pump for a long period as evaporation can lead to the formation of salt crystals which will scratch the piston and damage the high-pressure seal.

In the specific case of gradient HPLC pumps (pumps capable of delivering mixtures whose composition varies with time and discussed later), it is necessary that a pump be able to deliver a mixture of solvents, the composition of which changes with time. There are two approaches to this problem. First, the solvents may be mixed and then the required mixture is pumped through the system; this is called low-pressure mixing. The second option is to pump each solvent and then mix to the required composition under high pressure. There has been much debate over the relative merits of these two types of pumping system and each has its proponents. Irrespective of this, the key requirement is that the system is able to deliver accurately and reproducibly mixtures of two or more solvents at different compositions with time. Most frequently the mixtures used as mobile phases comprise two components, binary systems, but on occasion three or even four components are mixed; these systems are called ternary or quaternary gradients.

4.3.2 Autosamplers

In order to obtain good column performance it is essential that the sample be introduced onto the column in an appropriate manner. Ideally, the sample should be injected in a small volume of solvent so that the analytes are contained in a narrow plug as they reach the top of the chromatographic column, i.e. they are not overly dispersed. Any system should be capable of reproducibly introducing the sample in a narrow band, be capable of operating at high pressure and should be easy to use. Modern automated sample injectors, autosamplers, incorporate valves for injection. In one position, the valve directs the flow of mobile phase through the column whilst the sample is introduced into a loop which is held out of the line of flow. The valve is then switched and the flow passes through the loop en route to the column thereby sweeping the sample into the mobile phase and onto the column. This is shown in Figure 4.4. It is now the norm that sample injectors are automated which allows the injection of large numbers of samples without operator intervention. Typically today, samples are prepared during the day, injected unattended overnight and the data processed the following morning.

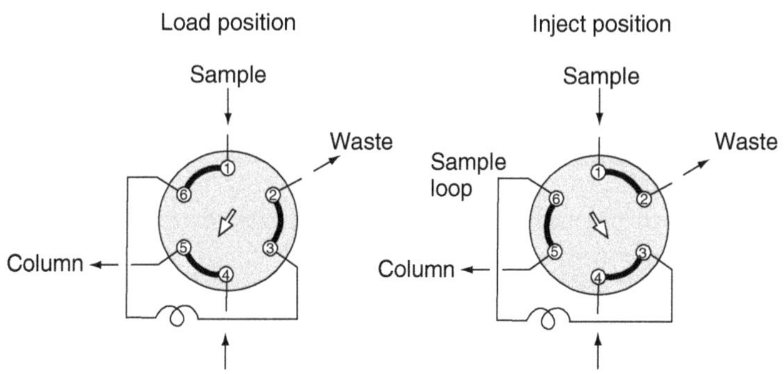

FIGURE 4.4 *Schematic representation of the two stages of the injection process.*

4.3.3 Columns

There are a myriad of different stationary phases which are today commercially available as HPLC columns. The most commonly used, however, are microparticulate, porous silica-based materials. Typically these are 3–5 μm spherical silica particles with internal pores of approximately 80–100 Å and offer efficiencies, *N*, in excess of 50,000 plates per metre. Frequently, the silica base has a surface-modifying chemical covalently bonded to it to alter the polarity and nature of the affinity by which the stationary phase binds analytes. The most common of these is an octadecyl (C18) alkyl chain in which case the surface is made very non-polar and separation occurs between this and a more polar mobile phase. This is known as reversed phase chromatography and will be discussed more fully later. To put in context the variety facing the chromatographer today, there are over 600 different reversed phase HPLC columns alone commercially available.

The most common format of the column is a stainless steel tube of 5–25 cm length with an internal diameter of 1–4.6 mm. The ends of the column contain stainless steel frits or meshes to retain the packing material. Low dead volume end fittings and short lengths of microbore tubing (i.d. 5,000–10,000 of an inch) are used to connect the column to the injector and the detector. It is worth noting that for spherical particles the stationary phase occupies only approximately 40 per cent of the volume of the column, so there is a degree of dead volume contributing to peak dispersion inherent in any column.

4.3.4 Detectors

There are a number of detectors which have found wide usage in HPLC, but the most commonly used in the pharmaceutical industry are UV absorbance, fluorescence, electrochemical, radiochemical and mass spectrometric detectors.

The most widely used detector of all is the UV absorbance detector. These detectors have high sensitivity for many drugs and metabolites but the analytes must absorb light in the UV/visible spectrum e.g. 190–600 nm. In modern UV absorbance detectors, the incident light is generated from a high intensity source such as a deuterium lamp and the wavelength of light required is then directed through the sample by the use of diffraction gratings, which deflect the light of the chosen wavelength according to the angle of the grating to the incident light. Light passes through the sample and a reference cell and is detected by a photomultiplier. The energy passing through each cell is compared electronically and the output is proportional to the sample concentration. The detector is, therefore, said to be concentration sensitive, that is, the detector response will be greater for a higher concentration of analyte in the flow cell and is governed by the Beer–Lambert law:

$$A = \epsilon c L$$

where, A is the absorbance, ϵ the molar absorptivity, c the concentration of the analyte in moles/L and L the cell pathlength. As can be seen, the longer the flow cell pathlength, the greater will be the detector sensitivity for any given concentration of analyte. Many cells have dimensions in the order of 1 mm i.d., 10 mm length with internal volumes of about 8 μL. Increasing the pathlength to further increase the response has an optimal point beyond which the increased volume of the cell becomes a factor adding to peak dispersion and thus lowering the sample concentration which has a detrimental effect on sensitivity.

A versatile extension of the applicability of UV absorbance detectors is the diode-array or rapid scanning detector. These detectors allow the collection of absorbance measurements at a range of wavelengths during the analysis of a sample. This offers the benefit of obtaining full spectral information for each analyte which can be of use qualitatively to determine whether a chromatographic peak is derived from the analyte or not. In the context of drug metabolism, very often the metabolism of a compound affects the functional groups which are part of the extremities of the molecule rather than the 'core' of the molecule which often includes the chromophore. Therefore, collection of UV spectra during the analytical run provides a means of determining whether a chromatographic peak results from a component which is drug related or not.

If the analyte of interest fluoresces there is the opportunity to use this characteristic as a means of detection. A particular molecule may absorb light at one wavelength and be energised to an excited state. The excited molecule may then release this energy as light at a different, longer wavelength in relaxing back to its ground state. This process is fluorescence. By exciting at one wavelength and monitoring the light emitted at the longer emission wavelength we have a very selective way of detecting analytes. The primary advantage of this technique is that it is not only very sensitive but also very selective, the compound has to not only excite at a specific wavelength but also emit at another specific wavelength. This is not only a key benefit but also its major drawback, as many analytes do not possess the ability to fluoresce. For fluorescence to be exhibited in a drug it is necessary that the drug molecule contains a fluorophore; this is usually a highly aromatic 'core' structure. As with the UV absorbance detector this detector is concentration sensitive. The fluorescence process is illustrated in Figure 4.5.

Another detection process which absolutely allows the determination of whether a peak is related to the drug of interest is radioactivity detection. Frequently, the study of a drug's metabolism involves the analysis of complex matrices such as plasma, urine, bile or faeces. These matrices contain many components, many of which exhibit substantial UV absorbance spectra of their own, making detection of one component alone, even after chromatographic separation, extremely difficult. By administering a radiolabelled version of the drug to the test species, a very easy way of deciding which chromatographic peaks relate to and/or are derived from the drug is available. Provided the radio-isotope is attached to the molecule in a metabolically stable position, one can reasonably assume that any peaks that are

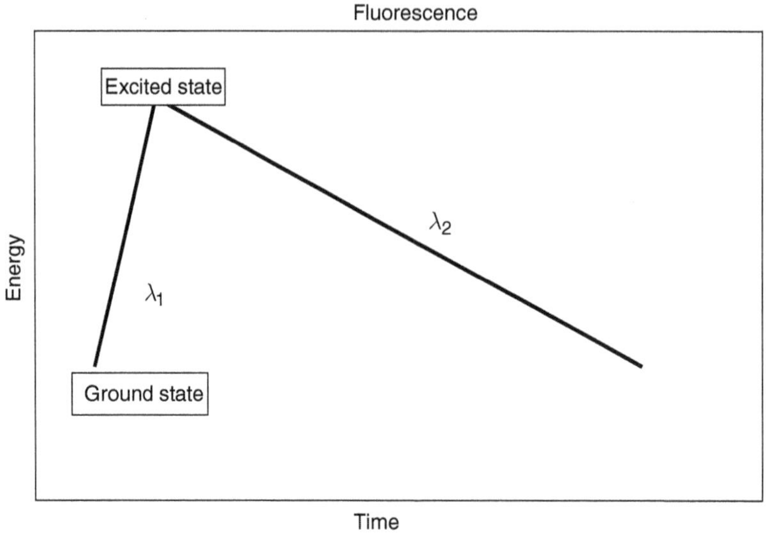

FIGURE 4.5 *Schematic representation of the fluorescence process, where λ_1 is the excitation wavelength and λ_2 the emission wavelength.*

detected by the radioactivity they exhibit are drug-related. Typically such detectors require a second pump which delivers scintillation fluids for mixing with the sample after the chromatographic separation has been performed on column.

Some drug structures contain moieties which are susceptible to oxidation or reduction. That is, the application of a voltage to the analyte as it passes through an electrochemical cell triggers a reaction to an oxidised or reduced species with the generation of an electrical current. This is the basis of electrochemical detection. Usually, either the current (amperometric detection) or the charge (coulometric detection) is detected. Not all molecules are susceptible to electrochemically induced reactions but some that are susceptible are listed in Table 4.1.

Often electrochemical detectors involve a graphitic carbon working electrode with a platinum auxiliary electrode and a reference electrode. Classes of drugs detected this way include the tricyclic antidepressants and the phenothiazines, many of which incidentally are also fluorescent.

The most widely applied use of electrochemical detection is in the oxidative rather than reductive mode as most modern HPLC is conducted in the reversed phase mode with largely aqueous mobile phases, which means that at substantial negative voltages a major problem is the reduction of oxygen in the mobile phase resulting in high background responses.

Recent years have seen the development of highly effective interfaces for coupling liquid chromatography to mass spectrometers. This has led to an explosion in the use of mass spectrometers as detectors for quantitative HPLC analyses as a result of the excellent sensitivity and selectivity of these instruments. A mass spectrometer can be

TABLE 4.1 *Molecules which are susceptible to electrochemically induced reactions*

Oxidation	**Reduction**
Phenolics	Ketones
Aromatic amines	Aldehydes
Dihydroxy (e.g. catechols)	Nitro compounds
Purines	Conjugated unsaturated systems
Heterocyclic rings	
Peroxides and hydroperoxides	

tuned to collect data from molecules or analytes of a specified molecular weight and furthermore, triple quadrupole mass spectrometers can be set up to fragment the analyte molecules and then detect a specific 'product' ion of a specified 'precursor' molecular mass. In practice, this means that the first quadrupole is used to select ions of the desired mass into the second quadrupole where the molecule is fragmented with a collision gas, then the third quadrupole selects only ions of a specified reaction product onto the detector. This is called selected reaction monitoring, SRM (or multiple reaction monitoring, MRM, if more than one analyte is involved such as a drug and an internal standard, a structurally similar compound added to samples at a constant amount to provide a reference for quantification). Although mass spectrometers are expensive, their extreme sensitivity and selectivity have seen them become often the detector of choice for quantitative bioanalysis (Figure 4.6). This topic

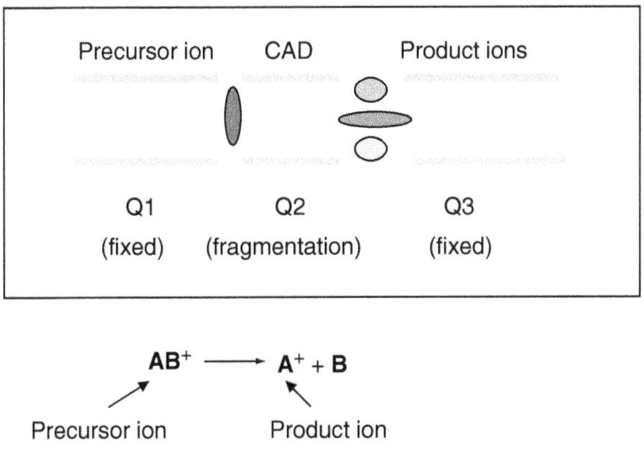

FIGURE 4.6 *Representation of the single reaction monitoring process in a triple quadrupole mass spectrometer. Q1 focuses only ions of a selected mass into Q2, the collision cell, where fragmentation is induced by collision with a gas, Q3 focuses only a specified fragment (product ion) through to the detector.*

is discussed in more detail in Chapter 5. The most widely used method of coupling HPLC to mass spectrometry for a wide range of typical drug analytes is atmospheric pressure ionisation using an electrospray mass spectrometer source. These systems can successfully cope with a limited volume of solvent; therefore, the eluent from the HPLC column may need to be split so that a flow rate of ~0.5 mL/min or less enters the mass spectrometer. As the solvent and the contained analytes enter the source, gases are mixed with the flow causing the formation of an aerosol. Voltage is applied to the stainless steel capillary through which the flow enters the source so that the droplets leaving the capillary are charged species. The addition of a nebulising gas encourages solvent evaporation and a decrease in droplet size – leading to a 'coulometric explosion' producing small ion droplets which enter the mass spectrometer. Obviously for this process, the key requirement of the analytes is that they are ionisable.

Another detection method which is increasingly being applied to liquid chromatography is nuclear magnetic resonance (NMR) spectroscopy. This technique is extremely information rich and is generally used for the determination of molecular structures rather than quantification. Although NMR can be directly coupled to the chromatograph the technique is insensitive compared to the other detectors discussed and is more often used off-line after collection of fractions from the column eluent. A further consideration is that NMR spectrometers, particularly the high resolution instruments contain very high field strength cryo-magnets and are not only very expensive but often need a specialised facility in which to house them. See Chapter 17 for a discussion of this technique.

4.3.5 Data handling systems

Historically, peaks arising from liquid chromatography detectors were displayed on pen recorders. The detector response was converted to a voltage output which moved the pens across a moving bed of paper in accordance to the size of the detector signal. However, in the modern pharmaceutical bioanalysis laboratory, most HPLC detector responses are captured electronically by computer-based systems. Frequently these systems are networked throughout a facility so that analysts can view their data from desks, remote from the actual chromatography laboratory. The programs contain algorithms which perform accurate integration of peaks, can produce calibration lines from the derived peak areas or heights and subsequently generate concentration results for the samples being analysed. Many of these systems are also capable of automatically calculating parameters such as k', N, As and Rs, which are useful for monitoring the performance of an assay. It is also a requirement that these systems maintain an audit trail, that is, modifications to the manner of data collection, integration or the contents of the calibration file and derived results are logged so that the integrity of the data is maintained.

4.4 Modes of liquid chromatography

4.4.1 Normal phase liquid chromatography

In normal phase chromatography the stationary phase is more polar than the mobile phase. Thus, polar analytes are more strongly attracted to the stationary phase and will elute from the column later than less polar analytes (e.g. metabolites) which will have a greater affinity for the less polar mobile phase. The types of attraction by which analytes bind to the stationary phases are dipole–dipole interactions and hydrogen-bonding. Figure 4.7 shows the interactions commonly involved in normal phase HPLC.

Once it has been decided to attempt a separation by normal phase liquid chromatography using, say, a silica column one can consider the stationary phase to be fixed. The most obvious way of affecting a polarity-based separation, therefore, becomes the relative polarity of the mobile phase. Table 4.2 shows the polarity of some commonly used solvents together with their relative polarity and eluting power. It should be remembered that in normal phase the more polar the mobile phase the greater the eluting power (known as the eluotropic strength) of the solvent or combination of solvents used, the faster analytes will be eluted from the column into the detector.

There are further factors pertaining to specific properties of the mobile phase solvents which may affect the relative affinities of the analyte for the stationary or mobile phase to a greater extent than a relatively small difference in polarity. For example, Dichloromethane is a good proton donor and will interact strongly with basic solutes such as amines. On the other hand, isopropyl ether is a good proton acceptor and will interact better with acidic functions.

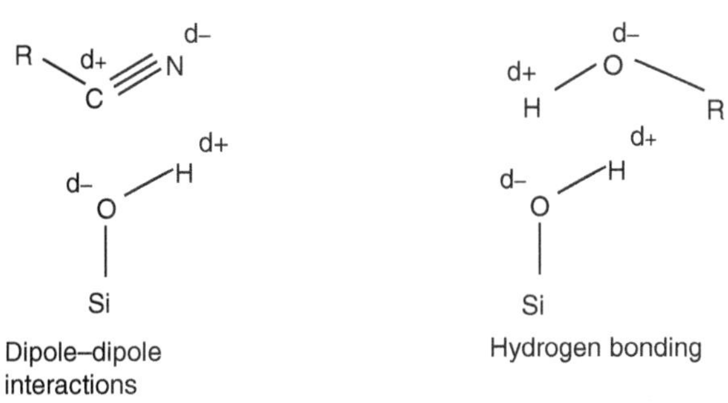

FIGURE 4.7 *Typical interactions in normal phase HPLC.*

TABLE 4.2 *The relative polarity and eluting power of polarity of some commonly used solvents*

Solvent	Increasing polarity	Increasing eluotropic strength
Hexane	↓	↓
Toluene		
Iso-propyl ether		
Dichloromethane (DCM)		
Tetrahydrofuran (THF)		
Ethyl acetate		
Ethanol		
Acetone		
Acetonitrile		
Methanol		
Water		

4.4.2 Reversed phase liquid chromatography

Reversed phase chromatography is the term applied to the situation where the mobile phase is more polar than the stationary phase. This is the opposite of the case in normal phase HPLC, which was developed earlier, hence the terms normal and reversed phase chromatography. The use of reversed phase chromatography has a number of advantages:

1 Reversed phase HPLC allows the use of binding interactions ranging from hydrophobic bonding to ionic interactions, and a mixture of these and polar interactions in between, offering a large range of selectivities.
2 The use of a more polar mobile phase compared to the stationary phase often involves the use of primarily aqueous mobile phases which are safer to use and easier to dispose of than the primarily organic mobile phases of normal phase HPLC.
3 Frequently, reversed phase HPLC separations are performed on stationary phases which are modified silicas and as silica is fairly reactive this allows for many variations in the nature of the stationary phase and so a wide range of selectivities are available. A further consideration which is key to the value of reversed phase HPLC in the area of pharmaceutical bioanalysis is that the retention is reversed compared to that in normal phase HPLC (i.e. the more polar the analyte, the faster it is eluted). Most drug metabolites are more polar than the drugs they derive from, therefore, the metabolites elute first. This is beneficial as it allows, in many cases, the use of the retention time of the parent drug compound as a definer of the end of the chromatography of interest for any given analysis. This mode of liquid chromatography is by far the most commonly used today.

Typically, in reversed phase chromatography the silica particles that are the backbone of the stationary phase are chemically reacted with a hydrocarbon to produce a non-polar surface. The most common bonded structure is an octadecyl hydrocarbon (C18 surface modifier). To consider the retention mechanism in reversed phase HPLC let us consider the stationary phase. The surface of the silica is covalently bonded to a long chain hydrocarbon which provides a very non-polar surface characteristic. This attracts and binds non-polar molecules or sub-structures of molecules whilst more polar moieties are less well, or not all, bound. Typically mobile phases are primarily aqueous with a degree of lesser polarity introduced by an organic solvent such as methanol or acetonitrile. With regard to Table 4.2, the solvents may be viewed as having reversed eluotropic strength. Thus, more polar analytes have a greater affinity for the mobile phase than the stationary phase and are eluted earlier than non-polar analytes. However, no matter how good the bonding chemistry of the surface modifier, not every surface silanol (Si—OH) is attached to a non-polar group. Thus, there are always some silanol functions on the stationary phase surface through which polar or even ionic binding may occur. Indeed, the nature of the stationary phase may be altered depending on the composition of the mobile phase. If we consider the unmodified silanol groups on the surface, these exhibit a degree of acidity. If the mobile phase pH is high the silanols will be ionised ($Si{-}O^-$) and ionic interactions will play a large role in binding of analytes. If, on the other hand, the mobile phase is more acidic, the silanol groups will be un-ionised and hydrogen bonding or hydrophobic interactions will be more important. These polar/ionic interactions can occur at the same time, as the hydrophobic binding processes depending on the analyte's molecular structure and are called secondary interactions (Figure 4.8). Such interactions can lead to a mixed mode of retention which can be very selective and, thus, useful in terms of selectivity or can be detrimental to the chromatographic

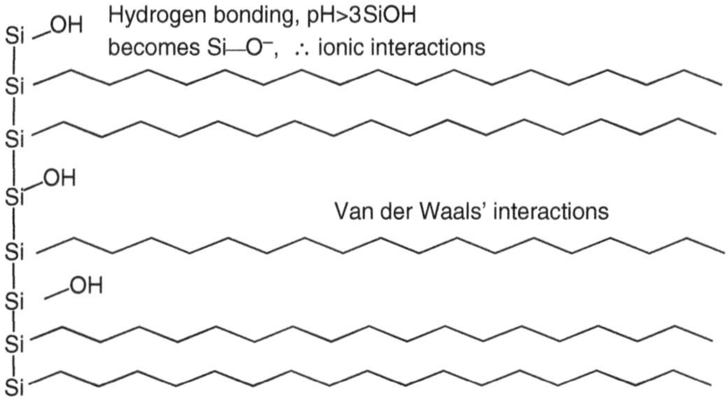

FIGURE 4.8 *Types of binding possible in reversed phase liquid chromatography on a bonded silica stationary phase.*

efficiency. For example, bases, as many drugs are, may be eluted from their hydrophobic binding sites only to experience a polar interaction with the silanol sites leading to additional binding and an appearance of *peak-tailing*, i.e. poor peak asymmetry.

As has been said, in reversed phase liquid chromatography, the more polar an analyte the earlier it will be eluted. However, very polar ionic molecules can be retained by use of an *ion-pair* reagent. For example, a basic drug structure that contains an amine may at the appropriate pH be positively charged. At the same pH an acidic reagent may be negatively charged. The two molecules will attract each other forming what is called an ion-pair. If the acidic moiety is attached to a hydrophobic structure (Figure 4.9) this will be attracted to the stationary phase. By this means very polar structures can be made to retain sufficiently in reversed phase HPLC to effect useful chromatography. Equally, an acidic drug can be ion-paired with a basic reagent in the mobile phase, such as tetrabutylammonium bromide.

4.4.3 Ion exchange chromatography

An alternative approach is to use ionic binding as the principal mode of retention by having an ionic stationary phase and ionic analytes and effecting elution by including a competitor ion to the analyte in the mobile phase. This is *ion exchange chromatography*. The most common retention mechanism involves a simple exchange of analyte ions and mobile phase ions with the charged groups on the stationary phase. Obviously, there are two modes, anion exchange and cation exchange (Figure 4.10). Analytes that interact weakly with the ion exchanger, the stationary phase, will be eluted more rapidly than those that interact strongly.

This type of chromatography is often used for the separation of organic acids and bases whose degree of dissociation into ionic forms is dependent on the pH. Higher pH will lead to greater ionisation of acids and less ionisation of bases which will lead to greater retention of the most acidic species.

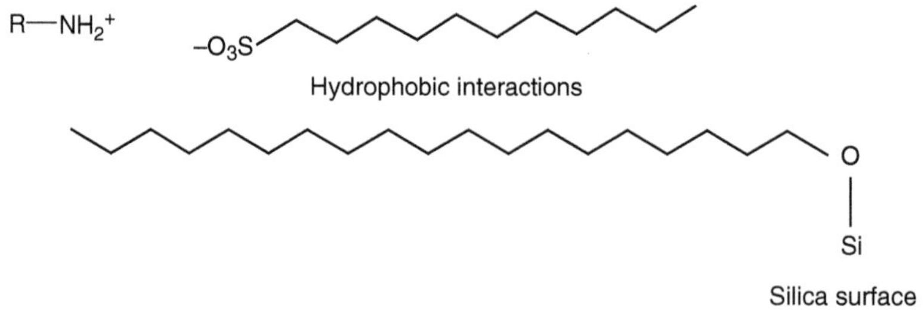

Figure 4.9 *Representation of the binding mechanism in ion-pair chromatography.*

Anion exchange:

X^-	+	R^+Y^-	$\rightleftharpoons$	Y^-	+	R^+X^-
Analyte ions		Stationary phase with mobile phase ions		Mobile phase ions		Bound analyte

Cation exchange:

$$X^+ \quad + \quad R^-Y^+ \quad \rightleftharpoons \quad Y^+ \quad + \quad R^-X^+$$

FIGURE 4.10 *Ion exchange.*

There are many other variations of HPLC, for example, using stationary phases with polarities intermediate between the very polar ionic or silica phases and the hydrophobic octadecyl phases; or size exclusion chromatography wherein only molecules below a certain size are able to penetrate the pores of the stationary phase and are retained. These all have their uses and full discussions on them are available elsewhere, but it should be remembered that the vast majority of pharmaceutical bioanalysis is carried out in the reversed phase mode on octadecyl bonded silicas.

4.4.4 GRADIENT HIGH-PERFORMANCE LIQUID CHROMATOGRAPHY

Thus far the chromatography discussed has involved a mobile phase with a constant composition throughout the separation process. The separation is said to be performed under *isocratic* conditions. For some cases, where a complex mixture requires separation or where a system is required that will not need altering to successfully chromatograph a wide range of compounds (a *generic* system), it is advantageous to be able to change the composition of the mobile phase during the course of a separation. This is called *gradient HPLC*. In this discussion only gradient HPLC in the context of reversed phase HPLC, which is its most usually applied mode, will be considered. Furthermore, this discussion will concentrate on mixtures of two solvents (*binary gradients*) which are most common although ternary or even quaternary gradients have found uses. A weak solvent, typically water or an aqueous buffer, is mixed with an organic solvent, such as acetonitrile, so that the percentage of the organic solvent in the mobile phase increases with time. That is, the solvent is a weak eluent at the start of the separation, but a strong one at the end. This allows the retention of polar analytes under the initial conditions and the elution at the final conditions of even quite highly bound hydrophobic analytes. Under the initial conditions, a given analyte, X, will exhibit a high k' value, whereas under the final conditions

X will have a low k' value i.e. its k' value will decrease as the gradient progresses. At some point the k' of X will decrease to the point where it begins to migrate along the column. For a more highly retained analyte, Y, this point will not be reached until later in the gradient and hence the analytes are separated. For each analyte eluting from the column, the end of the peak will be eluting under conditions whereby it is travelling faster than the front of the peak. This leads to reduced tailing and narrow peaks, which aids both resolution and sensitivity. The overall result is an extremely powerful system for analysing compounds of considerably differing polarities in a single separation. Figure 4.11 shows a typical gradient separation of a test mix of 13 compounds chosen to cover a wide range of polarities. This approach can provide highly efficient separations of many compounds in a single chromatographic run.

A further significant development which has recently led to even greater usage of gradient chromatography is *fast gradient* HPLC. As can be seen from the chromatogram in Figure 4.11, gradient chromatography has traditionally involved the development of a gradient over a period of 30–40 minutes which has resulted in some very fine separations. However, in the modern pharmaceutical bioanalytical facility, more and more samples from studies investigating increasing numbers of compounds need to be analysed rapidly, and this timescale

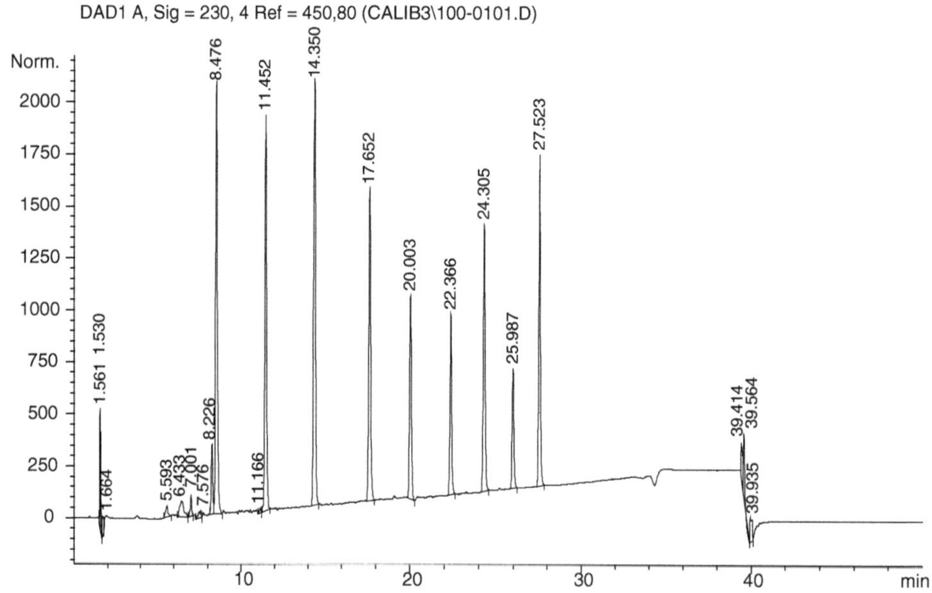

FIGURE 4.11 *25 μL injection of a test mix containing uracil, theophylline, acetofuran, acetanilide,* m-*cresol, acetopheneone, propiophenone, benzofuran, butyrophenone, valerophenone, hexanophenone, heptaphenone and octaphenone on a Supelco ABZ + 5 μm, 10 cm × 4.6 mm column at a flow rate of 1 mL/min. Gradient 0–95 per cent MeCN in 0.1 per cent aqueous formic acid over 35 min.*

is no longer acceptable for routine bioanalysis. Fortunately in gradient chromatography:

$$\text{Resolution} \propto \text{gradient time (i.e. the time to run the entire gradient)} \times \frac{\text{flow rate}}{\text{column length}}$$

This means that the column can be shortened and the flow rate increased (within pressure constraints) and the gradient time can then be reduced without loss of separating power. If we assume we have acceptable resolution and wish to maintain it, then the gradient time can be reduced 10-fold if the column length is reduced by a factor of 2.5 and the flow rate increased four-fold. These conditions do lead to higher operating system pressures but not higher than can be easily maintained by modern HPLC equipment. This approach has created the opportunity to do some very rapid separations of complex mixtures. The same mixture of analytes shown in Figure 4.11 is shown in Figure 4.12 separated under fast gradient conditions.

Obviously, this offers a lot of potential for higher throughput in modern pharmaceutical bioanalysis, whilst still offering the benefits of a method which is capable of application to a wide range of pharmaceuticals.

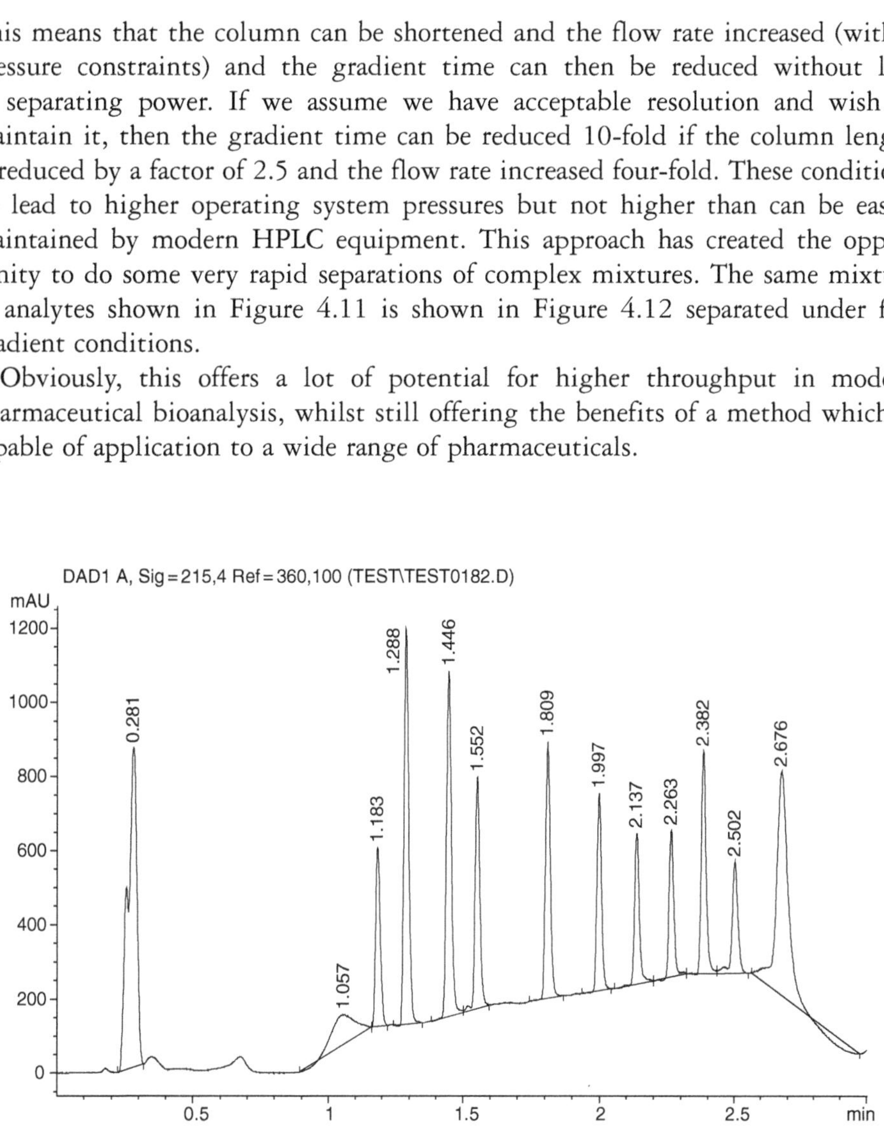

FIGURE 4.12 *An injection (1 μL) of an 11-component test mix onto a 50 × 2 mm Phenomenex Magellan C18. The column was maintained at 40 °C and eluted with a 0–95 per cent aqueous formic acid (0.1 per cent) and acetonitrile gradient over 2 min followed by a 1 min isocratic period of aqueous formic acid (0.1 per cent) at a flow rate of 800 μl/min. The column eluent was monitored by ultraviolet radiation at 215 nm.*

4.5 High-throughput bioanalysis

The advent of combinatorial chemistry approaches to drug synthesis has led to ever increasing numbers of candidate new pharmaceuticals entering the early stages of research and development. In consequence, there are increasing numbers of samples requiring bioanalysis per unit time. Not only is the number of samples increasing, but also the time available for method development is decreasing. Therefore, high throughput, generic strategies for bioanalysis are required to meet the demands of modern drug development.

In the Bioanalysis and Drug Metabolism Division of Glaxo Wellcome, we developed two key approaches to this problem. The first is the use of fast gradient chromatography as described above, following sample preparation by either solid phase extraction or protein precipitation. This is proving very successful for a large number of compounds of widely differing chemical structures.

The second approach we have developed is termed as ultra-high flow rate liquid chromatography and involves direct analysis of plasma samples without sample preparation. This is achieved by using large particle size (30–50 μm) stationary phases in contrast to conventional analytical columns, which are typically packed with 5 μm particles held in the column by 2 μm frits. Direct injection of plasma samples onto these columns quickly causes blocking. With the large particle sizes and the consequently larger (10–20 μm) column end frits this problem is removed. Also, with the large particle size stationary phases the back pressure generated is greatly reduced, so extremely high flow rates can be used. Typically, a standard system with a 1 mm i.d. column would be operated at 4 mL/min (for a conventional 5 μm stationary phase in a column of these dimensions, the normal flow rate would be 40–50 μL/min). This allows some very fast chromatography and using this approach a throughput of one sample every 1.2 minutes, equivalent to 50 samples per hour, can be achieved, with the only sample preparation being addition of internal standard solution. Indeed we have operated a system in which four such columns were operated in parallel, allowing a throughput approaching 200 samples per hour.

It should be noted that although the technique has some resolving power, it is not a high efficiency separation and plate counts, *N*, are low. As a result, a highly selective detector is required, normally a mass spectrometer operated in the MRM mode. Also, where there are metabolites which may breakdown back to the parent structure in the source of the mass spectrometer, such as *N*-oxides or glucuronides, it is necessary to check that these are chromatographically resolved from the parent under the conditions used before using this technique. However, within these limitations this technique offers the ability to analyse plasma samples for drug concentrations extremely rapidly and has found wide usage in our laboratories. Furthermore, a recent innovation has been the development of monolithic silica stationary phases, which allow high flow rates combined with high chromatographic efficiencies for the direct analysis of drugs in plasma samples. These columns comprise a single piece of silica with a defined bi-modal pore structure. Large macropores provide low flow resistance and permit the direct injection of plasma samples coupled with high flow rates and low back pressures, and small mesopores provide excellent diffusion characteristics leading to high efficiencies. Standard conditions for ultra-high flow rate liquid chromatography for direct pharmaceutical bioanalysis:

Column: 50 × 1 mm, 50 μm Octadecylsilane (ODS) or 50 × 4.6 mm Chromolith™ silica rod

Flow rate: 4 mL/min

Injection volume: 25–50 μL

Mobile phase: Solvent A: 0.1% aqueous formic acid
Solvent B: 5% 0.1% aqueous formic acid
95% acetonitrile

Gradient profile:

Time (mins)	%A	%B
0	100	0
0.2	100	0
0.8	0	100
0.9	0	100
1.0	100	0
1.2	100	0

Detector: Mass spectrometer in MRM mode with atmospheric pressure ionisation.

4.6 *Chiral HPLC*

Many pharmaceuticals are optically active. An optically active substance is one that rotates the plane of polarised light. Optically active drug molecules contain one or more *chiral* or *asymmetric* centres, carbon atoms to which are attached four different groups. For a structure containing a single chiral centre the molecule can exist as two non-superimposable forms which are mirror images of each other. These are called *enantiomers*. One enantiomer will rotate polarised light to the left, whereas the other will rotate it to the right. These are termed the *S*- and *R*-enantiomers, respectively. In many cases, only one of the enantiomers exhibits the desired pharmacological effect while the other may have no activity or worse, unwanted toxic activity. It is, therefore, necessary in drug development to be able to determine which stereochemical form the drug is in the body, how much of each form is present and whether one form inverts to the other. Analytical methods are, therefore, needed that are capable of resolving the enantiomers.

Enantiomers of the same molecule differ from each other only in the manner in which they rotate polarised light; all their other physicochemical properties are identical and conventional chromatography cannot separate them.

There have been two key approaches to this problem. The first has been to derivatise the drug, after extraction from the biological sample, with a stereochemically pure single enantiomer derivatising reagent. For example, amine-containing drugs can be derivatised with chiral acid reagents as shown below:

$$\text{S} - \text{reagent} + \text{S/R} - \text{analyte} \longrightarrow \text{SS} - \text{product} + \text{SR} - \text{product (diastereoisomers)}$$

The products containing two chiral centres are called *diastereoisomers*. These diastereoisomers have differing physicochemical properties and can be resolved on conventional chromatographic columns. This approach has been very successful.

The second approach has been direct chromatographic resolution of the two enantiomers. Direct chromatographic resolution of the enantiomers can be achieved in two ways: either by the use of a chiral mobile phase or a chiral stationary phase. The former of these is not widely used, as separation factors achieved are rarely sufficiently high, but the latter is now a well-established and widespread means of performing chiral separations.

There are many different chiral stationary phases commercially available offering a number of different separation mechanisms. One of the most commonly used 'family' of chiral stationary phases is the cyclodextrins. Cyclodextrins are toroidal-shaped molecules formed of glucose units. The most common are the α-, β- and γ-cyclodextrins containing 6, 7 and 8 glucose units, respectively. The molecules are shaped like truncated cones with an inner cavity the size of which depends on the number of glucose units in the molecule. Due to the orientation of the glucose units the interior of the cavity is relatively hydrophobic whereas the surface is hydrophilic. For chiral resolution, the analyte must enter the cavity such that its asymmetric centre, or groups near to it, interact with the surface hydroxyl groups, forming an *inclusion complex*. The separation is then based on a difference in the stability of the inclusion complex formed by each enantiomer of the analyte (see Figure 4.13).

Other types of chiral stationary phases include immobilised proteins, celluloses, macrocyclic antibiotics and immobilised metal co-ordinating ligands. These have different mechanisms of separation and are well described elsewhere.

4.7 *Future trends in HPLC*

HPLC, like any vibrant technique, is still evolving. The last few years have seen many new variations explored. The drive in the late 80s and early 90s was towards

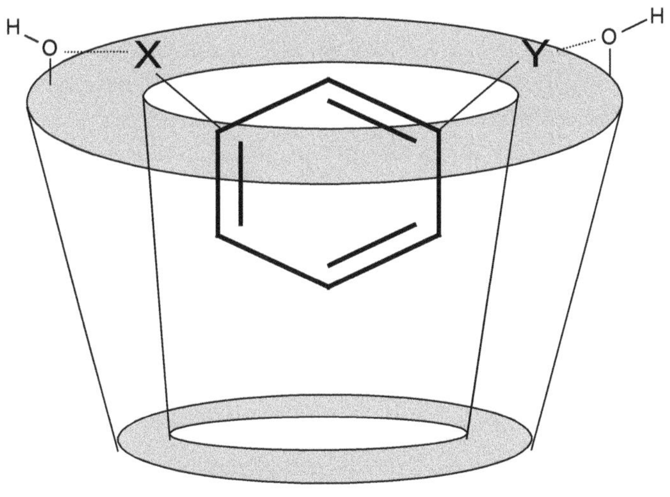

FIGURE 4.13 *Schematic representation of an inclusion complex in a toroidal cyclodextrin molecule. X and Y represent the groups at or near the chiral centre and interact with the surface hydroxyl groups of the cyclodextrin, whilst the hydrophobic part of the molecule sits within the cavity.*

ever more automation of the entire sample analysis process, including the introduction of robotic systems to automate all parts of the analytical procedure. Included in this has been a trend towards equipment which is compatible with the now widely used 96-well plate format for handling samples. Increased use of mass spectrometers has to some extent removed the need for extensive sample preparation and is also replacing many other detectors. However, the biggest trend which will affect HPLC in the pharmaceutical industry in the coming years is almost definitely, miniaturisation. The use of smaller scale HPLC has several distinct advantages.

First a typical, conventional HPLC column has an internal diameter of 4.6 mm and is operated at a mobile phase flow rate of approximately 1 mL/min. To maintain the same linear flow rate on a 1 mm i.d. column, the reduction in flow rate is proportional to the square of the radius of the column and the flow rate would, therefore, be reduced by a factor of approximately 21 to approximately 45–50 μL/min. Further reduction in the internal diameter of the column to the capillary scale (0.32 mm or less i.d. columns) results in flow rates of 5 μL/min. These days economic and environmental concerns regarding the disposal of waste solvents make such a significant reduction in the amount of HPLC waste mobile phase highly desirable.

Second, and more important, most detection systems are concentration-sensitive. That is, the size of response they exhibit is proportional to the concentration of analyte in solution reaching them. If a 0.32 mm column system is operated under conditions that show the same efficiency as a 4.6 mm column, then the peak width will be unchanged and the volume of mobile phase in which an eluting peak is contained will be also related to the square of the column radius. Changing from a 4.6 mm to a 0.32 mm i.d. column, therefore, offers a 207-fold increase ($4.6^2/0.32^2$)

in the concentration of an analyte in a peak as it reaches the detector. Even if the reduced column dimensions restrict the volume of sample that can be injected by 10–20-fold, there is obviously a significant gain in sensitivity that can be achieved this way. Alternatively, if the available sample volume is extremely small, then a miniaturised HPLC system offers the maximum sensitivity for chromatographic analysis of that sample.

A further benefit of miniaturised HPLC systems is that some mass spectrometer sources perform more efficiently at very low flow rates in terms of their ionisation rates, thus offering further gains in sensitivity when using these detectors. This includes techniques such as the rapidly emerging nano-spray LC–MS systems.

There are potential problems which need to be borne in mind when using micro-scale HPLC systems. The most important of these is that if the peak is eluting from the column in a volume of approximately 1 μL or less, it is vital that all extra-column volumes are minimised to avoid dispersion effects destroying the peak integrity and thus the sensitivity. This means that in the case of HPLC–MS, the column end needs to be as close to the source as possible and connected to it by no more than a short length of very narrow bore capillary tubing.

It should also be borne in mind that with UV absorbance detection systems the path length of the detector cell is proportional to the response and so minimising the volume puts constraints on the sensitivity of the detection system. The use of detector flow cells with narrow, long path length channels can help but is limited as too long a channel will lead to the danger of more than one peak entering the detector at any one time thereby destroying the resolution achieved by the chromatography.

Nevertheless, the potential gains in terms of environmental, economic and sensitivity factors, coupled with the wish for ever faster separations, are such that the future will see a swing away from columns of 1–5 mm i.d. and 10–25 cm length to columns of 50–320 μm diameter and 2–3 cm length and being operated with very fast micro-scale gradients. Indeed, many of the manufacturers of HPLC are already actively involved in the development of systems capable of meeting these requirements.

4.8 *Bibliography*

Krejčí, M. *Trace Analysis with Microcolumn Liquid Chromatography*. Publ. Marcel Dekker Inc.

Lough, W.J. (ed.) Chiral *Liquid Chromatography*. Publ. Blackie.

Snyder, L.R. and Kirkland, J.J. *Introduction to Modern Liquid Chromatography*. Publ. John Wiley & Sons Inc.

CHAPTER 5

Mass spectrometry and quantitative bioanalysis

Bob Biddlecombe, Sheryl Callejas and Gary Evans

5.1 *Introduction*

What is mass spectrometry? Mass spectrometry (MS) is based on the ionisation of molecules so that they become charged particles and can then be sorted according to their mass to charge ratio (m/z). The mass spectrometer is the instrument that provides the requisite functionality for this technique; however, there are several different types of mass spectrometers. The key to understanding advances in mass spectrometry is to appreciate the problem-solving nature of technological developments. Most of these advances are driven by the instrument manufacturers and have concentrated on improving methods of ionising molecules and the selectivity and sensitivity of detection. (For more detailed reading on mass spectrometery, see Bibliography.)

MS was originally used in conjunction with gas chromatography (GC) for the quantitative analysis of drugs. When liquid chromatography (LC) replaced GC as the preferred technique for bioanalysis, GC–MS continued to be used because of the difficulties encountered interfacing LC and MS. GC was used for volatile compounds or compounds which had been reacted with derivatising agents to render volatile products. These molecules were readily ionised by techniques such as electron impact (EI), and gas flow into the mass detector was advantageous for the technique. LC, however, introduced new problems, the molecules analysed were generally non-volatile and were not readily ionised. The mobile phase was liquid and present in more significant quantities than the analyte and was also incompatible with the high vacuum of a mass spectrometer. How to interface LC with MS provided a technological challenge which was successfully overcome by changing the ionisation techniques and the design of the mass spectrometer. In recent years these technological advances have made LC–MS the method which is now regarded as the standard method used for bioanalysis in pharmaceutical laboratories and clinical contract organisations. In this chapter we will review these developments and focus on the use of MS in quantitative analysis. MS is also a powerful tool for structural and molecular information and is used extensively in qualitative analysis and identification of metabolites. This is discussed in Chapter 17.

5.2 *The instruments*

There are a number of different mass spectrometers which are characteristic of the instrument manufacturer, ionisation technique or the instrument design (some instruments are designed so that they are optimised for particular applications). There are also technological differences in the mass analyser. For example, in sector instruments, ions are produced in the source of a mass spectrometer that is operating under vacuum. They are then accelerated by an electric field into a magnetic region. Scanning the magnetic field of the electromagnet sequentially focuses ions of differing mass at the detector. In contrast, quadrupole mass spectrometers operate by filtering masses through a radio frequency voltage field. Whilst there are differences in the instruments, the scientific principles and overall components are the same for all mass spectrometers. These are illustrated in Figure 5.1.

In each case there is a need to introduce the analysed sample into the mass spectrometer; in practice this is the interface with the chromatographic separation technique (primarily LC). The analyte molecule is then converted into an ionic compound by the ionisation process; following ionisation the ions are progressed to the mass analyser and ion detector. Each of these components is discussed in more detail in the following sections.

5.3 *Analytical interfaces*

There are a number of possible interfaces with LC and the main purpose is to evaporate the mobile phase and transfer the analytes to a gaseous phase suitable

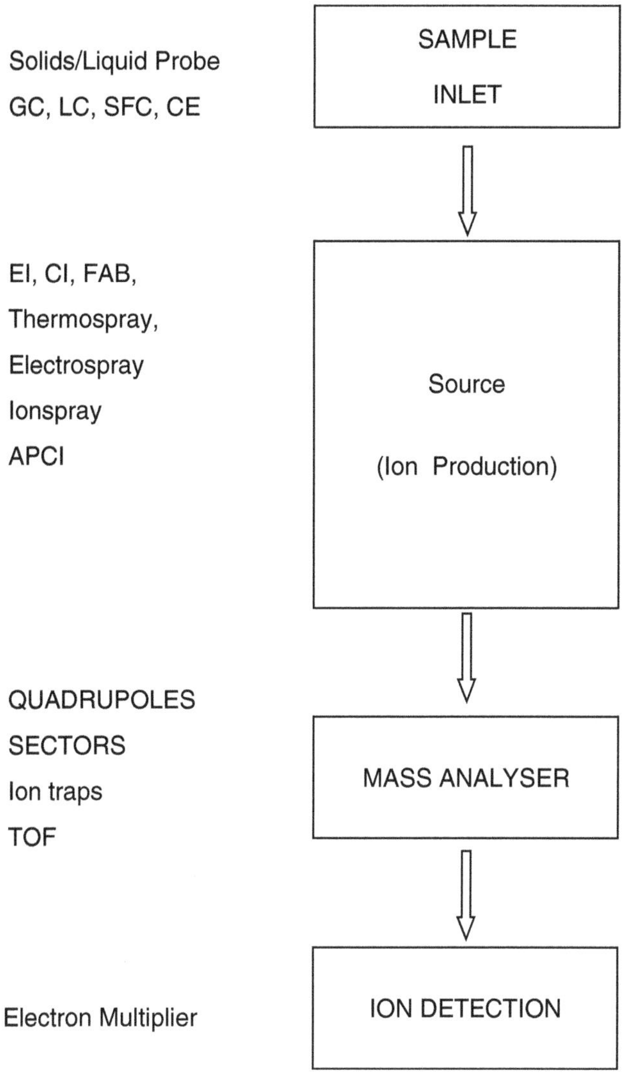

FIGURE 5.1 *Components of a mass spectrometer.*

for ionisation and to switch from the high or atmospheric pressures at which chromatographic separation was achieved to the lower pressures required for mass analysis. The main interfaces are described below.

5.3.1 Atmospheric pressure–chemical ionisation (APCI)

APCI creates gas-phase ions at atmospheric pressure. The ions produced pass through a series of channels into successive vacuum chambers. The eluant from the LC is sprayed into a heated chamber at a temperature of approximately 400 °C. The heat rapidly evaporates the liquid and solutes contained therein and does not appear to degrade most drugs and metabolites.

5.3.2 Electrospray (ES)

The ES interface produces gas-phase ions at atmospheric pressure. These pass into the vacuum system through a series of apertures separating successive vacuum stages. ES is composed of a hollow needle with a high electric potential through which the eluant flows. The high field at the tip of the needle produces a cone-shaped liquid meniscus from which a spray of highly charged droplets emerges. Subsequent evaporation of the droplets results in ion formation. Conventional ES operates at flow rates of 1–10 μL; higher flow rates can be achieved with alternative ES, ionspray (pneumatic assisted), ultraspray (ultrasonic assisted) and turbospray (thermally assisted).

5.3.3 Particle beam (PB)

The PB interface is designed to remove the mobile phase whilst transferring the majority of the analyte to the mass analyser. The PB conducts several functions: an aerosol generator serves to disperse the liquid eluant into a high surface area spray which passes into the heated desolvation chamber in which solvent-depleted solute particles are produced. The momentum separator serves to direct the aerosol through a series of apertures at atmospheric pressure into the low-pressure ion source.

5.3.4 Continuous flow fast atom bombardment (flow FAB)

The column eluant is directly introduced into the vacuum region of the MS through a probe at a very low flow rate of 5–10 μL. The eluant is mixed with a matrix material (glycerol, thioglycerol or nitrobenzyl alcohol) to facilitate the ionisation process. This mixture passes over the flattened end of the probe to form a very thin layer from where evaporation occurs and the low flow rates ensure that most of the solvent mixture evaporates in the ion source.

5.3.5 Thermospray

The thermospray vapouriser is a heated capillary tube through which the LC eluant passes and by controlling the temperature the complete eluant can be evaporated at the tip of the vapouriser. The thermospray is capable of controlling the evaporation of a wide variety of mobile phases. The vapourised solute is introduced into a reduced pressure spray chamber from which it passes into the high vacuum of the mass analyser.

5.4 *Ionisation*

There are several methods for producing ions in the source of a mass spectrometer. EI is a long established ionisation technique; however, a number of 'soft' ionisation techniques such as chemical ionisation (CI), fast atom bombardment (FAB), atmospheric pressure ionisation or ES are used. The latter two are the most important for modern quantitative LC–MS.

5.4.1 Electron impact (EI)

This was the commonest method of ionisation for GC–MS, as a great number of organic compounds were suitable for EI but it has limited use in LC–MS. To give an EI spectrum the compound must be volatile; specifically it must have a vapour pressure of at least 10^6 Torr. Ions are formed when a beam of electrons hits the sample molecules in the gas phase. This gives the sample molecules high energy, and fragment ions are formed. Unfortunately some compounds will fragment entirely and not produce molecular ions. EI can be performed by direct probe and GC–MS. PB is the only commercial LC–MS interface that produces EI spectra. A beam of solute particles enters the source of the mass analyser and impinges on the surface of the ion source. The ion source walls are heated to several hundred degrees facilitating the 'flash vapourisation' of the solute particles. Once in vapour phase the solute molecules are ionised by EI.

5.4.2 Chemical ionisation (CI)

CI can produce molecular ions for some volatile compounds that do not give molecular ions in EI. CI uses a reagent gas to transfer protons to the sample, usually producing $(M + H)^+$ quasimolecular ions. These ions have a tendency to fragment because they are even-electron species and excess energy is imparted to them. The reagent gas (methane, isobutane or ammonia) is present in the ion source, it is ionised by an electron beam and the resulting ions undergo a series of ion–molecule reactions to produce species such as CH_5^+ in methane. These reagent gases in a ratio of 106:1 to the sample then collide with sample molecules producing ions by proton transfer. CI has been used with PB and API interfaces for LC–MS.

5.4.3 Fast atom bombardment (FAB)

FAB is the most popular ionisation technique for non-volatile and/or thermally labile molecules. FAB has provided spectra for compounds which were unsuccessful for EI or CI. It works best for polar and higher molecular weight compounds such as peptides and ionic species. FAB utilises a beam of neutral fast moving atoms (xenon, argon) which impinge on a metal target coated with liquid matrix in which the sample has been dissolved. The impact of these atoms on the liquid surface transfers kinetic energy to the sample in a manner that results in the desorption of the sample ions into the gaseous phase. This process is gentle and little fragmentation occurs. FAB spectra are complex showing $(M + H)^+$ quasimolecular ions, fragments and cluster groups of the matrix and the sample plus matrix. Trifluroacetic acid can be added to the matrix to encourage formation of protonated ions. Some compounds give better negative ion FAB spectra where the quasimolecular ion is $(M - H)^-$. FAB has been used with the PB interface but is more commonly associated with the continuous flow FAB interface.

5.4.4 Electrospray ionisation (ESI)

Unlike most ionisation processes in MS which occur in the gaseous phase, ESI is the transfer of ions present in the liquid phase into the gas phase. A pre-requisite for ion production with ES is that the analyte exists in solution as an ion. ES can produce ions from 100 per cent aqueous solutions with no organic modifiers. Mobile phases may have volatile buffers such as ammonium acetate in moderate concentration. Many buffers especially those containing alkali metals will decrease sensitivity by competing for ionisation. ESI can also produce ions from 100 per cent solutions in organic solvents such as methanol and acetonitrile.

5.4.5 Atmospheric pressure chemical ionisation (APCI)

The LC eluant passes into a heated nebuliser or ionspray where it is mixed with a nebuliser gas; both these inlets are designed to provide soft ionisation of polar molecules. Ions are created at atmospheric pressure with little or no heating (API). Ionisation is accomplished with a source of electrons introduced with the heated spray. The electrons are supplied by a discharge source or 63 Ni beta emittor. These sources produce a rich stream of reagent ions resulting from interaction with the electrons. The reagent ions are produced by electron ionisation of the source gases; usually air or nitrogen is used. The ionisation of O_2 and N_2 by EI leads to the formation of hydronium ion water cluster $H_3O(H_2O)_n$. At atmospheric pressure there is significant interaction between reagent ions and analyte ions produced by the heated nebuliser. The gas-phase analytes will become and remain protonated if their proton affinity is greater than that of water (amines, for example, have a high proton affinity). The ionisation process is one of the most efficient with almost 100 per cent ionisation obtained under ideal conditions.

APCI is the method of choice for drugs and metabolites and has become the most widely used technology for high-throughput bioanalysis. The sensitivity, robustness and reliability of APCI are greater than those obtained with ES.

5.5 *Mass analysers*

All mass analysers determine the mass of an ion and mass to charge ratio and measure gas-phase ions. There are four main types of mass analysers:

5.5.1 Sector mass analyser

This is the traditional magnetic sector mass spectrometer in which ions created in the ion source are accelerated with high voltages into the analyser magnetic field. The radius of curvature in a given magnetic field of the sector is a function of *m/z* (mass to charge ratio). Ions of differing masses can be separated and detected by a single detector by varying the magnetic field or the source voltage to scan the mass range. Sector MS is capable of separating all ions all the time but can only detect one mass at a time.

5.5.2 Quadrupoles

A quadrupole MS consists of four parallel rods (quads) equally spaced around a central axis. Ions are introduced along the axis of the poles. The ions are accelerated at low voltages, and by applying different voltages to the different quads, conditions can be established in which only ions with a particular *m/z* ratio can pass through to the ion detector. Effectively only one ion is monitored; this is known as single ion monitoring (SIM) and is the most sensitive method for a single quad.

5.5.3 Ion trap MS

This mass analyser works by trapping ions and then detecting them based on their *m/z* ratios. The ion trap is a variation of the quad mass filter and uses the same principles to trap the ions. After trapping, the ions are detected by placing them in unstable orbits causing them to leave the trap. The ion trap is used in drug metabolism but are not as suitable for high-throughput bioanalysis as quads in a tandem MS.

5.5.4 Time of flight (TOF) analysers

These analysers are based on the fact that ion velocity is mass dependant. They consist of an ion source, a 'flight' tube and a detector. Each mass enters the flight tube at different velocities, small mass ions having a higher velocity. The mass ions separate as they pass down the tube and arrive at the detector. TOF has ideal characteristics for structural analysis and are often combined in modern MS with quads.

5.5.5 Tandem mass spectrometry

Tandem mass spectrometry also called mass spectrometry–mass spectrometry (MS–MS) because the instrument contains two mass spectral analysers in tandem; between the two analysers is a collision gas cell. Generally soft ionisation techniques do not cause fragmentation of the ionised particles. The basic approach of MS–MS is the measurement of mass to charge ratios of ions before and after fragmentation of the selected ion by collision with a high-pressure gas (normally helium). This collision process is called collision-induced dissociation (CID).

5.5.6 Mass detection

There are two main methods for ion monitoring: single ion monitoring (SIM) and selective reaction monitoring (SRM) or multiple reaction monitoring (MRM).

5.6 *Use of MS in quantitative LC–MS*

The improvements in LC–MS have been largely driven by instrument manufacturers and the characteristics are based on the commercially available instruments. In the past few years the main instruments used for high-throughput bioanalysis have been supplied by two vendors: PE Sciex and Micromass. These represent the API and ESI interfaces respectively. In addition to the technical developments, the cost and size of instruments including the required services have been significantly reduced with instruments becoming cheaper and smaller. Sciex MS caused a revolution in high-throughput quantitative bioanalysis by reducing significantly the time taken to analyse a single sample from 10–15 to 2–5 minutes. In addition the use of the tandem MS arrangement increased the specificity so that only minimal chromatographic separation was required.

The tandem MS arrangement allows the *m/z* relating to the analyte to be selected at the first quad and the *m/z* characteristic of the main fragment or daughter ion to be selected at the second quad. This provides for good selectivity and sensitivity without significant chromatographic separation required from endogenous material.

Although it is a soft ionisation technique if higher temperatures are used it can affect the decomposition of thermally labile molecules such as N-oxide metabolites and conjugates. If the spectrum indicates a loss of 16 amu (atomic mass units) this can indicate an N-oxide; however, if the conjugate reverts to the aglycone this can be difficult to detect. Molecular weight information is obtained from quasimolecular ions $(M + H)^+$ (positive mode) or $(M - H)^-$ (negative mode).

5.6.1 Optimising physical parameters for APCI

- Vary probe temperature – the formation of adduct ions may be reduced; however, high temperatures may cause problems if compound is thermally labile.
- Drying gas pressure – dependent on LC flow rates.
- Source temperature – dependent on flow rates and solvent composition.
- Cone voltage – high voltage will effect fragmentation and may lead to decreased molecular ion signal.
- More independent of buffer concentration than ESI.

Under APCI conditions a component with a molecular weight similar to the parent compound but at a different retention time is indicative of an N-oxide or conjugate.

5.7 *Developing an LC–MS assay method*

5.7.1 Example 1: a semi-automated method for the determination of fluticasone propionate (CCI187811) in human plasma using solid phase extraction and liquid chromatography tandem mass spectrometry

Fluticasone propionate (FP) is quantified in human plasma by automated solid phase extraction using a Packard MultiPROBE robotic sample handler and analysed by high-performance liquid chromatography (HPLC) with tandem mass spectrometric detection (LC–MS–MS) using selective reaction monitoring (SRM). Samples are spiked with internal standard, ^{13}C-labeled FP, extracted using C18 solid phase sorbent packed into columns in the 96-well plate format and eluted with methanol (Table 5.1). Extracts are reconstituted with methanol/buffer (50:50) after evaporation and submitted for analysis. Protonated molecules, MH^+, were used as precursor ions with the following SRM transitions being monitored for FP and [$^{13}C_3$]-FP, respectively: *m/z* 501 → *m/z* 313 and *m/z* 504 → *m/z* 313. A chromatogram of an extract of blank plasma is shown in Figure 5.2; compare with the chromatograms of the lowest and highest standards presented in Figures 5.3 and 5.4, respectively. A typical chromatogram obtained from a plasma sample taken from a patient receiving FP is illustrated in Figure 5.5. The calibration range for this method is 20–1,500 pg/mL from 0.5 mL plasma and the concentrations in calibration samples, quality control (QC) samples and study samples are determined using least-squares linear regression with a 1/*X* weighting factor (Figure 5.6).

HPLC Conditions	
Mobile phase	25 mM ammonium formate/methanol 20:80, 1 mL/min
Column	150 × 4.6 mm i.d. ResElut C8 BDS operated at 40 °C
Injection volume	80 μL
Split ratio	Between 5 and 10
Mass spectrometer parameters	
Mass spectrometer	PE Sciex API III+
Ionisation mode	Turbo ionspray
Polarity	Positive ion
Scan mode	Selected reaction monitoring (SRM)
Collision gas	Argon
Collision gas thickness (CGT)	250
Nebuliser gas	Zero grade nitrogen
Pause time	20 m
Acquisition time	4.5 minutes
Q2 settling	ON (1000 amu Q3 park mass)
The following transitions were monitored	
FP	*m/z* 501 → *m/z* 313 Dwell time: 250 ms
[$^{13}C_3$]-FP	*m/z* 504 → *m/z* 313 Dwell time: 250 ms

5.7.2 Example 2: sumatriptan (GR43175X) and rizatriptan (GR289537X) in human plasma

To support clinical trials, a generic SPE 'Triptan' liquid chromatographic tandem mass spectrometric method has been developed for the determination of Sumatriptan (GR43175X) and Rizatriptan (GR289537X) in human plasma.

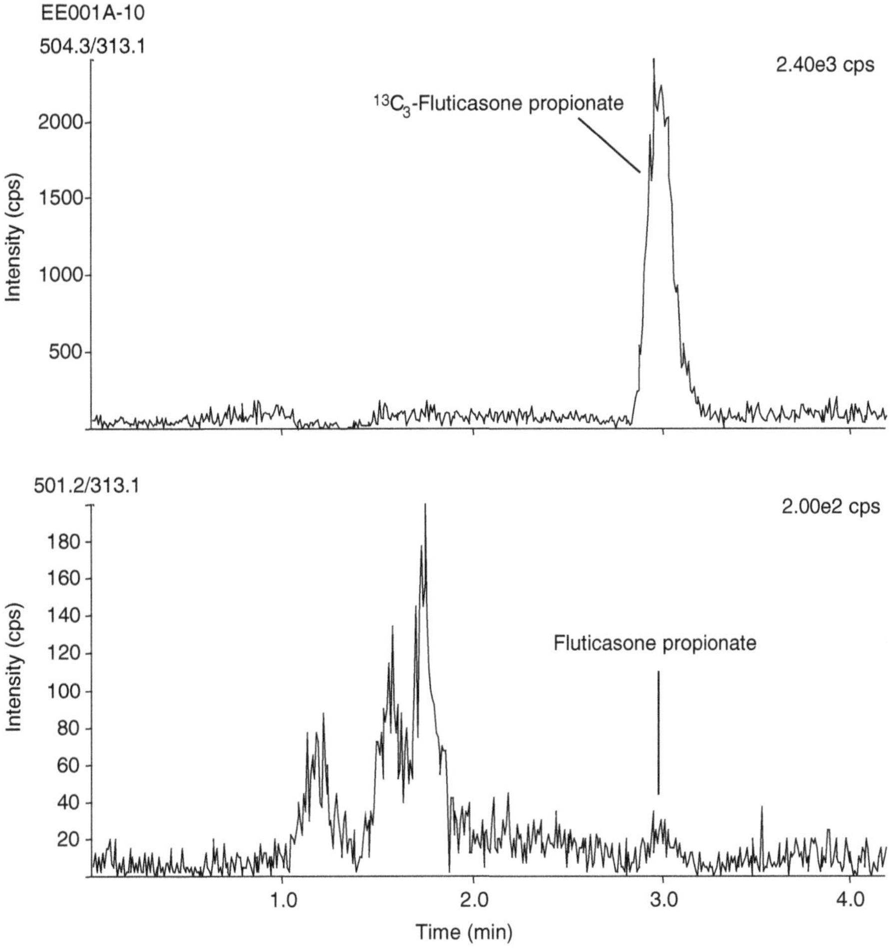

FIGURE 5.2 *Representative chromatogram of blank matrix.*

TABLE 5.1 *Sample preparation conditions*

Step	SPE process	Solvent	Volume (mL)	Bleed factor	Vacuum (s)
1	Condition	10% MeOH (v/v) aq.	0.1	50	10
2	Load	Sample ISTD	0.4	30	180
3	Wash	Water	0.2	10	30
4	Wash	Water	0.2	10	60
5	Elute	MeOH	0.2	30	90

Samples are spiked with internal standard, ^{13}C-labeled FP, extracted using C18 solid phase sorbent packed into columns in the 96-well plate format and eluted with methanol.

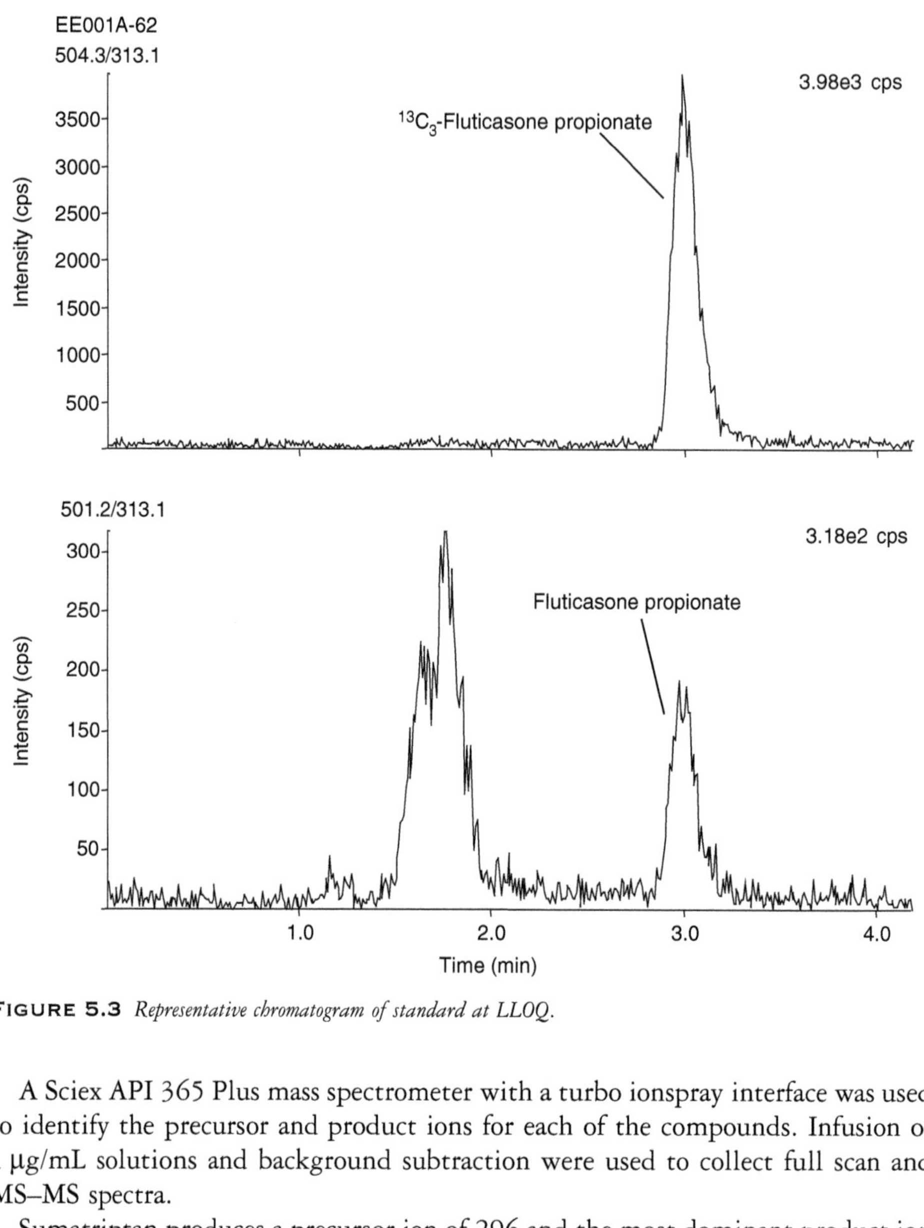

FIGURE 5.3 *Representative chromatogram of standard at LLOQ.*

A Sciex API 365 Plus mass spectrometer with a turbo ionspray interface was used to identify the precursor and product ions for each of the compounds. Infusion of 1 μg/mL solutions and background subtraction were used to collect full scan and MS–MS spectra.

Sumatriptan produces a precursor ion of 296 and the most dominant product ion of 58. The deuterated internal standard produces a precursor ion of 299 and a product ion of 61 (Figure 5.7).

Rizatriptan produces a precursor ion of 270 and the most dominant product ion of 201. The deuterated internal standard produces a precursor ion of 276 and a product ion of 207 (Figure 5.8).

An automated solid phase extraction (SPE) is performed using a zymate XP robot with a series of customised workstations (4). The method is internally standardised;

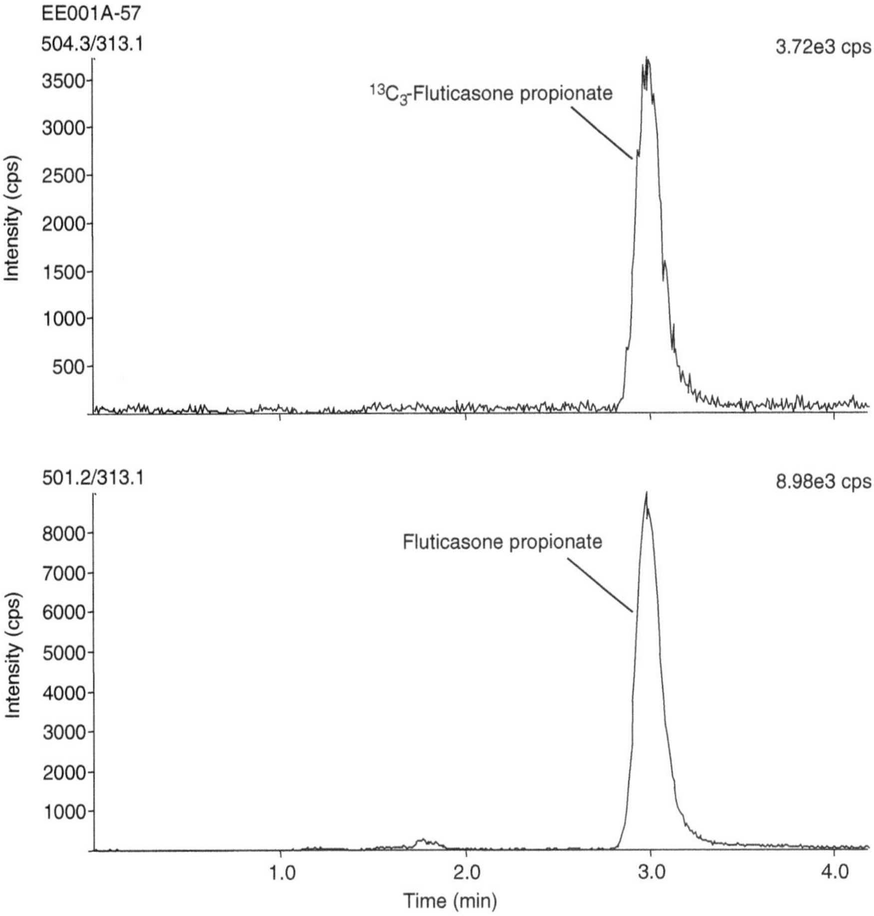

FIGURE 5.4 *Representative chromatogram of standard at ULOQ.*

for GR43175X, ISTD [2H3]-GR43175H is used and for GR289537X, ISTD [2H6]-GW289537C is used.

To start with, a 5 mg Oasis extraction block and 96-well collection plate are housed in the carousel and this is accessed by a zymate XP robot for sample preparation. The SPE station conditions the Oasis block ready for sample loading. A Multiprobe (a four-probe aspirating and dispensing station) transfers the internal standard and sample to the Oasis block. The SPE station then washes the block and elutes the samples into a 96-well collection plate (Figure 5.9).

The resulting extracts are evaporated to dryness under a stream of heated nitrogen and reconstituted with 90:10 0.1 per cent formic acid (aq):acetonitrile. The plate is then transferred to the automated plate sealer where it is sealed with aluminium and polypropylene plate ready for mass spectrometric analysis.

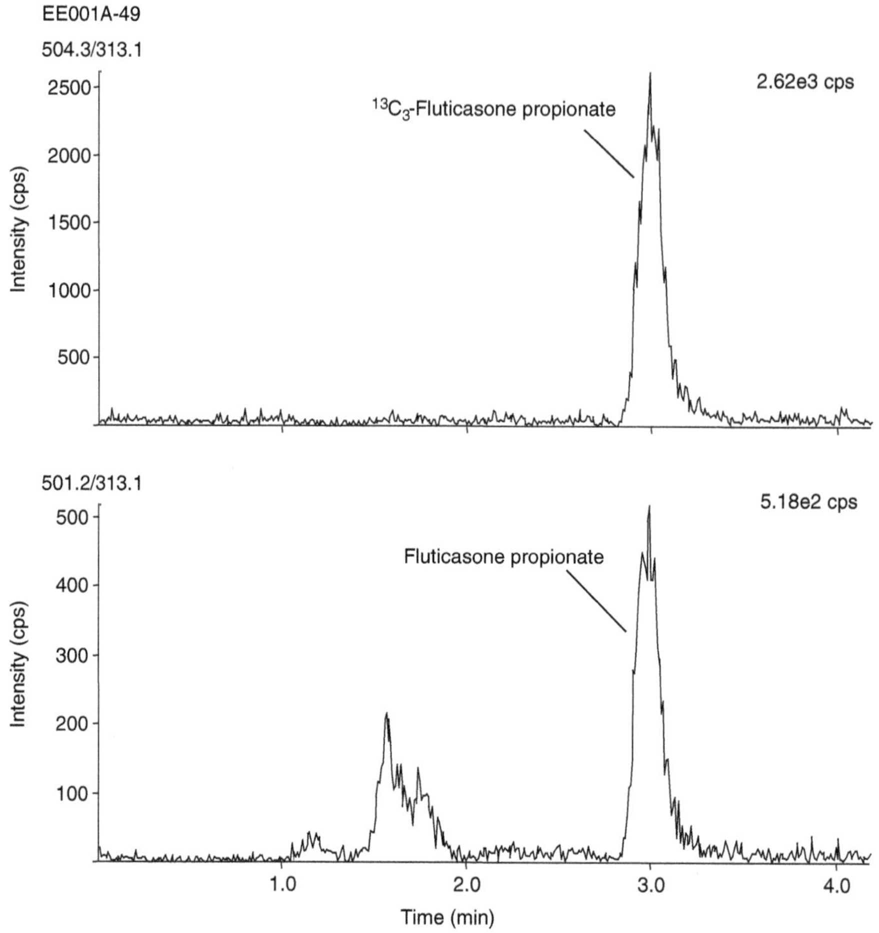

FIGURE 5.5 *Representative chromatogram of subject 27683.*

Samples are analysed using HPLC under gradient conditions. 20 μL of sample is injected onto a 5 cm × 2.1 mm i.d. ODS3 column (5 μm) and the analytes are eluted using a combination of two mobile phases: A = 0.1% formic acid; B = 95% acetonitrile: 4.9% water: 0.1% formic acid (Table 5.2).

Typical chromatograms for blank plasma, lower limit of quantification (LLOQ) and upper limit of quantification (ULOQ) are illustrated in Figure 5.10. Data is acquired using Multview and processed using Macquan. Peak area ratios are used to construct a calibration line with a linear regression fit and a $1/X$ weighting factor. Typical calibration lines, range 0.1–20 ng/mL, are shown in Figures 5.11 and 5.12 for Sumatriptan and Rizatriptan, respectively.

The accuracy and precision of Sumatriptan and Rizatriptan in human plasma was determined using spiked validation control samples spiked at 20, 10, 1.0, 0.25 and 0.1 ng/mL. These were analysed in replicates of six on four separate occasions and the agreement between the measured and nominal concentrations of validation control samples assessed. Results are shown in Tables 5.3 and 5.4. This method has successfully been used to support several clinical studies.

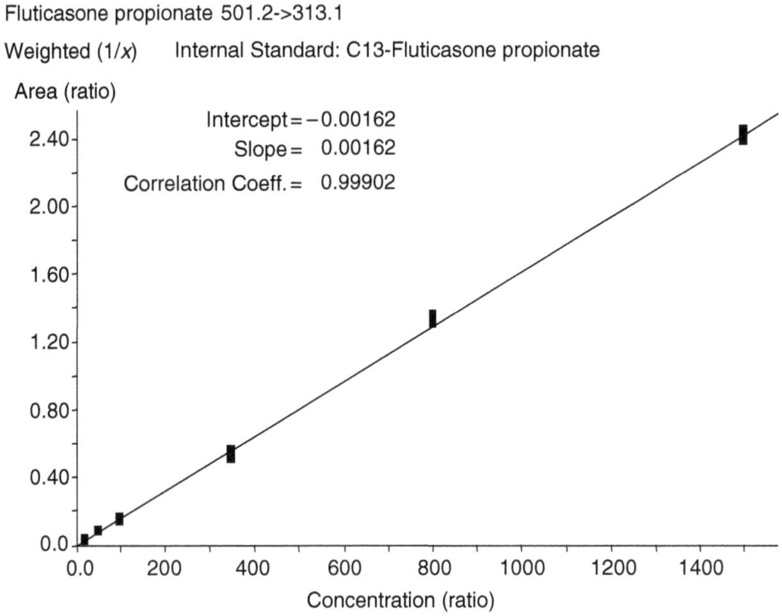

FIGURE 5.6 *Representative calibration curve for fluticasone propionate.*

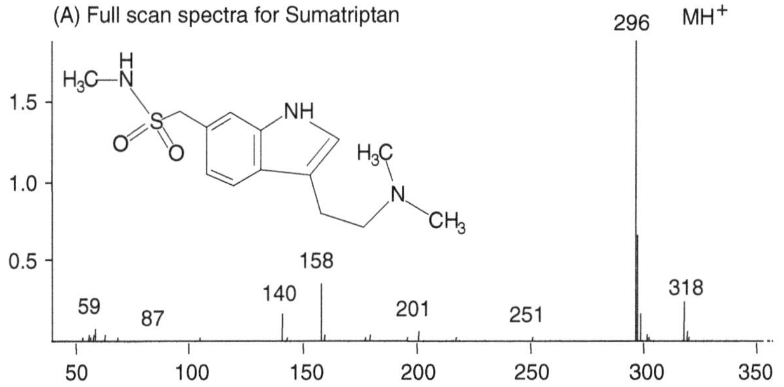

FIGURE 5.7 *MS–MS spectra for Sumatriptan.*

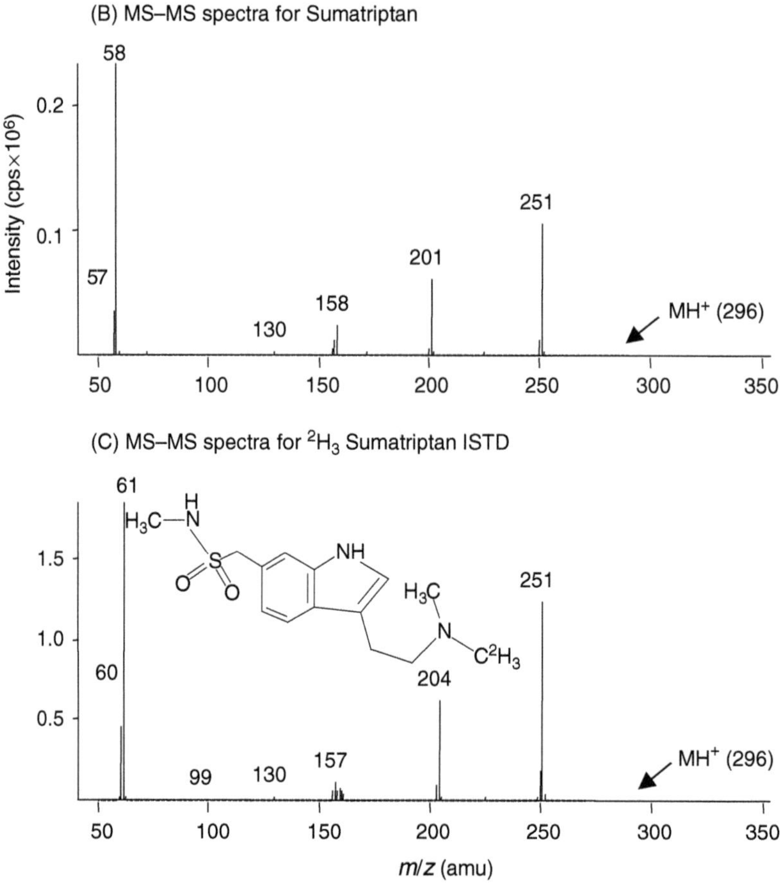

FIGURE 5.7 *(Continued).*

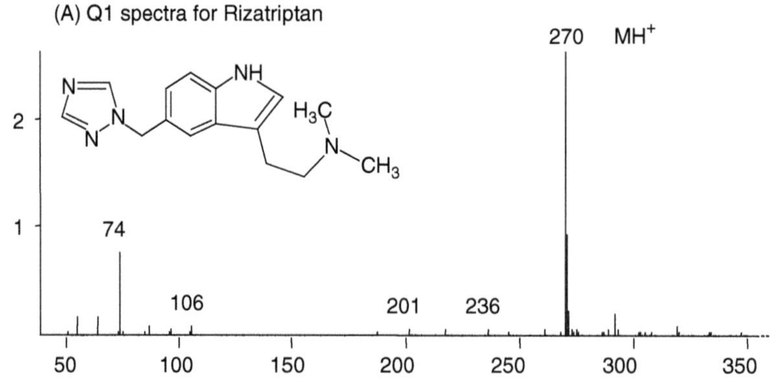

FIGURE 5.8 *MS–MS spectra for Rizatriptan.*

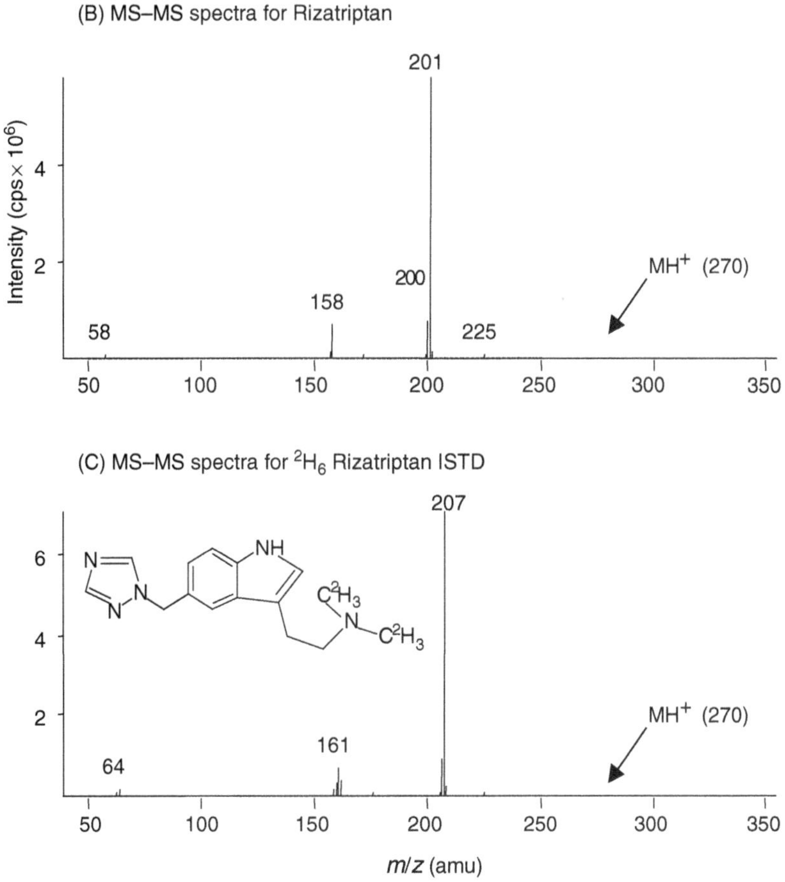

FIGURE 5.8 *(Continued).*

TABLE 5.2 *Samples are analysed using HPLC under gradient conditions. 20 μL of sample is injected onto a 5 cm 2.1 mm i.d. ODS3 column (5 μm) and the analytes are eluted using a combination of two mobile phases: A = 0.1% formic acid; B = 95% acetonitrile:4.9% water:0.1% formic acid*

Start (min)	Duration (min)	Flow (μl/min)	Profile	% Solvent A	% Solvent B
−0.1	0.1	800	0	100	0
0	2.0	800	−2	0	100
2.0	0.1	800	−10	100	0
2.1	1.9	800	0	100	0

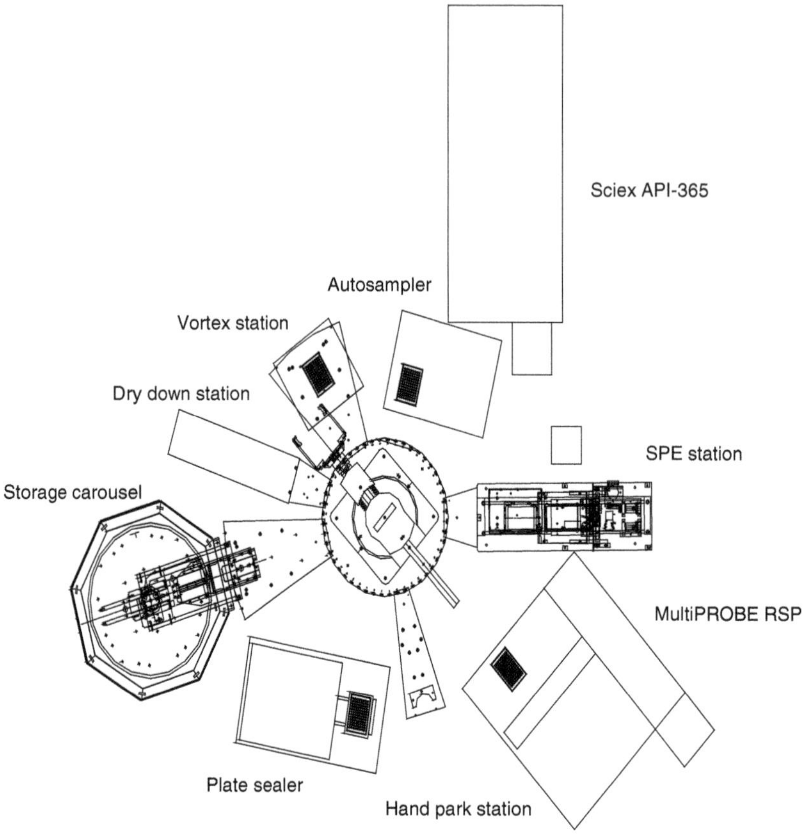

FIGURE 5.9 *Schematic representation of Zymark Zymate sample preparation system.*

TABLE 5.3 *Assay validation results for Sumatriptan assay*

	VC1	VC2	VC3	VC4	VC5
Target and actual VC concentrations for Sumatriptan					
Target VC	20	10	1	0.25	0.1
Number	24	24	24	23	22
Mean	20.5066	9.6593	1.0078	0.2235	0.0933
Standard deviation	0.4048	0.2538	0.0372	0.0176	0.0088
Accuracy					
%Bias	2.5%	−3.4%	0.8%	−10.6%	−6.7%
Precision: 1-way ANOVA on log-transformed data					
%CV					
Intra-assay	2.0%	2.6%	3.8%	7.1%	8.5%
Inter-assay	Negligible	0.7%	Negligible	2.4%	4.7%
Overall	2.0%	2.6%	3.8%	7.5%	9.8%

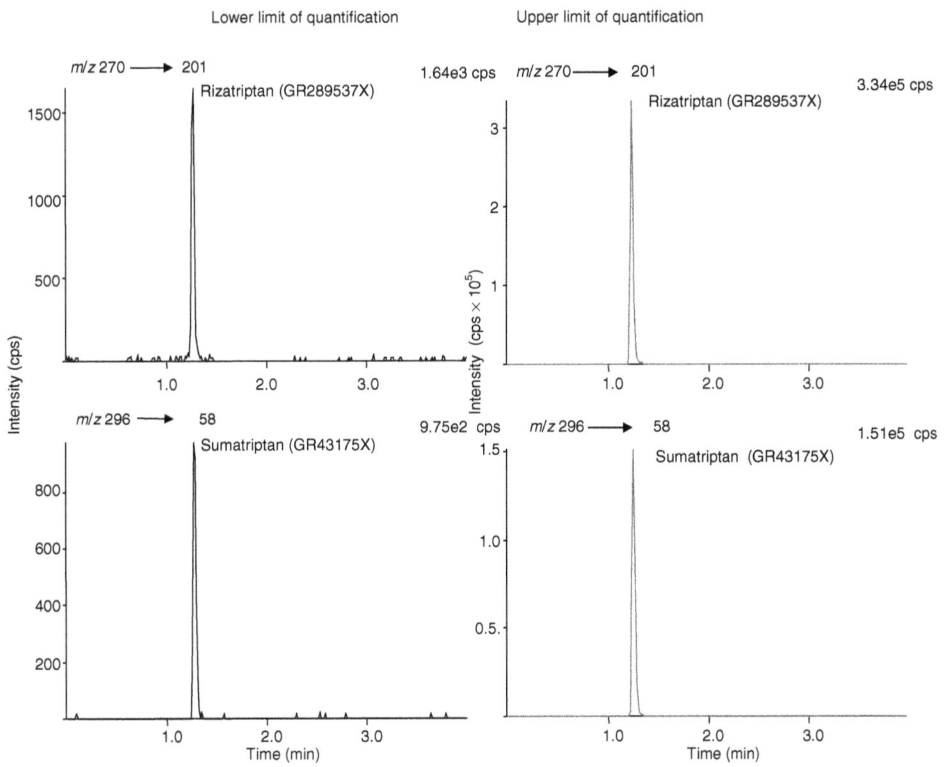

FIGURE 5.10 *Lower and upper limits for Sumatriptan and Rizatriptan assays.*

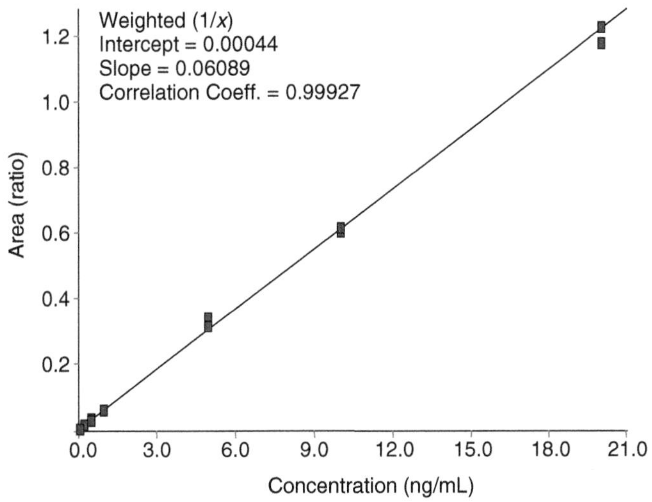

FIGURE 5.11 *Calibration line for Sumatriptan.*

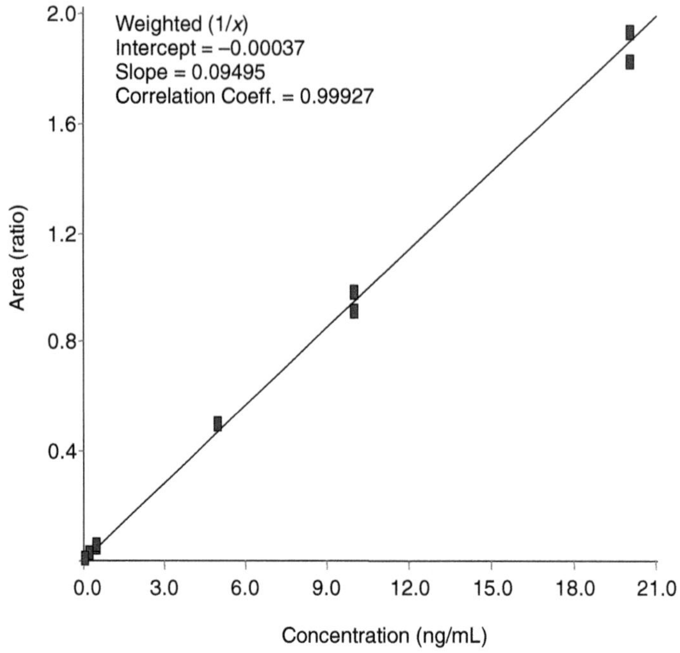

FIGURE 5.12 *Calibration line for Rizatriptan.*

TABLE 5.4 *Assay validation results for Rizatriptan assay*

	VC1	**VC2**	**VC3**	**VC4**	**VC5**
Target and actual VC concentrations for Rizatriptan					
Target VC	20	10	1	0.25	0.1
Number	24	24	24	23	22
Mean	19.570	9.781	1.068	0.222	0.103
Standard deviation	0.772	0.301	0.037	0.015	0.009
Accuracy					
%Bias	−2.1%	−2.2%	6.8%	−11.3%	2.7%
Precision: 1-way ANOVA on log-transformed data					
%CV					
Intra-assay	2.2%	1.7%	3.3%	6.6%	8.1%
Inter-assay	3.7%	2.9%	1.5%	Negligible	3.6%
Overall	4.3%	3.4%	3.6%	6.6%	8.9%

5.8 *Bibliography*

Biddlecombe, R.A. (1999) An automated approach to sample preparation in high throughput bioanalytical laboratory. MipTec-ICAR Conference, Montreux.

5.8.1 Mass spectrometry textbooks

Desiderio, D.M. (1994) *Mass Spectrometry Clinical and Biomedical Applications*. Vol. 2, Plenum Press.

Niessen, W.M.A. and van der Greef (1992) *Liquid Chromatography–Mass Spectrometry*, Marcel Dekker.

Venn, R.F. (2000) Principles and Practice of Bioanalysis. Taylor & Francis.

Willoughby, R., Sheehan, E. and Mitrovich, S. (1998) *A Global View of LC/MS*. Global View Publishing, Pennsylvania.

CHAPTER 6

Immunoassay in pharmacokinetic and pharmacodynamic bioanalysis

Richard Nicholl, Paul Linacre and Bill Jenner

6.1 *Summary*

This chapter outlines the general concept of immunoassay as a bioanalytical tool and describes the modern application of the technique in a bioanalytical department within the pharmaceutical industry.

The various types of immunoassay procedure are described in the context of the requirements for the development and optimisation of an immunoassay method. This includes the generation of polyclonal and monoclonal reagent antibodies and the selection of a suitable label.

Once a method has been developed it is essential that it is validated in terms of accuracy, precision, sensitivity, specificity, linearity and analyte stability, and this important requirement is described both for methods developed in-house and for commercial kits.

Although still used for the bioanalysis of small molecule drugs where appropriate, the current major application for immunoassay is in the measurement of biomarkers. The various types of marker and their importance are described and illustrated with a specific example (determination of Cox-2 selectivity in human blood).

The chapter includes a brief description of immunoassay data processing, the important points that must be considered here, and a summary of assay automation possibilities.

The other important current application of immunoassay in bioanalysis is in the measurement of biological drugs (biopharmaceuticals). The important issues that relate to the use of immunoassay in this area are described together with an actual example of an application of the technique in support of a bio-pharmaceutical product.

6.2 *The role of immunoassay in drug discovery and development*

Within the pharmaceutical industry, immunoassay has traditionally been used for the analysis of small and large drug molecules in biological fluids to support pre-clinical and clinical drug discovery and development programmes. In the 1980s radioimmunoassay (RIA) was the major form of immunoassay used but this has largely given way in the 1990s to techniques involving spectrophotometric detection such as enzyme-linked immunosorbent assay (ELISA) or time-resolved fluorescence immunoassay (TRFIA). Until the 1990s high-performance liquid chromatography (HPLC) was the main alternative technique for the bioanalysis of drugs but often it could not match the sensitivity or throughput of immunoassays. Therefore, choice of technique was made on a case by case basis depending on the structure of the drug, availability of suitable expertise and resource, and desired limit of quantification.

There are many examples of successful drug development programmes where immunoassays have been used as the bioanalytical tool of choice such as ranitidine (Zantac), acyclovir (Zovirax and Valtrex) and lamotrigine (Lamictal). Lamotrigine is still being quantified by immunoassay in post-marketing studies.

The advantages of immunoassay as a bioanalytical technique include the ability to achieve very sensitive assays with very small sample volumes. In addition, there is generally no need for a sample preparation or extraction step prior to analysis and samples can be assayed directly in an appropriate matrix. Once established, immunoassays are easily automated and are high-throughput methods that do not require expensive instrumentation. However, there are disadvantages of immunoassays, most notably the perception that immunoassays for drugs are intrinsically non-specific, particularly with respect to metabolites. This is not entirely true as specificity is dependent on appropriate assay development, particularly with respect to antiserum generation. Another major disadvantage is the comparatively long assay development time, which is usually some months, with no guarantee of success.

In recent years LC–MS–MS technology has improved to such an extent that it has become the technique of choice for small molecule drug and metabolite analysis throughout the pharmaceutical industry, largely replacing immunoassay and HPLC. These considerable improvements have led to the potential for extremely short assay development time (days), improved sensitivity (comparable to immunoassay) and extensive automation of the tedious and time-consuming extraction procedures. The question therefore must be asked is there still a role for immunoassay in future drug discovery and development programmes? The answer to this question is most definitely yes and the reasons for this are as follows.

First, there are many exciting developments ongoing in the commercial immunodiagnostic industry which will undoubtedly impact upon immunoassay use in drug discovery and development. Such efforts include the simultaneous determination of related analytes in multi-analyte immunoassays, development of ultrasensitive immunoassays (e.g. immuno-PCR) and the continuously increasing number of commercial assays and antisera for novel biomarkers. The measurement of biomarkers in drug discovery and development is becoming increasingly important and as many of these markers are macromolecules, such as proteins, immunoassay is usually the technique of choice. This developing area is discussed in detail later in the chapter.

Second, immunoassay has an important role supporting the increasing number of biological drug discovery and development programmes, e.g. therapeutic monoclonal antibodies and vaccines where it is often the only appropriate analytical technique.

Finally, immunoassay development and application may still be useful for some small molecule drugs such as in the analysis of established drugs, mainly in the later stages of clinical development. This strategic use of immunoassay can free-up valuable LC–MS–MS resource and instrumentation or can provide a cost-effective alternative to outsourcing the method. The relatively long immunoassay development time may not be an issue at this stage of drug development, and the availability of an LC–MS–MS assay provides a simple means of evaluating the specificity of the immunoassay by simply cross-validating the two methods.

To summarise, it is clear that immunoassay will have a major role to play in bioanalysis in the future and instead of diminishing in importance it is staging somewhat of a renaissance.

6.3 *Principles of immunoassay*

Immunoassay is an analytical tool that relies on the ability to generate a response as a result of an antibody–antigen interaction. An antigen is a molecule that can be bound by a specific antibody and is capable, either directly or indirectly of eliciting an immune response when injected into a living host. Part of this immune response results in the production of high-affinity antibodies which bind specifically to the antigen. In nature this is designed to aid in the removal of foreign molecules from the host but specific and high-affinity antigen–antibody interactions can be exploited to quantify molecules by means of an immunoassay. Since the discovery of immunoassay over 40 years ago this technology has been very widely exploited for the bioanalysis of both small and large organic molecules.

In general immunoassays fall into two broad categories, competitive and non-competitive. In a competitive assay, analyte (antigen) in a sample competes with a constant amount of labelled analyte for a limiting amount of antibody. Increasing amounts of analyte in the sample will result in less-labelled antigen being bound by the antibody. Before measurement of the labelled fraction bound to the antibody, separation of antigen–antibody complex and free-labelled antigen is achieved by one of a number of methods including activated charcoal, polyethylene glycol (PEG), and a secondary antibody which binds to the primary antibody. In RIA the label is a radioactive form of the analyte (usually ^{3}H or ^{125}I) which can be determined in the antibody-bound fraction by scintillation or gamma counting (see Figure 6.1).

Alternatively, an enzyme conjugate, where a suitable enzyme such as alkaline phosphatase has been covalently attached to the analyte whilst retaining its catalytic activity, is used as the label (enzyme immunoassay, EIA). The amount of enzyme in the bound

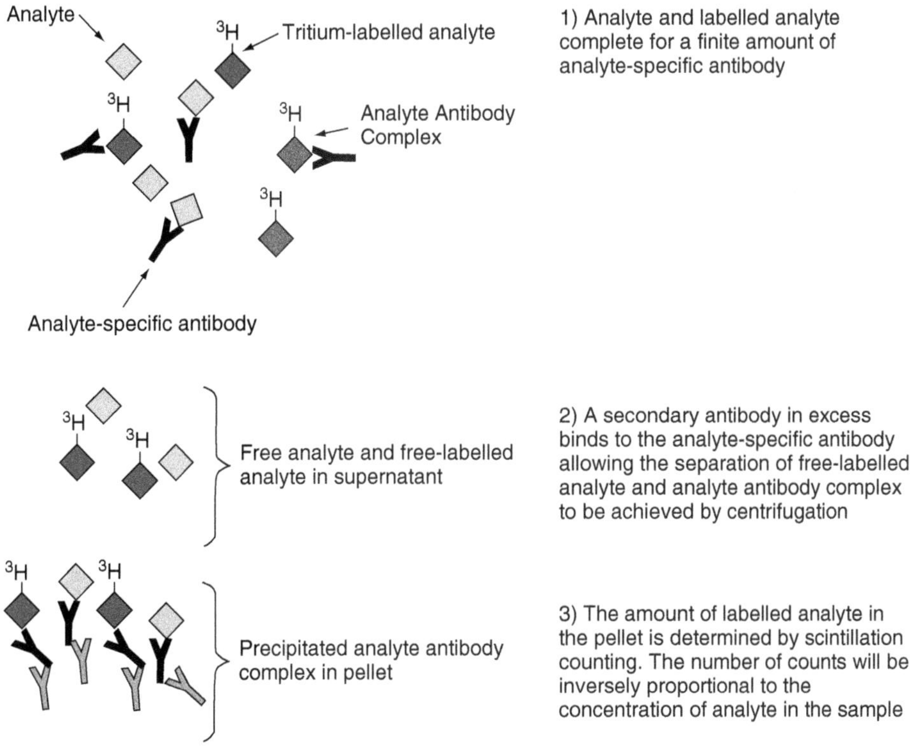

FIGURE 6.1 *An RIA utilising a second antibody to enable separation of bound and free fractions.*

fraction (using a separation system that retains the bound fraction in the supernatant) is determined by the addition of a substrate resulting in the formation of a coloured product. The intensity of the colour is determined spectrophotometrically.

A non-competitive immunoassay, in effect, involves the capture of all the analyte in the sample by excess antibody. The capture antibody is usually immobilised on a solid phase such as a polystyrene bead, a coated tube or more commonly the surface of a microtitre plate resulting in the most popular immunoassay format currently used, ELISA. Following washing of the solid phase a secondary antibody, which is also specific for the analyte but at a different site (epitope) and is typically conjugated to an enzyme, is added. The secondary antibody binds to the captured analyte forming a 'sandwich'. Further washing to remove unbound secondary antibody and addition of enzyme substrate result in the development of colour, the intensity of which is directly proportional to the concentration of analyte in the sample (Figure 6.2). Because this 'sandwich' assay format is dependent on the analyte being large enough to accommodate two different antibody molecules it is usually only applicable to macromolecule analytes.

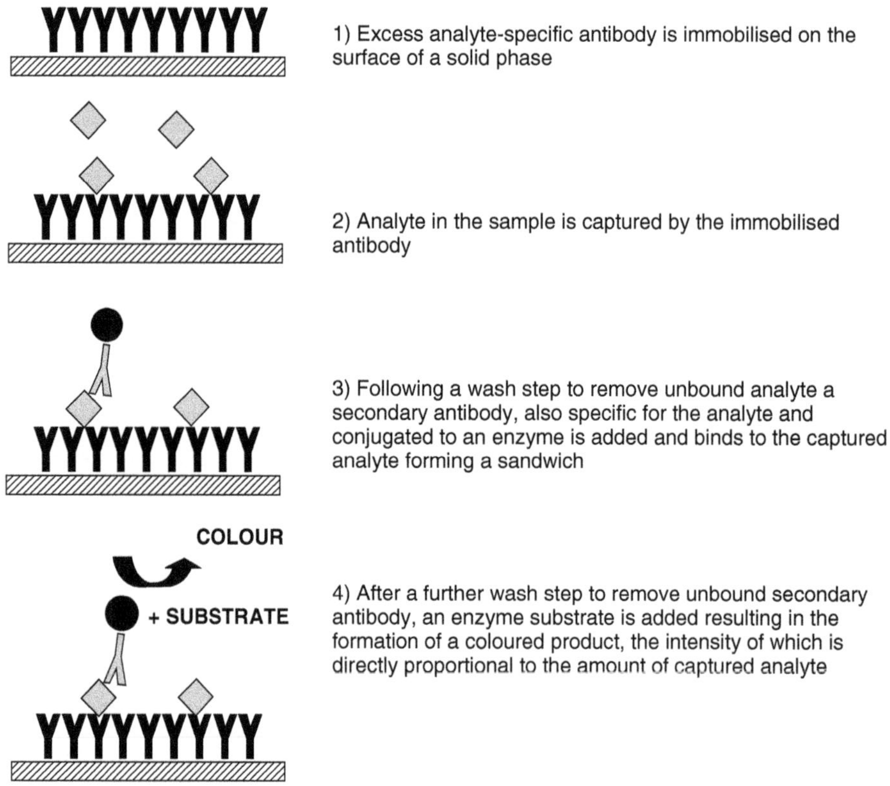

1) Excess analyte-specific antibody is immobilised on the surface of a solid phase
2) Analyte in the sample is captured by the immobilised antibody
3) Following a wash step to remove unbound analyte a secondary antibody, also specific for the analyte and conjugated to an enzyme is added and binds to the captured analyte forming a sandwich
COLOUR
+ SUBSTRATE
4) After a further wash step to remove unbound secondary antibody, an enzyme substrate is added resulting in the formation of a coloured product, the intensity of which is directly proportional to the amount of captured analyte

FIGURE 6.2 *A non-competitive ELISA format.*

6.4 *Assay development*

The first consideration in assay development and optimisation should be the intended application of the assay as this will influence the development goals such as desired accuracy, precision and sensitivity.

Immunoassay, compared to other bioanalytical techniques, requires a relatively long time for assay development. The step that takes by far the most time is generation of the reagent antibody, be it monoclonal or polyclonal, which can take a number of months with no guarantee that a suitable reagent will be produced. There are often commercially available immunoassay kits and/or reagent antibodies that can be used directly, or adapted for use in the analysis of biomarkers. These kits and reagent antibodies therefore save a lot of time and effort and if applicable would be used in preference to developing assays in-house. For novel biomarkers, academia may be the best source of antibody reagents.

There are a variety of immunoassay types (e.g. RIA, ELISA) and a number of formats for each, and it is therefore not possible to describe the development of all of these here. There are many excellent books and references which describe the assay development process for immunoassays in detail. The following section will briefly describe production of antisera, introduce the different types of label (often called tracer) available and list the steps necessary for assay development and optimisation.

6.5 *Production of reagent antibodies*

The antiserum is the key reagent in any immunoassay as it governs the selectivity, sensitivity, precision and accuracy of the method. Macromolecules, such as high molecular weight foreign proteins and polypeptides, are naturally immunogenic whereas lower molecular weight haptens (<2,000 Daltons) will require coupling to a protein to make them immunogenic.

A decision is required regarding production of monoclonal or polyclonal antiserum. As a rule of thumb, monoclonals are best suited for large molecules for use in two-site sandwich assays (one monoclonal to capture the molecule of interest and a second against a different non-overlapping epitope) and polyclonals for small molecules. For competitive immunoassay formats such as RIA, polyclonals are often superior because of their generally greater affinity.

For monoclonal antibody production the standard method involves a series of immunisations of mice with antigen over the course of several weeks to enhance the activation and proliferation of mature B cells producing antigen-specific antibodies localised within the splenic capsule. Several mice are usually immunised, and serum is periodically tested to determine antigen-specific antibody titre. When a suitable titre is achieved, spleen cells are removed and somatically fused with immortal hybridoma or myeloma cells which are diluted and cultured in microtitre plates. Once the desired antibody-secreting wells are identified, the cells are expanded and antibody harvested. The time frame for generating monoclonal antibodies is generally 3–9 months but an alternative more rapid method is now available using a novel repetitive, multiple-site immunisation strategy called RIMMS. RIMMS can produce reagent antibodies in a month.

Polyclonal antibodies can be generated in a number of species with rabbits and sheep being the most commonly used. Generation of polyclonal antisera is less labour intensive than generation of monoclonal antibodies. In short, animals are immunised (prime) with the immunogen in a suitable adjuvant (material to enhance the immune response, e.g. Freund's) and then after a delay are boosted several times over a number of months and serum harvested when a suitable titre has been achieved. Immunisation and boosting are usually carried out intradermally, intramuscularly or subcutaneously.

Reagent antibodies can also be produced using molecular biology techniques without the use of animals but currently these are not widely used in the pharmaceutical industry.

6.6 *Selection and production of label*

Labelling of reactants is one of the most critical factors of immunoassay development and can be relatively labour intensive and technically difficult for those new to immunoassay. For these reasons commercial sources of label are generally sought and only if these are not available would labels be developed in-house.

A number of different labels have been used in immunoassays but there are essentially four types of label commonly used in the pharmaceutical industry:

- Radiolabels
- Enzyme labels
- Fluorescent labels
- Chemiluminescent labels.

Choice of label is dependent on the assay requirements (e.g. high sensitivity), ease of availability (e.g. commercial source), detection capabilities, site radioactivity regulations and restrictions (may preclude use of radiolabels) and experience of the bioanalyst.

6.6.1 Radiolabels

Radiolabels were used in the very first immunoassays and despite a decline in their usage there are still many assays using a radiolabel as a tracer. It is possible to radiolabel the antigen as used in traditional RIAs or the antibody as used in immunoradiometric assays (IRMAs). There are several radioisotopes that could theoretically be used but in practice it is only ^{125}I, and to a lesser extent tritium (^{3}H), that are commonly used. The latter, however, has found favour in the pharmaceutical industry for small molecular weight drugs where bioanalytical sensitivity requirements are often relatively modest (>1 ng/mL).

All molecules of interest contain hydrogen atoms, and it is usually possible to synthesise a version of the molecule in which one or more of these atoms have been replaced with tritium to create a tracer. However, one major limitation is the preparation of the label which requires specialist input from a radiochemistry perspective. In addition, separation of the antibody-bound and free fractions of the analyte and the counting times required to achieve acceptable precision can also be bettered by alternative labels. There is however, the possibility of developing homogeneous RIAs suitable for tritium tracers by utilising Amersham's scintillation proximity assay (SPA) technology. SPA also provides the opportunity for using radiolabels in microtitre plate immunoassays.

In contrast to tritium tracers, it is far easier to prepare iodinated tracers, and specialist input may not be necessary provided that adequate facilities are available. The vast majority of commercial RIAs or IRMAs use ^{125}I as a tracer as it is generally the only suitable radiolabel for proteins. An additional advantage of iodinated tracers is the higher specific activity which gives the potential for more sensitive assays and simpler, more rapid radioactivity counting. Iodination procedures can either be direct, where the analyte (or an analogue) is labelled by replacing an atom of hydrogen with ^{125}I, or indirect by linking a suitable pre-iodinated molecule (radio-tag) to the analyte. The main disadvantages of iodinated tracers are safety issues such as monitoring exposure, monitoring contamination and stringent disposal procedures. In addition, the labels have a relatively short shelf-life due to the short half-life of ^{125}I with labels only really being viable for a few months at best before re-synthesis is required.

6.6.2 Enzyme labels

Enzyme labels were introduced into immunoassays in the early 1970s and have now become established as the most versatile and popular class of label. Enzymes are covalently coupled to a protein (e.g. an antibody to the analyte of interest) and enable amplification of a signal by creation of a coloured product from a substrate. The most commonly used enzyme labels are horseradish peroxidase and alkaline phosphatase. A wide range of antibody–enzyme conjugates are available commercially that can be used as detection reagents in ELISAs and therefore there is usually no need for label production during assay development. The main advantages of enzymes as labels are their availability, suitability for microtitre plate-based assays and the fact that they are measurable by many methods with very high sensitivities. The main disadvantage is their size; large enzyme-containing complexes diffuse slowly leading to longer incubation times and may bind non-specifically to reaction vessels.

6.6.3 Fluorescent labels

The use of time-resolved fluorescence has provided a viable alternative to radiolabels and enzyme labels for immunoassays, with the potential for lower background values and greater sensitivity. Perkin Elmer Life Sciences (formerly Wallac Ltd) provides readily available commercial kits and reagents for this assay technology as dissociation-enhanced lanthanide fluorescence immunoassay (DELFIA®). The technology uses chelates of the lanthanide metal ions which have long-lived flourescence under some circumstances. In DELFIA these lanthanide metal ions, particularly Europium, are used to label the molecule of interest. Preparation of fluorescent labels, other than those available commercially, can be accomplished in-house with limited training, and the assays are ideally carried out in microtitre plate format.

6.6.4 Chemiluminescent labels

Chemiluminescent labels are extremely popular in the immunodiagnostic industry with a wide range of kits and analysers available, mainly to support clinical chemistry applications. At present, the labels are not widely used in conventional bioanalysis departments other than in EIAs to quantitate enzyme labels (e.g. horseradish peroxidase, alkaline phosphatase).

6.6.5 The streptavidin–biotin system

The streptavidin–biotin (or avidin–biotin) system is widely used in immunoassay. Streptavidin is a binding protein isolated from *Streptomyces* that has an extremely high affinity and specificity for the water-soluble vitamin B6, biotin. Avidin is a protein found in egg white that has similar properties to streptavidin but is more prone to non-specific binding. Biotin is relatively polar and thus can be easily coupled to antibodies, and streptavidin (or avidin) can be coupled to solid phases, fluorochromes and enzymes. Streptavidin is a tetramer and has four biotin-binding sites per molecule. Therefore, use of the streptavidin–biotin system in immunoassay can greatly improve sensitivity of the assay by dramatically amplifying the signal.

6.7 *Assay development and optimisation*

After generation or purchase of reagent antibodies and a suitable label there are a number of further steps required to develop and optimise an immunoassay. Assay development work will be affected by a number of variables some of which are listed here:

- Quality of antiserum and label
- Type of buffer
- Protein additives
- Incubation volume
- Concentration of reactants
- Plate coating conditions (if appropriate)
- Time and temperature
- Separation step selected
- Sample matrix.

There are obviously specific challenges and issues for each assay format and label type but the following five phases are applicable to most formats:

1 Selection of operating conditions and reagents, e.g. assay format, buffer to be used, commercial enzyme-label, production of plate conjugate for ELISA, etc.
2 Selection of initial assay conditions (e.g. incubation temperature) and separation system (if appropriate).
3 Assessment and selection of antisera with respect to specificity, titre and potential sensitivity.
4 Introduction of matrix to determine matrix effects on the assay.
5 Optimisation of assay conditions to obtain the desired sensitivity, specificity, precision and accuracy and to limit non-specific interference.

It is important to note that matrix is not introduced until a working assay has been established in buffer to avoid complicating the assay development process.

6.8 *Assay validation*

The published proceedings from the Crystal City Conference on the validation of bioanalytical methods have been generally accepted as guidelines in the pharmaceutical industry. However, it is clear that these proceedings do not adequately address the special issues pertaining to the validation of immunoassays (e.g. non-linear calibration curves) and therefore there is a clear need for specific guidelines. To this effect there has been an excellent review recently published in the *Journal of Pharmaceutical and Biomedical Analysis* (Findlay *et al.*) and also a specific conference was held in March 2000 on the validation of assays for macromolecules (sponsored by the American Association of Pharmaceutical Scientists, AAPS). There is a workshop report arising from the meeting which will form the basis of guidelines specific to the validation of methods for the bioanalysis of macromolecules.

The validation requirements and assay acceptance criteria for immunoassays will vary depending on the analyte and the intended application of the method. For example, an immunoassay method intended for use for the analysis of a drug in pre-clinical safety or clinical evaluation would require a full validation package as well as cross-validation to a reference method. In contrast, an immunoassay for use in exploratory discovery, when rapid turnaround of results is required, does not need to be fully validated provided that the users are satisfied that the method is suitable for the intended purpose. If an immunoassay has been purchased as a kit then the objective is to verify performance of the kit rather than to validate it from scratch.

Immunoassays are generally less precise than chromatographic assays and therefore the criteria for accuracy and precision for assay acceptance may need to be more lenient than for chromatographic assays.

6.9 *Immunoassays developed in-house*

The purpose of assay validation is to establish confidence that the result obtained in each assay will always reflect the 'true' value. To do this a series of assays are carried out to determine a number of criteria as described below.

Accuracy is a measure of how close the observed result is to the 'true' value. It can be determined by 'spiking' reference analyte material into control biological matrix to create a series of validation controls (VCs) each with a known concentration of analyte. The reference analyte stock solution should be different to that used to prepare the assay standards. In addition the VCs should reflect the anticipated concentration range of the unknown samples and should span the assay standard curve. The VCs are assayed in replicates of six in a three to six separate assays. From the observed results for each VC within and between assays and calculating the percentage difference from the known concentration of analyte, a percentage bias can be obtained which indicates the inter- and intra-assay accuracy of the method.

Precision is a measure of the ability of an assay to reproduce an observed result. VCs should be prepared and assayed in the same way as that described in the determination of accuracy. The mean and standard deviation within and between assays should be determined and the percentage coefficient of variation of the mean (CV) calculated. The CV provides an indication of the variability and therefore the inter- and intra-assay precision of the method. Precision is independent of accuracy and a method can be inaccurate but reproducible and vice versa.

Specificity is defined as the ability of the assay to distinguish the analyte from other substances in the sample. This is a particularly important factor in the validation of an immunoassay as these assays are perceived as being less specific than physicochemical techniques. This latter perception is because it is possible for an antibody to bind to a number of different molecules if the latter all share some of the same structural features. The best way to determine whether an assay is specific for the analyte is to cross-validate it where possible with a gold standard technique such as MS. However, the use of MS will not be possible if the analyte is a macromolecule. The alternative is to carry out accuracy measurements in the presence of potential cross reactants; these could include drug metabolites, co-administered drugs or molecules which are structurally related to the analyte.

The limits of quantification are defined as the lowest and highest concentrations of the analyte that can be determined with both acceptable accuracy and precision. These values are determined by using VCs at concentrations near the expected limits of the assay.

The stability of the target analyte in biological matrix should be determined for various storage conditions over the period of time that the samples are likely to be stored prior to analysis. The effect of multiple freeze-thaw cycles on the analyte should also be investigated as in most cases samples need to be stored frozen prior to assay.

If a sample extraction step is required prior to assay the analyte recovery should be determined. This is important because a low extraction recovery could reduce assay accuracy, sensitivity and precision. Recovery is checked by passing a known concentration of the analyte in the appropriate biological matrix through the extraction procedure and determining the amount of analyte recovered. This is usually expressed as a percentage of the concentration of the analyte originally spiked into the biological matrix.

Linearity of dilution has to be assessed to make sure that if a sample containing a high concentration of the analyte is diluted into the range of the assay the correct result is obtained. Effects of biological matrices are diminished with increasing sample dilution in assay buffer, and this may cause the apparent concentration of the sample to increase or decrease. To determine whether matrix interference occurs, a VC with a high concentration of the analyte should be assayed undiluted and then at increasing dilutions in assay diluent until the lower limit of quantification of the assay is reached. The results when corrected for dilution should be the same as the result obtained for the undiluted VC. If this is not the case then samples must be diluted in blank sample matrix and an equal volume of blank matrix incorporated into the calibration curve.

The above list of considerations is not exhaustive and constitutes the minimum investigations that should be carried out when attempting to validate an immunoassay. When carrying out these investigations it is important to have as good a knowledge of the assay system and analyte as possible and to have already established that the assay is fully optimised and performing reliably. Potential problems with the assay can be predicted and validation experiments carried out to determine the limits of the assays' use.

6.10 *Commercial kit immunoassay*

The objective of the validation is to verify that the performance of the method in-house is satisfactory for the intended purpose and in agreement with the claims of the manufacturer.

Commercial immunoassay kits will contain an instruction booklet or kit insert that will detail the use of the kit. This booklet usually contains information on assay performance, the detail of which varies from kit to kit and manufacturer to manufacturer. Some kits are well established and accepted by regulatory authorities as 'gold standard' analytical methods whereas others are less well characterised and are intended for 'research purposes only'. It is the suitability and performance of the latter category that usually requires the closest scrutiny. The validation is also particularly important if the kit is modified in some way, e.g. it is to be used for a different matrix to the one stipulated by the manufacturer.

The validation assays should be designed to assess the following:

- Accuracy
- Precision
- Specificity and matrix effects
- Elements of stability
- Linearity of dilution (as necessary)
- Equivalence of clinical material to that in the kit (as necessary)
- Recovery (as necessary).

Most kits will contain all reagents necessary for the assay. In some circumstances it may be necessary to prepare standards using clinical trial material instead of using the calibration standards provided in the kit. This is important when the analyte being measured and the standard in the kit are not equivalent (e.g. different binding affinities).

In common with in-house developed immunoassays, the preparation of VCs is required and these VC samples should be prepared in the biological matrix for which the method will be validated. A vast majority of commercial kit immunoassays will be for the determination of biomarkers. Unlike conventional drugs, biomarkers are usually present endogenously in the matrix of interest which causes additional complications during assay validation. Essentially, the analyst has two choices: attempt to remove the endogenous analyte prior to VC preparation, or not to remove it before adding a known amount of analyte and correct the data accordingly. For example, some analytes can be removed by stripping the matrix (e.g. charcoal for low molecular weight analytes) or affinity purification using antibodies (for immunogenic large molecular weight analytes).

6.11 *Data handling*

At the endpoint of an immunoassay an appropriate instrument will capture label signals such as optical densities or counts derived from radioisotopic decay. It is then necessary to process these raw data and produce a standard curve allowing the interpolation of unknown sample concentration. This can be simply carried out by plotting the standard curve manually using graph paper. However there are certain characteristics of an immunoassay standard curve that make this difficult and it is also not a practical approach in terms of reproducibility or high throughput in the bioanalytical laboratory.

There is a non-linear relationship between the measured response in the assay and the analyte concentration with the result that immunoassay standard curves tend to be sigmoidal. There is no universal mathematical function that will uniquely fit the best curve through the standard points, so care must be taken to avoid the introduction of bias. An additional problem is that there is greater error associated with the standard points at the extremes of the calibration curve where it becomes asymptotic, than in the central linear region of the curve. For these reasons computer software is used which offers a choice of curve fitting procedures based on either the 'best fit' through the actual standard points produced (e.g. spline fit) or on a mathematical model which reflects the physical principles underlying immunoassays (e.g. four-parameter logistic fit). The latter are generally preferred as they are less subject to bias resulting from any inaccurate standard points. MultiCalc, produced by Perkin & Elmer Life Sciences, is an industry standard immunoassay data processing software package which has a range of curve fitting options that can be applied to the raw data. Examples of standard curves produced using Multicalc are shown in Figures 6.3 and 6.4.

6.12 *Automation*

Automation allows higher sample throughput, potentially increases assay precision, negates the need to manually assay high-risk samples from infected patients and also frees scientists from having to spend large amounts of time carrying out routine analysis. Hospital Clinical Chemistry Laboratories, where very large numbers of samples are analysed on a routine basis, have been taking advantage of automated immunoassay systems for some time. These have tended to centre on large dedicated autoanalysers such as the Abbott Laboratories AxSym, which can carry out many of the standard clinical biochemistry tests. Samples are collected, labelled with a barcode and loaded onto the analyser. The barcode carries all the information required for the analyser to carry out the requested analysis using a common immunoassay format and report the results to a database of patient results. The analyser will also periodically run quality control samples and carry out appropriate calibration. In this way thousands of samples can be analysed per day. However, the modern bioanalytical facility within a drug

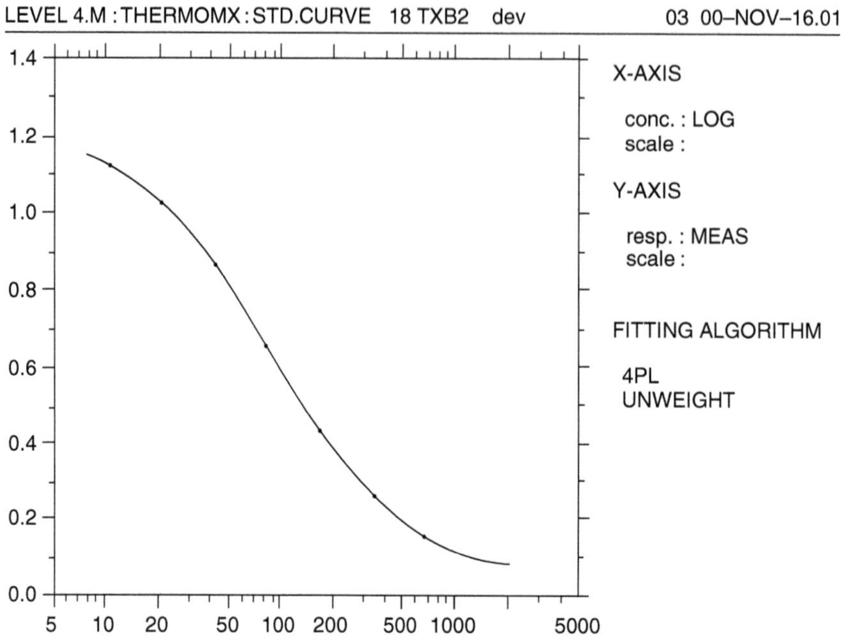

FIGURE 6.3 *Competitive EIA using four-parameter logistic curve fitting procedure (unweighted).*

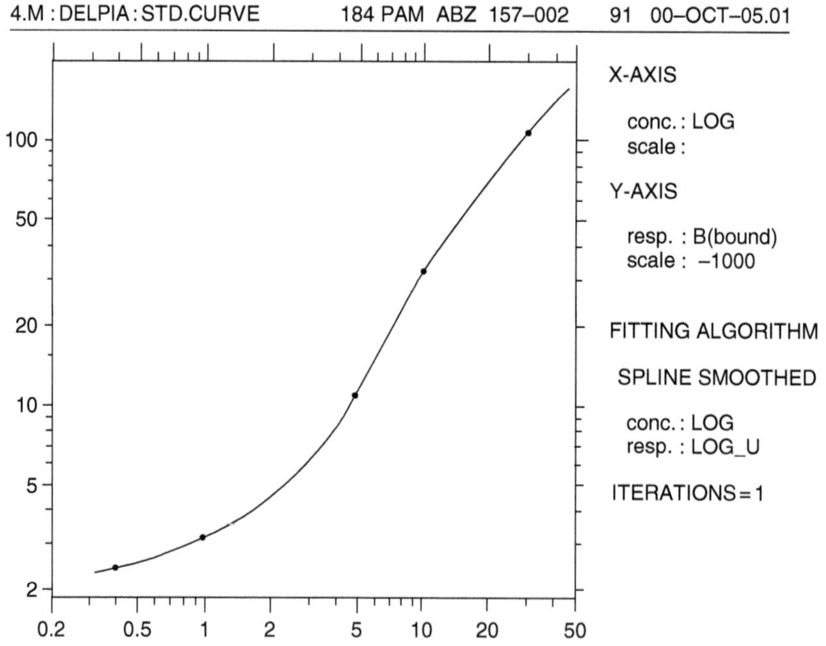

FIGURE 6.4 *Non-competitive DELFIA using a smoothed spline curve fitting procedure.*

discovery and development department requires a much more flexible approach to immunoassay automation. This is because the types of assay carried out change regularly as new candidate drugs are evaluated and new analytes are identified. Unlike the situation in a clinical chemistry facility there is no standard set of long-term routine tests, constituting the majority of the workload. Also, within a bioanalytical immunoassay lab an array of assay formats (EIA, RIA ELISA) would be carried out in different sized tubes and in a variety of microtitre plates. For this reason robotic sample processors have been chosen for automating the majority of immunoassays in the bioanalytical facility as these instruments provide the most flexibility.

Robotic sample processors such as the TECAN genesis (see Figure 6.5) or the Packard Multiprobe enable immunoassays developed in a variety of formats to be automated relatively quickly. In the past only homogeneous assays which did not require a separation phase were amenable to full automation. However plate washers, incubators and plate readers can now be added to a system allowing entire heterogeneous assay procedures to be carried out by the robot. The development of scheduling software has been a further bonus as it is now possible to carry out a number of different assays at the same time on the same robot.

6.13 *Biomarkers*

Biomarkers are becoming increasingly important in the pharmaceutical industry to aid the efficient development of new therapeutics. Biomarkers provide information

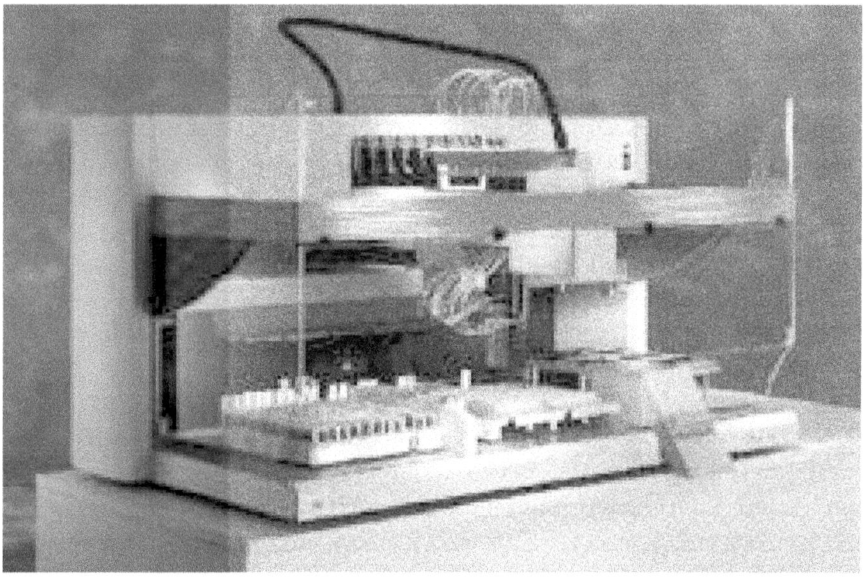

FIGURE 6.5 *TECAN genesis robotic sample processor.*

on drug mechanisms and potential efficacy and can aid in study design and appropriate dose selection. With many complex chronic disorders such as stroke, chronic obstructive pulmonary disease (COPD) and osteoarthritis, it would be necessary to treat thousands of patients over a number of years to prove the efficacy of a candidate drug. Measurement of appropriate biomarkers of drug efficacy or safety can substantially shorten this clinical drug development time or the time taken to reach a critical decision point in drug discovery. Indeed, the information provided by a good biomarker, or a panel of biomarkers, in any clinical development programme contributes to informed decisions on progressing the best drug candidates into full development quickly. The converse is also true; the poorer molecules can be de-selected more rapidly freeing up valuable resource and saving money.

The terms biomarker and surrogate endpoint are now widely accepted and the term surrogate marker, which is often used generically for all types of marker, is discouraged. Some definitions have been developed by a working group of the National Institutes of Health Director's Initiative on Biomarkers and Surrogate Endpoints and are provided below.

- A *Biomarker* is a characteristic that is objectively measured and evaluated as an indicator of normal biological processes, pathogenic processes or pharmacologic responses to a therapeutic intervention.
- A *Surrogate* endpoint is a biomarker that is intended to substitute for a clinical endpoint.
- A *Prognostic marker* is a test or set of tests which indicates the likely progression of a specific disease.
- A *Diagnostic marker* is a test or set of tests that determines the presence or absence of a specific disease.

There is a 'hierarchy' of validity in association with clinical disease that grows from a biomarker through a surrogate to a prognostic. A given test or set of tests thus may 'mature' through this progression as the supporting clinical validation becomes progressively stronger.

Physiologic functions and imaging have been used as surrogate endpoints for some time (e.g. electrocardiograms, blood pressure, X-ray) but it is for the determination of macromolecular biomarkers in biological fluids, for example cytokines or eicosanoids, that immunoassay is important.

In the drug discovery and development arena, biomarkers are currently commonly measured by immunoassay. This is because macromolecules in biofluids are generally not amenable to bioanalysis at high sensitivity using chromatographic approaches but elicit a good immune response for the generation of reagent antibodies for immunoassay development. This has been exploited by commercial suppliers and a vast array of commercial immunoassay kits or antisera are available which can be utilised when appropriate.

A case study is summarised below which illustrates the usefulness of measuring biomarkers (thromboxane B2 and prostaglandin E2) by immunoassay in support of a drug discovery project.

6.14 *Case study: determination of COX-2 selectivity in human blood*

Non-steroidal anti-inflammatory drugs (NSAIDs) are used extensively as analgesics; however, their use is associated with side effects. The mechanism of action of the NSAIDs is through their inhibition of the enzyme cyclooxygenase (COX) which is involved in the metabolism of arachidonic acid with subsequent prostanoid formation. COX has two isoforms, COX-1 which is constitutive and COX-2 which is induced during inflammation. A currently accepted hypothesis is that COX-2 inhibition provides the anti-inflammatory activity of NSAIDs, whereas COX-1 inhibition is responsible for most of their adverse effects such as disruption of the cytoprotection of the stomach, kidney function and platelet aggregation. COX-1 and COX-2 are structurally distinct, therefore the development of drugs that selectively inhibit COX-2 might lead to a new generation of anti-inflammatory drugs with increased tolerability.

The aim of this work was to determine the COX-2 selectivity of the NSAID Naproxen and a selective COX-2 inhibitor Celecoxib (Searle) in human whole blood *in vitro* according to a published method (Brideau *et al.*, 1996). This could enable the establishment of a model system for the evaluation of candidate COX-2 inhibitors in drug discovery.

To determine COX-1 activity, control human blood was collected from a number of healthy volunteers and test compound (Naproxen or Celecoxib) added at a range of concentrations to separate sub-samples. After incubation, serum was harvested and samples were assayed for thromboxane B2 (TxB_2) using a commercial enzyme-immunoassay.

To determine COX-2 activity heparinised whole blood samples (from the same volunteers and occasions as for COX-1 activity) were sub-divided and a range of test compound (Naproxen or Celecoxib) concentrations added. Lipopolysaccharide (LPS) was added to all samples to stimulate an inflammatory response, following which plasma was harvested for prostaglandin E2 (PgE_2) analysis using a commercial enzymeimmunoassay.

The inhibitory potency of the test compounds was expressed as an IC_{50} value. This is defined as the concentration of the compound required to inhibit either the LPS-induced PgE_2 release (measure of COX-2 inhibition) or clotting-induced TxB_2 release (measure of COX-1 inhibition) by 50 per cent. The selectivity ratio of inhibition of COX-1 versus COX-2 was calculated by comparing respective IC_{50} values.

The results shown in Table 6.1 demonstrate that the COX-2 selectivity of the NSAID Naproxen was poor compared to Celecoxib as indicated by the relatively

TABLE 6.1 *COX-2 selectivity*

		IC_{50} (nM)		
Compound	**Volunteer**	**COX-2 (PgE_2)**	**COX-1 (TxB_2)**	**Selectivity ratio**
Naproxen	1	12000	72000	6
	2	10900	10100	1
	3	55000	100000	2
	Mean	–	–	3
Celecoxib	1	120	10600	88
	2	400	50000	125
	3	140	65000	464
	4	300	8000	27
	Mean	–	–	176

low selectivity ratios of the former compared to the latter. Early clinical data has indicated that the selective COX-2 inhibitor Celecoxib has fewer adverse effects than non-selective NSAIDs.

This whole blood assay can be used *in vitro*, as described in this example, to determine the COX-2 selectivity of compounds in the drug discovery phase as well as *ex vivo* during clinical development.

6.15 *Biological drugs*

Although most drugs in the discovery and development portfolios of the major pharmaceutical companies are small molecules there is a significant and growing interest in biological drugs. These products, which are also often referred to as biotechnology products or biopharmaceuticals, embrace gene therapy products, peptides, monoclonal antibodies, vaccines, enzymes and other biologically active proteins. Although some biological drugs have been on the market for many years (e.g. interferon, insulin) there has been a massive growth in development of these products in recent years with many new products now on, or about to enter, the market.

With the exception of gene therapy products, immunoassay techniques are the method of choice, and often the only viable methods available, for the bioanalysis of these complex macromolecules. In some cases, immunoassay is used to measure concentration (more correctly immunoreactive concentration), but in other cases it is used indirectly as an endpoint in a bioassay to measure the biologically active concentration, or potency, of the drug. In addition to the measurement of the parent drug in biofluids there is often a requirement to measure other analytes either expressed or induced by the treatment. This is because many of these biological products, since they are recognised as a foreign protein by the treated individual, induce an immune response leading to the production of antibodies against the parent drug. In some cases this is a desirable response (e.g. vaccines, development of anti-idiotype networks) but in other cases it is undesirable (e.g. production of neutralising antibodies) as it abrogates the drug's activity. It is often very important to measure and characterise these immune responses to biological drugs and immunoassay; usually ELISA is the primary technique used.

Although many of the validation requirements of immunoassays in general are relevant to the bioanalysis of biological drugs, there are some additional requirements that must be considered in the bioanalysis of these molecules. For instance, in pharmacokinetic studies it must be considered whether a bioassay, which would measure the biologically active molecule in the bio-fluid of interest, might be more appropriate than measuring immunoreactive concentration by immunoassay. In the latter case, the immunoassay may be measuring degraded and inactive forms of the drug in addition to the parent molecule and in general there is no way of knowing if this is the case.

Another example where additional or different validation criteria are required is in the measurement of the antibodies produced against biological drugs. The methods used need to be able to clearly distinguish between neutralising and non-neutralising antibodies and in the case of the former, since they are clinically very important, the validation study must also demonstrate that the assay is able to detect all classes of antibodies and all antibody affinities likely to be present in an antibody positive sample.

Wellferon, an interferon alpha preparation, provides an example of where immunoassay has been used for the bioanalysis of a biological drug. This example also illustrates some of the typical challenges that often have to be overcome in developing and validating bioanalytical techniques for measuring complex biological molecules.

Wellferon™ (interferon α-N1) is a highly purified mixture of at least nine subtypes of human interferon alpha (h)IFNα produced from a human lymphblastoid cell line. This preparation had been on the market for several years for the treatment of hairy cell leukaemia and for certain patients with chronic active hepatitis B. However, when a new master cell bank was laid down to replace the original it became necessary to conduct a clinical study to demonstrate bioequivalence of the products from the two master cell banks. The ideal way of establishing clinical bioequivalence for this type of product is to use a relevant bioassay to compare the biological activity of Wellferon in blood following administration of the two preparations to healthy volunteers on a cross-over basis. However, in this case, this was not a viable proposition because there was no suitable bioassay with adequate precision and accuracy available. The best alternative approach was to use a pseudo-pharmacokinetic endpoint by using a commercial immunoassay kit to compare immunoreactive concentrations of IFNα, derived from the two Wellferon preparations, in serum.

The most suitable analytical method was the Amersham Biotrak™ kit for the determination of human IFNα in serum. The method is a solid phase ELISA, which utilises an antibody for human recombinant interferon alpha (h)IFNα bound to the wells of a microtitre plate for capture of interferon alpha in the sample. The captured interferon alpha is then detected by means of a labelled second antibody, also specific for the analyte and, under normal circumstances, the concentration of IFNα in the sample is read off a standard curve, prepared with standards of recombinant IFNα supplied in the kit.

Although the immunoassay utilises antibodies raised against recombinant human IFNα it has been shown to be suitable for the quantitation of both recombinant and natural (e.g. Wellferon) preparations of IFNα. However, there is a complication in that it was demonstrated that different subtypes of Wellferon had markedly different affinities for the anti-IFNα antibodies in the kit. As the relative subtype composition and specific activity of Wellferon can vary significantly from batch to batch, within the specification of the product, different batches of Wellferon would have different analytical responses when measured using the method. There was therefore a high probability that if the method had been used to compare the concentration of IFNα in serum in a bioequivalence study of two different Wellferon preparations then the preparations would not have been demonstrated to be bioequivalent.

In an attempt to overcome the potential difficulties in the measurement of IFNα derived from Wellferon it was decided that the two batches of material to be compared in the clinical bioequivalence study would have been used to prepare the respective standards for the analyses of the blood samples resulting from the administration of each preparation. This enabled the concentration data to be normalised with respect to variations in sub-type and specific activity between the two batches of Wellferon being compared. This strategy was successful as it enabled bioequivalence of Wellferon derived from the new and original master cell banks to be established.

Vaccines constitute another class of bio-pharmaceutical product where immunoassay plays a major role in their pre-clinical and clinical development. Most vaccines are used prophylactically for the prevention of infectious disease and their efficacy depends on the production of an adequate humoral immune response (seroconversion) to the bacterial or viral antigen used for immunisation. This is characterised by the production of specific antibodies to the antigen and the development of immunological memory so that when the individual is later exposed to the appropriate disease-causing organism expressing the antigen a protective immune response can be rapidly mounted to combat the disease. The concentration (titre) of specific antibodies is usually determined by ELISA and for most vaccines there is a range of commercial diagnostic kits and dedicated instrumentation available.

In addition to prophylactic vaccines there is increasing interest in the development of immunotherapeutic vaccines. These will essentially be used for treating already infected patients by enhancing the patient's existing immune response. In addition to the humoral response generated these vaccines enhance the cellular (T-lymphocyte) immune response which is essential in clearing the existing infecting organism. Immunoassay also plays an important part in measuring this cellular immune response and one of the methods that is currently used is ELISpot.

ELISpot is essentially a variant of ELISA in which the proportion of T-lymphocytes that have been induced to respond to the viral or bacterial antigen used for immunisation can be determined. This is done by counting the number of cells capable of secreting a cytokine on stimulation by the antigen *in vitro*. The method involves the addition of a lymphocyte suspension prepared from the blood of a vaccinated individual to a microtitre plate coated with antibodies to an appropriate cytokine such as gamma-interferon (IFN-γ). The antigen is also added and the plate is incubated. Cells that are specific for the antigen respond by producing cytokine on their surface and this binds to the antibody on the plate in close proximity to the secreting cell. After washing, a second antibody detection system is used as in an ELISA assay. However, in this case a number of coloured spots are detected on the bottom of the plate wells, each spot corresponding to a single positive (antigen specific) cell. By counting the number of spots an assessment can be made of the extent of the specific cellular immune response in that individual. The principles of ELISpot are illustrated in Figure 6.6.

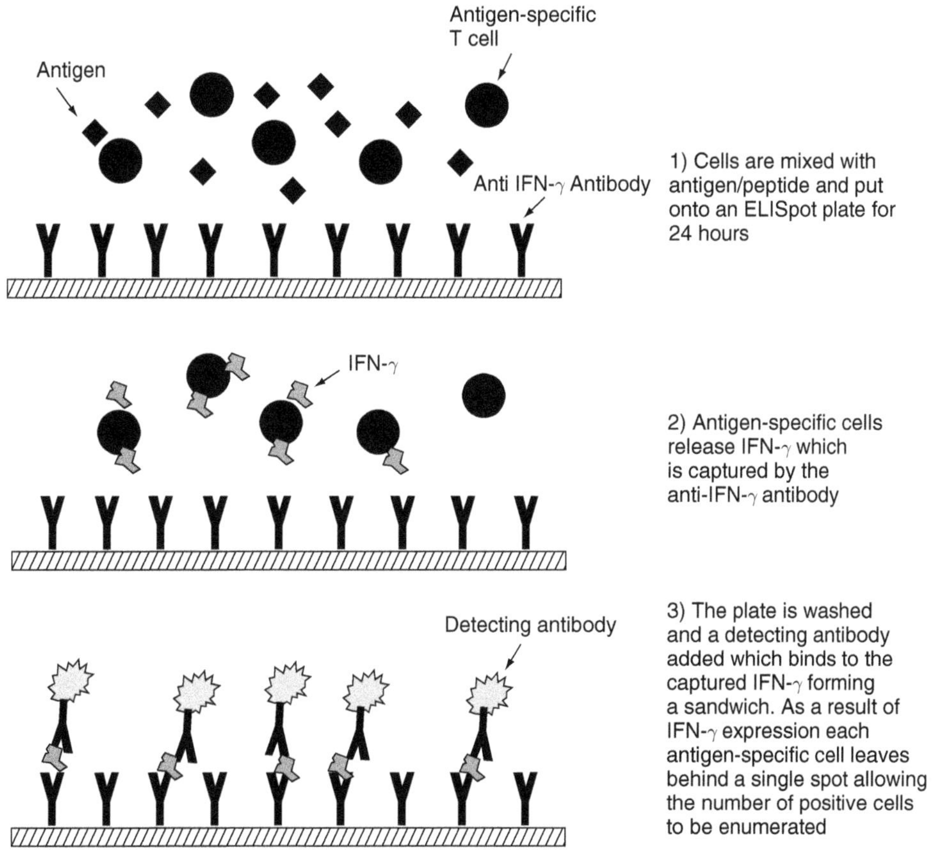

FIGURE 6.6 *Measurement of the cellular immune response by ELISpot.*

6.16 References

Biomarkers definitions working group (2001) Biomarkers and surrogate endpoints: preferred definitions and conceptual framework. *Clin. Pharmacol. Ther.* 69, 89–95.

Brideau, C. *et al.* (1996) A human whole blood assay for clinical evaluation of biochemical efficacy of cyclooxygenase inhibitors. *Inflamm. Res.* 45, 68–74.

Findlay, J.W.A., Smith, W.C., Lee, J.W., Nordblom, G.D., Das, I., DeSilva, B.S., Khan, M.N. and Bowsher, R.R. (2000) *J. Pharm. Biomed. Anal.* January.

CHAPTER 7

Pre-clinical pharmacokinetics

Sheila Schwartz and Tony Pateman

7.1 *Introduction*

When a patient is given a new medicine the doctor will instruct them how often the medicine should be taken, for example 'take a tablet three times a day' and any other conditions 'to be taken with food'. These are not arbitrary traditions but important instructions, which have a firm scientific basis. These dosing regimens are important in developing new medicines as potential advantages, which a new drug can provide over its competitors. How are the dosage regimens decided and what factors are important? These questions are examined in this chapter on pharmacokinetics.

Pharmacokinetics (PK) is a term applied to the quantitative study of the *in vivo* disposition of a xenobiotic, usually a drug. A good definition of PK is 'what the body does to the drug'. Typically pharmacokinetics describes how the concentrations of a drug in plasma change with time following a known dose being given by a specific route. The 'true' pharmacokinetic data on a drug molecule, obtained following intravenous dosing, provides an understanding of how readily the drug can distribute in the body, the ability of the body to eliminate the drug and how rapidly the drug leaves the body.

Additionally dosing the drug by the oral route provides information on how rapidly and how much of this dose reaches the systemic circulation. Thus intravenous and oral pharmacokinetic parameters of a molecule provide a great deal of information about its disposition. The many routes of administration and elimination are illustrated in Figure 7.1. How pharmacokinetic information is obtained and interpreted is described in this chapter.

The study of PK is an important component of both the research and development phases in the discovery of new drugs. In research, chemical compounds will be screened in various biochemical and pharmacological tests to find compounds which show a positive effect. Typically the compounds will be categorised based on the biological or pharmacological potency with the compounds, which are most active at the lowest concentration, regarded as the most promising lead compound. However, *in vitro* potency is not the only factor required by a good drug because many compounds which are potent *in vitro* are inactive *in vivo*. It is critically important that pharmacokinetic properties are given just as much weight as

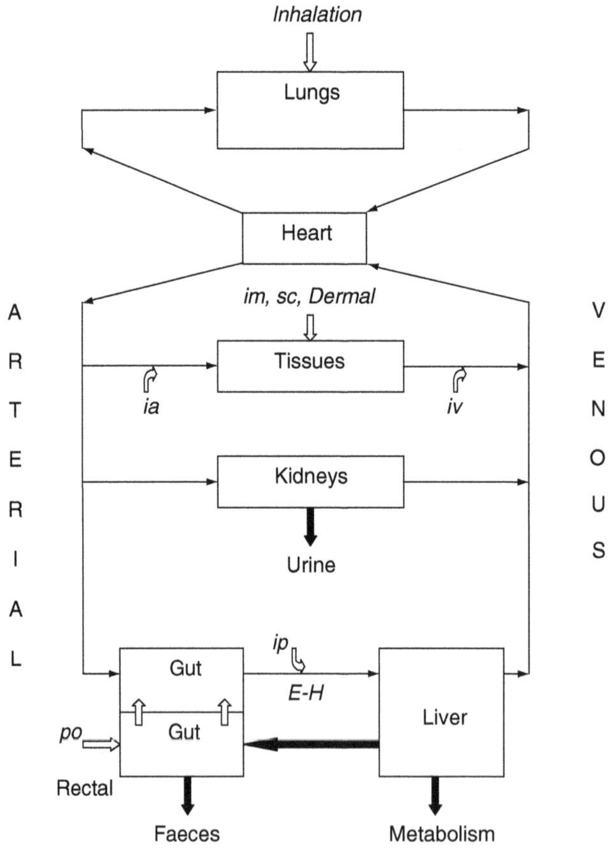

FIGURE 7.1 *Schematic representation of routes of administration and elimination.*

efficacy. Good efficacy but poor PK is unlikely to lead to a successful medicine, and failure during the development phase due to inappropriate PK is both expensive and inefficient. The understanding of *in vivo* biological results is greatly enhanced if the disposition of the molecule is understood. A poor *in vivo* result may be due to inappropriate plasma concentrations rather than a poor model, or a molecule lacking in potency. Relating plasma concentrations to effect (pharmacokinetic/pharmacodynamic or PK/PD modelling) is covered in Chapter 8.

In pre-clinical development, PK has a key role to play in understanding the safety of the drug molecule. This manifests itself primarily in toxicokinetic studies in support of safety evaluation, which will be covered in Chapter 9. In addition during the development process detailed pharmacokinetic studies are performed to characterise the molecule to a level that satisfies the regulatory authorities.

Finally, through species comparisons and scaling, forecasts of the likely clinical parameters are made from the pre-clinical data. These forecasts are an invaluable contribution in designing efficient clinical trials and for evaluating the likely commercial and clinical success of the molecule.

7.2 *Pharmacokinetic parameters*

Pharmacokinetic parameters describe the exposure, distribution and time course of the drug in the body, and are generated from systemic drug concentration versus time data. Parameters of exposure are related to drug concentrations circulating in the blood, serum or plasma, and are usually expressed as an amount of drug per unit of volume. For simplicity the parameter descriptions in this chapter will relate to plasma, but they can be similarly applied to blood or serum.

When a drug is administered intravenously it enters the systemic circulation without an absorption phase, and drug is distributed from the blood to the tissues and organs. The blood levels obtained following intravenous administration provide the definitive PK of a compound reflecting the distribution and elimination phases.

7.3 *Bioavailability*

When a drug is administered by a route other than intravenous it has to pass absorption and metabolic barriers before it reaches the general circulation system. If a compound is poorly absorbed or extensively metabolised before it reaches the general circulation then only a fraction of the dose administered will reach the systemic circulation. Blood samples are taken for pharmacokinetic analysis from the systemic circulation; consequently they will only reflect the fraction of the drug reaching the systemic circulation. Bioavailability is the measure of the dose fraction available systemically after an extra-parenteral dose. For a compound to have good bioavailability, it must have good absorption and low clearance.

As a 'rule of thumb', low bioavailability results in high inter-subject variability and increases the difficulty in selecting the appropriate dosage level. As shown in Figure 7.1 when a drug is absorbed from the gastrointestinal tract the blood flow passes through the liver before reaching the general circulation. If a drug is cleared by metabolism the concentration of the drug in blood entering the liver is higher than the concentration in blood leaving the liver. This phenomenon is known as first pass metabolism, and removal of the drug by the liver is called hepatic clearance. Blood (plasma) levels taken for pharmacokinetic analysis inevitably reflect the level of drug in the general circulation consequently, when the plasma levels after oral administration are compared to those following intravenous administration (measure of bioavailability of the drug: see Section 7.5.10), the values are lower for oral administration because of the amount of drug removed in the 'first pass' through the liver. High hepatic clearance leads to low oral bioavailability, even if the drug is well absorbed.

7.4 *Calculation of pharmacokinetic parameters*

The main parameters of exposure are C_{max} (maximum plasma concentration – example: ng/mL) and AUC (area under the plasma concentration–time curve – example: ng.h/mL). Distribution parameters describe the extent of drug distribution and are related to body volumes (example: mL or litre), and time course parameters are related to time. For a comprehensive discussion about pharmacokinetic concepts see clinical pharmacokinetics: concepts and applications (Rowland and Tozer, 1989).

These pharmacokinetic parameters are calculated from mathematical formulae, and specific computer programs are usually used to do this (e.g. WinNonlin^{TM}). The parameters may be estimated by compartmental or non-compartmental approaches (or model-dependent and model-independent, respectively).

The plasma concentration and time point data may be fitted to a compartmental model using specially designed pharmacokinetic modelling programs (e.g. WinNonlin^{TM}). Modelling of data is based on an iterative process providing a solution to non-linear regression problems. The concept of 'compartments' is a hypothesis for the input, distribution and elimination of the drug from the body, and does not represent true bodily compartments. In general, non-compartmental PK is more than adequate to describe the time course of novel compounds in animals and is the method most often used in pre-clinical discovery. Schematic representations of the one- and two-compartment models are shown in Figures 7.2 and 7.3, respectively. Intravenous dosing provides the definitive PK of any compound. Parameters may also be derived after an oral dose, or a dose from any other route of administration,

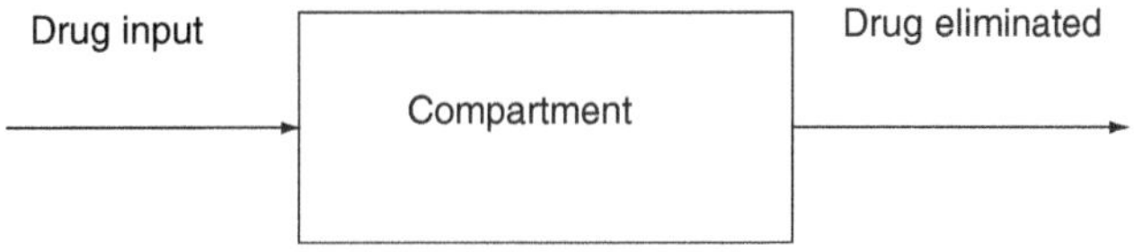

FIGURE 7.2 *Schematic representation of a one-compartment open model.*

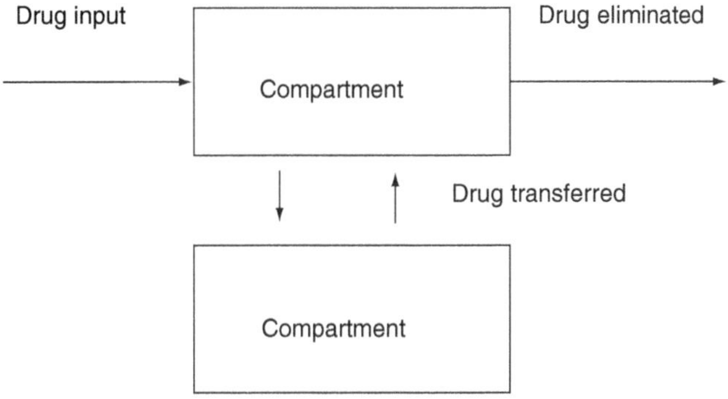

FIGURE 7.3 *Schematic representation of a two-compartment open model.*

but in these cases, parameters would need to be adjusted for the fraction of the dose absorbed because not all dose taken enters the systemic circulation.

This chapter will focus on describing the basic formulae for the parameters but will not endeavour to educate the reader in the mathematical derivations. For a comprehensive understanding of the derivation of the formulae, refer to PK (Perrier and Gibaldi, 1982).

7.4.1 Half-life

Half-life is the time taken for the drug concentration in plasma to be reduced by half. This parameter is important because it helps define how often a drug should be administered. If a drug is dosed once every three half-lives, the ratio of peak to trough concentrations will be around 10-fold. In addition there will be no significant accumulation during the dosing regime. Thus, provided the safety profile of a molecule will allow it, an 8 hour half-life is ideal for once a day dosing. If the therapeutic window is small, a longer half-life or more frequent dosing will reduce the peak to trough ratio, but will lead to some accumulation during the initial doses. This in turn may necessitate an initial loading dose (e.g. two tablets at once and one tablet a day thereafter). If the half-life is too short the dosing frequency may have to be increased to provide an appropriate safety/efficacy profile, and this may be less attractive commercially. Conversely, if the half-life is too long, it will be difficult to reverse the drug action should an adverse event occur.

If the drug is administered by intravenous infusion or a slow release formulation a steady state can be achieved where the systemic drug concentration remains constant when the rate of absorption/infusion is equal to the rate of elimination. One example of this situation is the administration of anaesthesia.

The plasma time profile may be multiphasic with several different 'half-lives' over the elimination phase. It is difficult to define the terminal half-life without measuring the complete time course, and the measurements are often restricted by the sensitivity of the assay method used. Which half-life is important is dependent on the pharmacological activity of the drug. It is possible that the pharmacological duration of action may be long, despite a short half-life, in which case frequent dosing will not be required. This will be discussed further in the PK/PD chapter.

7.4.2 Clearance

Total plasma clearance is the volume of plasma cleared of drug per unit time. Clearance determines the overall exposure that the body receives from a drug. Furthermore, clearance determines the rate of dosing required to maintain a given average plasma concentration. Thus a high clearance may lead to low exposure and low plasma average concentrations during chronic dosing. A high dose will be required to compensate for this, which will be a burden on cost and patient acceptability.

There may be instances when high clearance is a very desirable property. For example, inhaled products for topical action in the lungs will have the best safety profile if a high clearance results in low systemic exposure. Clearance would be considered to be high if blood clearance approached hepatic blood flow indicating that the only factor limiting the rate of clearance was blood flow. A drug which is cleared by the liver passes from the blood into the liver cells where metabolism of the drug occurs. If the compound is only slowly metabolised then the rate of metabolism is the rate-limiting process and the clearance will not be significantly affected by blood flow.

The other major route of clearance is renal where the drug is eliminated by the kidneys and excreted in urine. This clearance can also be related to blood flow; however, it is also affected by the rates of glomerular filteration and active secretion or reabsorption. Renal clearance would be classed as low if significantly less than glomerular filtration rate.

It should be noted that whilst pharmacokinetic parameters are not physiological measurements these physiological values can be useful in interpreting the values obtained. Table 7.1 shows some typical physiological flow rates in various species (some data taken from Davies and Morris, 1993).

TABLE 7.1 *Typical physiological flow rates*

	Body weight (kg)	Hepatic blood flow (mL/min/kg)	Glomerular filtration rate (mL/min/kg)
Mouse	0.02–0.025	90	14
Rat	0.25	55	9.0*
Marmoset	0.3		2.9*
Rabbit	2.5–3	71	3.1
Cynomolgus monkey	4–5	44	2.1
Dog	10–12	31	3.3*
Man	70	21	1.8

Data taken from *Pharm. Res.* 10, 1093–1095 (1993) except values marked with asterisk.
*in-house data.

7.4.3 Volume of distribution

The volume of distribution describes how well the drug distributes in the body. If the volume of distribution is too low, a molecule with an intracellular site of action, such as an antiviral agent, may not reach high intracellular concentrations even if the plasma concentrations are high. Conversely a molecule such as an antibiotic that acts in the extracellular space may suffer if wide distribution leads to low fluid concentrations. A volume of distribution of 0.07 L/kg or less generally suggests that the drug is confined to the systemic circulation. A volume of distribution of 0.25 L/kg may indicate that the drug reaches interstitial fluids, but does not penetrate cells. A large volume of distribution of 0.6 L/kg or more suggests that the drug is well distributed, but does not necessarily mean the drug enters all cells. The large volume may be due to uptake by a specific tissue or membrane, for example, highly lipophilic compounds are known to distribute into lipids in cell membranes and fat stores; these effectively form slow release depots of the drug and prolong the plasma levels. Table 7.2 shows typical physiological volumes, which may be applied as 'rules of thumb' to describe how well a particular drug is distributed.

TABLE 7.2 *Typical physiological volumes*

Plasma volume	Blood volume	Extracellular water	Total body water
4%	7%	26%	60%

7.5 *Parameter derivations*

7.5.1 C_{MAX}, T_{MAX}

The maximum plasma drug concentration (C_{max}) and the time taken to reach C_{max} (T_{max}) are obtained directly from the observed concentration–time data. The plasma concentration at the intercept (C_0) is a hypothetical concentration relevant only for an intravenous dose. It is derived by extrapolation from the first measured plasma concentrations to time zero based on the slope derived from regression of the initial two or three time points. Figure 7.4 shows a representation of a plasma concentration–time curve showing C_{max} and T_{max} for an oral dose.

7.5.2 Terminal phase rate constant (λ_z) and half-life ($t_{1/2}$)

The terminal phase rate constant (λ_z) is estimated by linear regression of logarithmic transformed concentration versus time data:

$$\lambda_z = \text{slope} \times -2.303$$

The terminal half-life ($t_{1/2}$) is calculated as follows:

$$t_{1/2} = \frac{\ln 2}{\lambda_z}$$

where ln 2 equals 0.693. The elimination may be monophasic (a single phase of elimination) or biphasic (comprising an initial or distribution phase and a terminal or elimination phase). These are illustrated in Figures 7.5 and 7.6.

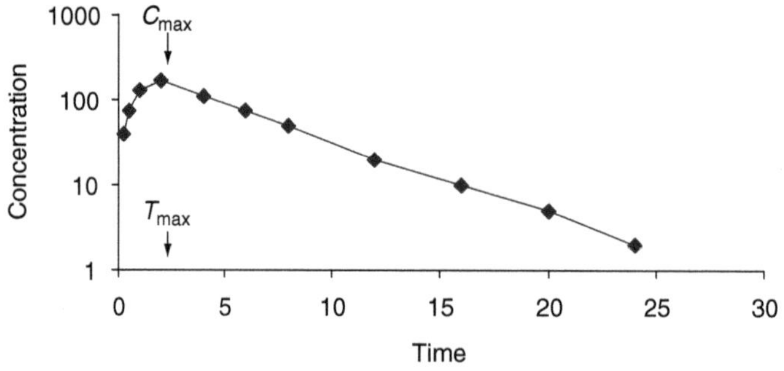

FIGURE 7.4 *Representation of a plasma concentration–time curve showing* C_{max} *and* T_{max} *for an oral dose.*

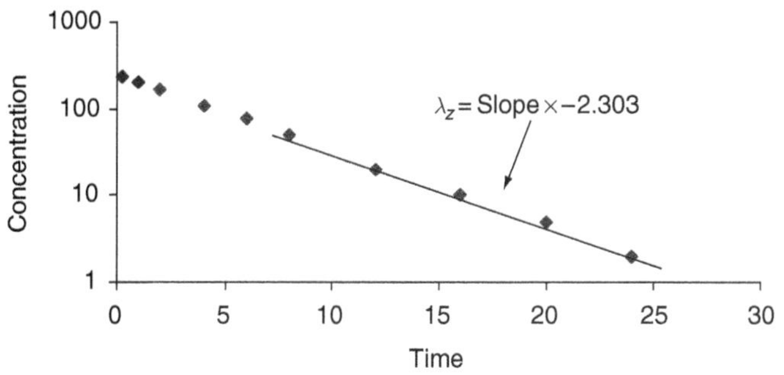

FIGURE 7.5 *Plasma concentration–time curve showing a monophasic elimination.*

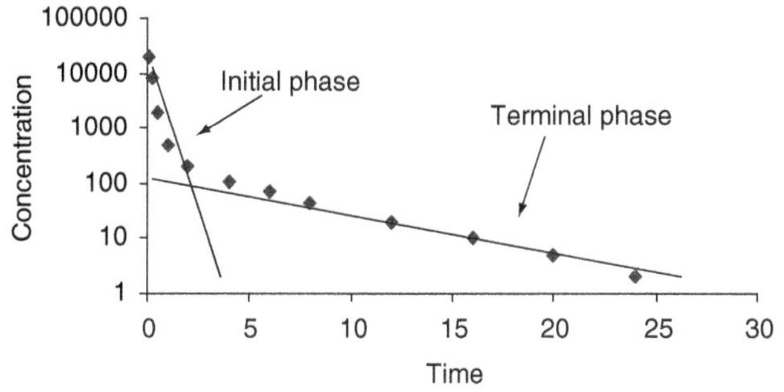

FIGURE 7.6 *Plasma concentration–time curve showing a biphasic elimination.*

7.5.3 Area under the plasma concentration–time curve (AUC_{last} and AUC_{∞})

The AUC from zero time to the time of the last quantifiable concentration (AUC_{last}) is calculated by the linear trapezoidal rule, or a combination of linear and logarithmic trapezoidal methods. These are illustrated graphically in Figure 7.7.

The linear trapezoidal method alone may be used if the time between terminal sampling times is less than the terminal half-life of the drug. However, this is rarely the case with pre-clinical data, as in the interest of reducing animal usage and stress, relatively few time points may be collected from animals.

(a) Linear trapezoidal area method

The trapezoidal area between the two data points (t_1, C_1) and (t_2, C_2), where $t_2 > t_1$ and $C_2 \geq C_1$, is given by:

$$AUC_{t_1-t_2} = 0.5 \times (t_2 - t_1) \times (C_1 + C_2)$$

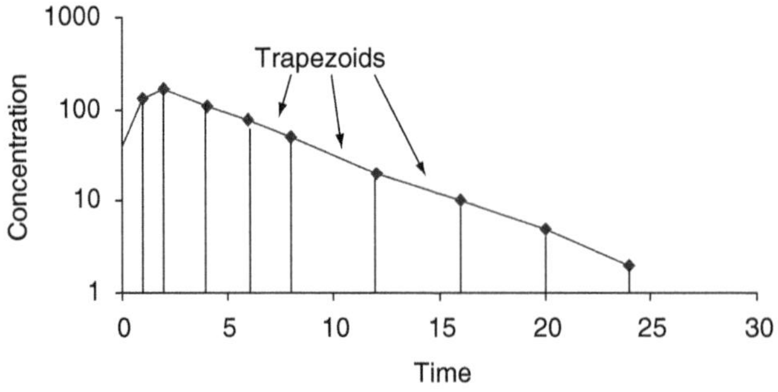

FIGURE 7.7 *Area under the plasma concentration–time curve showing the constituent trapezoids.*

where concentrations have been sampled at intervals greater than the elimination half-life, a combination of the linear and logarithmic trapezoidal rules can minimise overestimation of the AUC, which is a factor of exponential elimination. The linear trapezoidal method is employed when the plasma concentrations are rising and the logarithmic trapezoidal method when the concentrations are declining.

(b) Logarithmic trapezoidal area method

The trapezoidal area between the two data points (t_1, C_1) and (t_2, C_2), where $t_2 > t_1$ and $C_2 < C_1 (C_2 > 0)$, is given by:

$$AUC_{t_1-t_2} = \frac{(t_2 - t_1) \times (C_1 - C_2)}{\ln(C_1/C_2)}$$

Extrapolation of AUC_{last} from zero time to infinity (AUC_∞) is calculated as follows:

$$AUC_\infty = AUC_{\text{last}} + \frac{C_{\text{last}}}{\lambda_z}$$

where C_{last} is the last observed quantifiable concentration.

The percentage of AUC_∞ obtained by extrapolation ($\%AUC_{\text{ex}}$) should be less than 20 per cent for reasonable confidence in the extrapolated parameter. The $\%AUC_{\text{ex}}$ can be calculated as follows:

$$\%AUC_{\text{ex}} = \frac{(AUC_\infty - AUC_{\text{last}})}{AUC_\infty} \times 100$$

7.5.4 Clearance (CL)

The total plasma clearance (CL) is calculated as follows:

$$CL = \frac{Dose}{AUC_{\infty}}$$

or for continuous infusion

$$CL = \frac{R_o}{C_{ss}}$$

where R_o is the infusion rate and C_{ss} the plasma concentration at steady state.

7.5.5 Volume of distribution (V)

Volume of distribution, in non-compartmental PK, may be estimated as follows. The volume of distribution immediately after an intravenous bolus dose is:

$$V = \frac{Dose}{C_o}$$

The volume of distribution associated with the elimination phase can be estimated from the clearance and elimination rate constant:

$$V_z = \frac{CL}{\lambda_z}$$

7.5.6 Statistical moment theory ($AUMC_{last}$ and $AUMC_{\infty}$)

The plasma concentration–time curve can also be regarded as a statistical distribution curve, and statistical moment theory may be applied to the derivation of parameters. Although not generally quoted in pharmacokinetic interpretation, the area under the first moment curve can be used to estimate the volume of distribution at steady state.

The area under the first moment of the plasma (serum or blood) concentration–time curve ($AUMC$) from zero time (pre-dose) to the time of last quantifiable concentration ($AUMC_{last}$) may be calculated as shown below.

The linear trapezoidal method alone may be used if an appropriate sampling scheme (i.e. sampling time intervals $\leq$ to the elimination half-life) has been employed. The trapezoidal area between the two data points $(t_1, t_1 \times C_1)$ and $(t_2, t_2 \times C_2)$, where $t_2 > t_1$ and $C_2 \geq C_1$, is given by:

$$AUMC_{t_1-t_2} = 0.5 \times (t_2 - t_1) \times (t_1 \times C_1 + t_2 \times C_2)$$

If sampling intervals are longer than the half-life of elimination of the drug, a combination of the linear trapezoidal method (employed when the plasma concentrations are rising) and the logarithmic trapezoidal method (employed when the concentrations are declining) should be used.

The trapezoidal area between the two data points $(t_1, t_1 \times C_1)$ and $(t_2, t_2 \times C_2)$ where $t_2 > t_1$ and $C_2 < C_1 (C_2 > 0)$, is given by:

$$AUMC_{t_1-t_2} = \frac{(t_2 - t_1) \times (t_1 \times C_1 - t_2 \times C_2)}{\ln(C_1/C_2)} - \frac{(t_2 - t_1)^2 \times (C_1 - C_2)}{(\ln(C_1/C_2))^2}$$

$AUMC$ from zero time to infinite time ($AUMC_\infty$) may be calculated as follows:

$$AUMC_\infty = AUMC_{\text{last}} + \frac{(t_{\text{last}} \times C_{\text{last}})}{\lambda_z} + \frac{C_{\text{last}}}{\lambda_z^2}$$

where C_{last} is the last observed quantifiable concentration.

The percentage of $AUMC_\infty$ obtained by extrapolation ($\%AUMC_{\text{ex}}$) may be calculated as follows:

$$\%AUMC_{\text{ex}} = \frac{(AUMC - AUMC_{\text{last}})}{AUMC_\infty} \times 100$$

If the percentage of $AUMC_\infty$ obtained by extrapolation constitutes more than 50 per cent of the total, caution must be exercised if subsequent parameters are estimated using these values (e.g. MRT, V_{ss}).

7.5.7 The mean residence time (*MRT*)

The *MRT* similarly is rarely used for interpretative purposes in pre-clinical evaluation. *MRT* for an intravenous bolus dose can be calculated as follows:

$$MRT_{\text{iv}} = \frac{AUMC_\infty}{AUC_\infty} - \frac{T}{2}$$

The *MRT* following an intravenous infusion may be calculated as follows:

$$MRT = \frac{AUMC_\infty}{AUC_\infty} - \frac{T}{2}$$

where T is the infusion time.

7.5.8 Volume of distribution at steady state (V_{SS})

The volume of distribution at steady state (V_{ss}) provides us with a more homogeneous measure of volume, as it is not dominated by the distribution in the initial or terminal phases. It is calculated as follows:

$$V_{ss} = CL \times MRT$$

7.5.9 Renal clearance (CL_R)

If sufficient urinary excretion data are available, the renal clearance (CL_r) may be calculated as follows:

$$CL_r = \frac{Ae_\infty}{AUC_\infty}$$

where Ae_∞ is the total amount of unchanged drug recovered in the urine.

7.5.10 Bioavailabiliy (F)

The fraction of an oral dose that reaches the systemic circulation unchanged is calculated as follows:

$$F = \frac{AUC_{\infty po}}{AUC_{\infty iv}} \times \frac{Dose_{iv}}{Dose_{po}}$$

multiplied by 100, this is also referred to as 'bioavailability'.

7.6 *Study design and data handling in pre-clinical drug development*

7.6.1 Study design

The objective of the pre-clinical pharmacokinetic study is to evaluate the PK of the developmental drug in the animal species used in safety studies. The dose level is often selected as the lowest dose used in toxicology studies, another toxicity test dose or a pharmacologically therapeutic dose. Single dose pharmacokinetic studies provide the definitive pharmacokinetic profile in the pre-clinical species and systemic exposure to metabolites with the use of a radiolabel.

It is important to perform the pharmacokinetic assessment at a dose level that is within the range of linear kinetics (i.e. not where elimination is saturable) as many drugs will exhibit non-linear kinetics over a wide dose range. This is because the mechanisms for drug clearance can be saturated by, for example, metabolic clearance. Metabolism is a biological process mediated by enzymes, and the rate of metabolism is related to the concentration of the drug substrate and amount of enzyme available. It is also dependent on blood flow and the intrinsic rate of metabolism of the compound. Some compounds may act as inducers or inhibitors of their own metabolism. At higher doses the metabolism may be rate limiting, and greater levels of unchanged drug may reach the systemic circulation. Likewise mechanisms involved in renal clearance notably glomerular filteration and active secretion can be saturated at higher doses resulting in decreased clearance of unchanged drug. These situations are further complicated if the pharmacological action of the drug results in a decrease in blood flow.

Absorption of drug may also be concentration dependent and in some cases the drug formulation, dissolution and solubility factors lead to a decrease in the percentage of the dose which is absorbed.

Generally non-linear kinetics is only observed in the dose ranges used in pre-clinical toxicity studies which are much greater than those used in human studies.

Intravenous data is required to obtain the definitive clearance and volume of distribution data. Oral and intravenous data together provide a measure of the bioavailability of the drug.

During a single dose pharmacokinetic study, blood should be collected over a period of at least four half-lives of the drug if the terminal half-life is to be accurately determined.

'Mean profiles' in which the plasma time profile is constructed from blood samples taken from different animals are typically used for small animals and may be conducted using a destructive (single time point from each animal) or composite design (several samples taken from different animals at different times). The reason for this is the difficulty in obtaining sufficient sample volume for analyses if all samples were taken from an individual animal (see, the toxicokinetics, Chapter 9).

The nominal times when plasma samples are taken are used to calculate the mean and standard deviation (or median and range) drug concentrations at each time point for each period and dose.

Individual profiles are more typical for larger animals which may be serially bled. Blood sampling times should be designed to minimise large gaps between time points (i.e. where concentrations are not detectable at 24 hours, consideration should be made to include a 12 or 16 hour time point).

Before a pharmacokineticist can begin to estimate the pharmacokinetic parameters, it is important that the data is inspected to ensure no gross deviations from the protocol have occurred. For example, on occasion, the actual sampling times during a pharmacokinetic study may deviate from the target sampling times.

Deviations of greater than 5 per cent between the target sampling time and the actual sampling time should be taken into account especially for drugs with rapid absorption/distribution rates. If the rate of change in the plasma time profile is rapid then a significant difference between the nominal time and the actual time can give errors in the calculated pharmacokinetic parameters. In these cases, the actual sampling times should be used in the individual concentration–time profiles. Otherwise, it is sufficient to use the target sampling times for the analysis.

A common question for the novice pharmacokineticist is 'how should values below the quantitation (BQL) limit be handled?'. Non-quantifiable values are treated differently by various scientists; either being considered to reflect zero, or the actual limit of quantification, or even some value half way between. One recommendation for handling of BQL data is as follows:

1 BQL values at early time points, when appreciable absorption will not have occurred, should be set to zero.
2 When two consecutive BQL values are encountered, all subsequent non-BQL values should be excluded from the pharmacokinetic analysis.
3 When a BQL value occurs between two adjacent non-BQL values, it may be more appropriate to exclude it from the pharmacokinetic analysis.

Descriptive statistics (median, range or mean $\pm$ *SD*) are often used to summarise the data. To calculate the mean plasma concentration in the presence of BQL values, the BQL values should be set to zero. If the mean value calculates to a value below the quantitation limit the mean should be reported as BQL.

The bioanalytical method is important as it underlines the integrity of the pharmacokinetic evaluation. While the method must be demonstrated to be valid, a formal validation report is not required for pre-clinical studies. The method of validation includes analyte stability, specificity, precision, accuracy and sensitivity. A calibration line with appropriate limits of quantification is defined. It may be necessary to quantify metabolite as well as parent compound, and this should optimally be done with the same assay.

7.7 *Application of PK in drug discovery*

7.7.1 Pharmacokinetic screening methods during lead optimisation

When designing a new drug, the desirable pharmacokinetic profile of the compound can be predicted from deficiencies in existing medicines or based on the required pharmacological target. On discovery a number of compounds will be screened to select those whose pharmacokinetic characteristics are closest to those desired. This process is called lead optimisation. The pharmacokinetic parameters investigated are half-life, clearance, volume and bioavailability. In the past, significant numbers of molecules have failed in the early stages of clinical development due to inappropriate pharmacokinetic properties, and the aim of lead optimisation should be to reduce this attrition rate.

Until recently the time taken to conduct a pre-clinical pharmacokinetic study was too slow to allow a pharmacokinetic screen to be used on the critical path of lead optimisation. Much of the bottleneck was with bioanalytical methods. Advances in the use of LC–MS–MS in bioanalysis have changed the situation radically. Rapid development and use of sensitive methods for many compounds per week is now a reality. Decisions now have to be made on how best to use this new technology. Conventional pharmacokinetic studies may not be appropriate in a lead optimisation programme. There must be a balance between compound throughput and the depth of information gained. There are a number of study designs now in general use.

Conventional studies will provide detailed characterisation of the pharmacokinetic parameters of molecule, but are relatively time-consuming. They are most appropriate for characterising lead molecules, or differentiating within a limited group of molecules in which small differences could be significant.

For the selection of the best molecules during a lead optimisation programme, it may only be necessary to rank molecules according to specific pharmacokinetic parameters. For example, if high oral bioavailability is required for a series of compounds that is known to be well absorbed, it is not necessary to dose by both oral and intravenous routes. A simple intravenous screen for low clearance will identify the best and worst compounds. Furthermore, to rank compounds according to clearance an estimate of plasma concentrations at two, or at most, three time points may be all that is needed. Whilst an *AUC* based on these limited points would not give an accurate measure of clearance, it will, with the right study design, correlate with clearance and hence be a reliable ranking tool. Both of these approaches reduce analytical and *in vivo* workload, and if terminal bleeds are involved animal numbers are also reduced.

Another approach currently being explored by a number of pharmaceutical companies is N-in-One dosing. Individual animals receive a cocktail of up to around ten compounds in a single dose formulation. The specificity of the LC–MS–MS bioanalysis then enables a plasma concentration–time profile and associated pharmacokinetic parameters to be obtained for each individual compound. To minimise drug–drug interactions, the doses are kept low, and to monitor such interactions a standard compound is included in each cocktail. Whilst this system is not foolproof it can dramatically increase throughput, reduce animal numbers and produce valid and useful PK screening information. Clearly the risk of interactions is ever present, and the method should be validated for any compound class prior to use in a decision-making role.

A further increase in throughput, mirrored in a further reduction in the detail of the PK output, can be obtained by incorporating the limited time point approach into N-in-One studies. The clear disadvantage of N-in-One studies is the potential for drug–drug interactions. If this precludes their use in a particular chemical series, some gains in throughput can still be obtained by N-in-One assays. In this study design, animals only receive one compound in a dose, but plasma samples from animals that have received different compounds are pooled prior to LC–MS–MS assay. Whilst the *in vivo* workload is not reduced, the sample processing and Mass Spec time are markedly reduced, leading to greater efficiency in the lab. Of course there is still a chance of interactions during LC–MS–MS analysis but these are usually both predictable and avoidable. In a lead optimisation environment, N-in-One bioanalysis should be the norm for all PK work so as to make best use of the resource available.

In summary, there are a number of ways to increase PK throughput by using novel study designs of N-in-One dosing, N-in-One analysis and limited sample time PK. The decision on whether to use any of these, or to use conventional study design, must be made on the balance between throughput on the one hand and accuracy and confidence in the PK parameters on the other.

7.8 *Interspecies scaling*

The PK of a novel compound in humans may be forecast by allometric scaling of pre-clinical data. This is a method of interpolation and extrapolation based on the anatomical, physiological and biochemical similarities in mammals. Mathematical analysis of pre-clinical pharmacokinetic data may permit the extrapolation of animal data to human data, and thus predict pharmacokinetic parameters and therapeutic dose levels in man. The two approaches described below are particularly successful if the major route of elimination of the test compound is as unchanged drug in the urine or if hepatic clearance is high.

In conjunction with non-clinical PK–PD data (see PK–PD chapter), the scaled parameters can be used to forecast effective doses for humans. This is important both in early discovery when the suitability of lead compounds for clinical effectiveness needs to be judged, and during drug development when the dose levels for early clinical studies need to be estimated.

Once the pharmacokinetic parameters and dose levels for early human studies have been predicted, data may be simulated to show the exposures at the selected dose levels. The exposure cover generated from the toxicology studies should be compared to the predicted exposures in man to aid in assessing risk. The exposures in the toxicology species should be higher than the predicted exposure in humans at the recommended dose levels for early human studies and ultimately for therapeutic use (see toxicokinetics, Chapter 9).

Two methods of interspecies scaling will be described here, simple allometry and flow-based scaling.

(a) *Simple allometry*
All available pharmacokinetic data from research or ADME (absorption, distribution, metabolism and excretion) studies should be used for the scaling; the more species the better. Experience has shown that it may be a disadvantage to use toxicokinetic data for scaling. This is because there is usually a smaller number of time points available from these types of studies, and more complex kinetics (like biphasic elimination) may not be evident from the profile. A simple allometric approach may be used to scale to humans using the formula $y = aW^b$, where y the pharmacokinetic parameter in question, a the value at the intercept at 1 kilogram, W body weight, and b the slope of the regression line. This is illustrated in Figure 7.8.

Based on the above example, parameter estimates for humans were $t_{1/2} = 2.6\,\mathrm{h}$, $\lambda_z = 0.27\,\mathrm{h}$, $CL = 0.21\,\mathrm{L/h/kg}$ and $V = 0.77\,\mathrm{L/kg}$.

(b) *Flow-based scaling*
Flow-based scaling is based on the premise that in all species the volume of distribution (L/kg) of a given molecule is the same, and that clearance is the same fraction of either glomerular filtration rate (renally cleared) or liver blood flow (hepatic clearance). This fact allows us to forecast the human pharmacokinetics from pre-clinical studies in only one or two species by comparing physiological flows in different species.

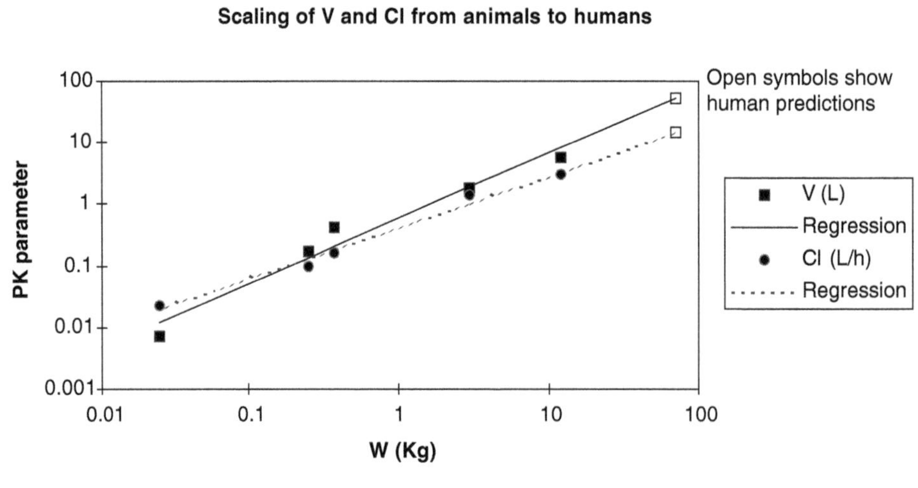

FIGURE 7.8 *Simple allometric scaling of clearance and volume.*

Using this technique for a renally cleared compound:

$$half/life_{\text{man}} = \frac{half/life_{\text{animal}} \times GFR_{\text{animal}}}{GFR_{\text{man}}}$$

where *GFR* is glomerular filtration rate (mL/min/kg). The calculation is the same for hepatically cleared compounds using liver blood flow. The inverse equation is used for clearance.

The outcome of this is that the half-life in man is most likely to be around three-fold higher than that in rat and dog. Clearly significant differences in intrinsic clearance of moderately cleared molecules can render this model (as with graphical models) erroneous. Nonetheless, experience has shown that the forecast is more often right than not. The advantage of being able to scale with data from only one or two animal species is evident as human forecasts can be made from the very first pre-clinical pharmacokinetic study on a compound. In addition, if the human forecasts vary widely from different species they would be viewed with more uncertainty than if they were all similar.

7.9 *References*

Davies, B. and Morris, T. (1993) *Pharm. Res.* 10, 1093–1095.

Perrier, D. and Gibaldi, M. (1982) *Pharmacokinetics*, 2nd edn. Marcel Dekker Inc.

Rowland, M. and Tozer, T.N. (1989) *Clinical Pharmacokinetics: Concepts and Applications*, 2nd edn. Lea & Febinger.

WinNonlin™ Pharsight Corporation, 800 West El Camino Real, Mountain View California 94040.

CHAPTER 8

Pharmacokinetic/ pharmacodynamic modelling in pre-clinical drug discovery

Tony Pateman

8.1 *The importance of pharmacokinetic/pharmacodynamic modelling*

A concentration is only worth measuring if it produces an effect! The derivation of pharmacokinetic (PK) parameters from plasma concentration data and how these parameters relate to the disposition of the compound under study has been discussed earlier. However, PK studies serve little purpose if the compound is biologically inert. PK studies are performed because it is assumed that the parameters obtained are relevant to the *in vivo* activity of the compound. Perhaps the duration of action can be determined from the half-life? Perhaps the volume of distribution can be related to access to a receptor? In reality these relationships may not be straightforward. A short half-life does not necessarily equate to a short duration of action. A large volume of distribution does not ensure access to intracellular receptors. For PK parameters to be related to biological activity the relationship between the plasma concentrations (PK) and the effects (pharmacodynamics or PD) must be established through PK/PD modelling.

8.2 *Advantages of incorporating PK/PD modelling in the drug discovery process*

PK and metabolic screens are now an integral part of the drug discovery process. However, the interpretation of these screens is difficult if it is not known how the PK parameters in animals, along with *in vitro* metabolic stability data, relate to the required clinical activity in man. If the clinical target, in terms of PK and efficacy, is understood, the required pre-clinical properties of the molecule can be estimated by coupling PK/PD parameters and interspecies scaling. By performing these simulations to set the criteria for candidate selection, the chances of success in the clinic are enhanced. For example, within our own company a PK/PD study identified high protein binding as a problem in translating good *in vitro* potency of an inhibitor into good *in vivo* efficacy, and this information was then used to steer the lead optimisation process.

An understanding of the PK–PD relationship allows the importance of PK properties to be rationalised. In the drug discovery process, a project team may strive to achieve a molecule with a particular half-life, without knowing whether they must achieve that particular value or whether something rather shorter would do. PK/PD will enable this decision to be made, and this can potentially save months of unnecessary refinement of a molecular series. For example, the duration of action of an irreversible neutrophil inhibitor was shown to be governed by the turnover of neutrophils and was not related to the half-life of the inhibitor.

Understanding the sensitivity of PD to changes in PK can also clarify the relevance of potential drug–drug interactions. A PK interaction need not be a problem if it has an insignificant effect on PD. Likewise, disease and ageing may affect PK, but this may not necessarily translate to an affect on PD. It must always be remembered that PK is a surrogate for PD and not a goal in its own right.

The slope of the PD concentration response curve can have a significant impact on the suitability of a compound class to its disease target. A steep response curve will give a rapid onset and termination of activity, a desirable property of an anaesthetic perhaps. It will also make the PD very sensitive to small changes in PK. A shallow response curve would be more suited to diseases, such as high blood pressure, where safe chronic dosing is required.

The PK–PD relationship may not be an obvious one. There may be a delay between the PK profile and the effect, such as is seen for the effects of corticosteroids on cortisol levels. However, such relationships can usually be modelled, and the relevance of PK understood. Furthermore, if the relationship between plasma concentrations and centrally mediated effects of a drug can be modelled we can obviate the need, during drug development, for measuring levels of compound in the brains of animals or the cerebrospinal fluid in man.

Many of our receptor targets mediate more than one physiological function. For example, the adenosine A1 receptor controls cardiovascular, metabolic and central nervous system (CNS) functions. Understanding the *in vivo* PK–PD relationship for all of these processes allows us to optimise a molecule to a particular physiological target.

Finally PK/PD has a unifying effect on the scientific disciplines with the drug discovery process. Pharmacokineticists need to work closely with both *in vivo* and *in vitro* pharmacologists, and with clinical pharmacologists to provide the link between pre-clinical and clinical efficacy.

8.3 *PK/PD in the drug discovery process*

8.3.1 The changing role of DMPK in drug discovery

When drug metabolism and pharmacokinetics (DMPK) was first recognised as a key discipline within the pharmaceutical industry, its function was reserved for the development process. The driving force was from the regulatory bodies who recognised the need to understand the disposition of drug molecules in order to understand and interpret safety and efficacy studies (both animal and clinical). Soon after, many companies recognised that understanding more about drug disposition prior to the development phase was advantageous to the process. However, the bioanalytical tools available at the time (e.g. HPLC/UV) meant that disposition studies could only be performed on a limited number of compounds due to the time taken in methods development. Consequently DMPK studies usually took place on a limited number of compounds prior to full development. As the data was generated so late in the discovery process, any shortcomings in the disposition of a molecule could not be fixed as the chemical programme had focussed for a long time on one chemical series. The widespread use of LC/MS has changed the situation radically. Sensitive and specific assays can now be developed rapidly, and providing DMPK support to the discovery process at the earliest stages of lead optimisation is a reality. The consequence of this is that decisions on entire discovery programmes can now be made based on DMPK criteria. For that reason it is imperative that those scientists supplying that support can fully interpret the meaning and relevance of their data. As stated in the introduction, PK alone is not a reliable indicator of a compound's suitability for the market place. To make the right decisions, the link between PK and PD must be understood.

8.3.2 PK/PD in a research strategy

A typical way in which PK/PD can be incorporated into the research process is outlined below. It is very important to recognise that the purpose of this strategy is to make the right decisions and reduce the risk of taking an inappropriate molecule through to the expensive process of drug development. Usually the PK/PD models will be far from perfect, and the study design may not be ideal. The understanding of the biological processes involved in the PD response may be far from clear. It is therefore important to take a pragmatic approach to PK/PD, using the simplest of models and a study design commensurate with making the right decision. Remember always that forecasting what will happen in patients (the ultimate goal) is an imprecise science not only from the point of view of PK and PD, but also in selecting the appropriate pre-clinical disease models.

8.3.3 Defining the PK target

Many companies are now using *in vitro* metabolic screens at an early stage of the selection process. Traditionally compounds with high turnover are rejected in favour of metabolically stable molecules. An understanding of the PK–PD relationship will enable a reasoned judgement on compound selection/rejection to be made. Lack of stability may not necessarily be a problem. Likewise, the relevance of *in vitro* permeability screens, such as MDCK cell monolayers, is clearer if the physiological location of the target receptor is known. Both of these concepts combine *in vivo* to determine clearance, volume and half-life. In addition, the requirement for good oral bioavailability is not always given. A compound acting on the gastrointestinal (GI) tract may work either topically or systemically, and it is important to understand which applies to a given compound class. Conducting PK/PD studies on representative molecules from a given compound series at an early stage of the discovery process enables these issues to be resolved, and hence the screens can be interpreted correctly. At the same time a greater understanding of the PD model is obtained.

Once the relevance of PK parameters has been established from the PK/PD studies, the hypothesis should be regularly tested to ensure continued validity. PK/PD studies using molecules with widely differing properties (clearance, volume, physicochemistry) maintain confidence in the model.

Throughout the pre-clinical discovery process the assumption is made that data has some relevance to patients, and invariably an animal model is utilised at some stage. Traditionally, PK in man has been forecast from pre-clinical data using allometric scaling of the PK parameters. The addition of PK/PD to the project knowledge base enables this to be taken one step further. If the PK–PD relationship in animals has been defined, along with *in vitro* comparative data on the receptor binding in animals and man, it is possible to forecast not only the PK but also the magnitude and duration of pharmacological effect in man. Throughout this process it is assumed that the forecasts to man have some chance of success. As with all extrapolations, these forecasts must be viewed with caution, recognising the assumptions made on the way. None-the-less, forecasting based on PK/PD knowledge provides the best chance of selecting the most appropriate molecule for progression into the clinic.

8.3.4 PK/PD in pre-clinical drug development

In its broadest sense, PK/PD has for many years been an integral part of the pre-clinical package in the form of toxicokinetics (see toxicokinetics chapter). Parameters of exposure such as AUC and C_{max} are related to general toxicological findings. This chapter will, however, focus on PK/PD relating to specific pharmacological events. The utility in the discipline of safety pharmacology is obvious. If the relationship between plasma concentrations and both wanted and unwanted effects can be modelled, a very clear understanding of the potential acute therapeutic window in man can be obtained. The dosage regime can be optimised to maximise safety. In addition, comparative studies with several compounds of the class can aid in selecting the safest. However, getting PK/PD data that can be used in this way presents significant practical difficulties. Not the least is the fact that taking sufficient blood samples routinely from animals involved in cardiovascular or behavioural studies may impact on the very pharmacological events that are under study. For this reason anything other than the simplest of PK/PD models may not be practical.

8.4 *Principles of PK/PD modelling*

8.4.1 Data requirements

Both plasma concentration and effect data versus time are required. The PK data should preferably be in the form of a compartmental model, although non-compartmental analysis may be adequate. Importantly the time points may need to be different for the PK and PD measurements. The drug concentration samples should be taken to fully characterise the PK profile. The effect measurements should be taken at times that characterise the full range of the PD response. Ideally, all should be done simultaneously in the same animal. However, this is often impractical for a number of reasons:

1 The dose that produces the desired PD response may give plasma concentrations that cannot be detected. In this case a higher dose should be given for the PK determination, and linearity of PK assumed.
2 Taking blood samples may affect the response.
3 Insufficient samples for drug analysis can be taken from the animal in the PD model. Under these circumstances separate PK studies should be

carried out, taking into account route, formulation, species, strain and anaesthetic state.

8.4.2 The sigmoid E_{max} model

For most purposes the most complex PD model required in drug discovery is the sigmoid E_{max} model. In this, plasma concentrations are related to effect by the following equation:

$$\text{Effect} = \frac{E_{max} \times C^N}{EC_{50}{}^N + C^N} + E_0$$

This represents the following relationship between effect and concentration and is illustrated in Figure 8.1.

E_{max} is the maximum effect that can be produced by the drug, at infinite concentration (all receptor-mediated responses have a maximum!).
EC_{50} is the concentration of drug that produces 50 per cent of the maximum effect. E_0 is the effect produced in the absence of drug (placebo or baseline noise). N is the slope of the response curve. A large value of N (e.g. >1) gives a rapid transition from minimum to maximum effect with concentration. The converse is true for a small value of N (e.g. <1).

Between 20 and 80 per cent maximum response, the effect is approximately proportional to log concentration. This will be of no surprise to pharmacologists, who have been doing two-point log dose response curves within the 20–80 per cent range for many years.

If the *in vivo* PD response curve can be defined, the effect versus time profile can be modelled for various PK scenarios, and appropriate decisions made. For a

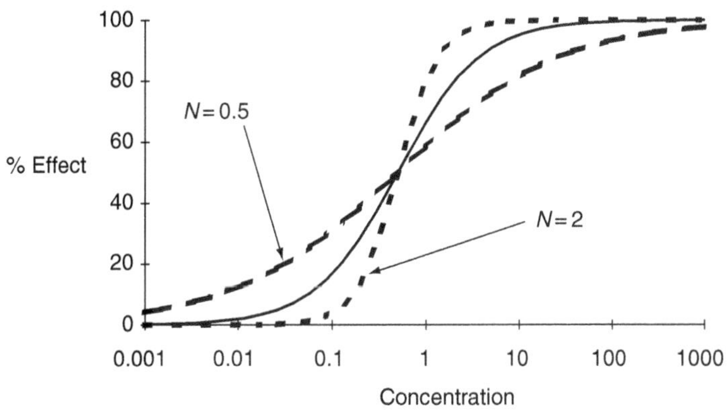

FIGURE 8.1 *Sigmoid E_{max} model.*

detailed review of PK/PD modelling, with examples of the use of WinNonlin™ the reader is referred to Gabrielsson and Weiner (1997).

8.4.3 Delayed response

Very often a simple plot of effect versus concentration, as shown above, does not yield a graph that can be used predictively. This may be because there is a delay between the concentration and the effect as shown in Figure 8.2.

This situation is often referred to as counter-clockwise hysteresis. The arrow on the graph indicates the third dimension of time. Clearly there is not a single solution to this concentration–effect relationship, as the same effect is produced by widely differing concentrations depending on whether the measurements are taken sooner or later after drug administration. The situation can be further visualised as shown in Figure 8.3. In this example the EC_{50} could be either 75 ng/ml or 15 ng/ml depending on when it was measured.

Currently two methods are available in WinNonlin™ for modelling the sigmoidal PD relationship to plasma concentrations when the response is delayed relative to the plasma concentrations. These models can then be used predictively.

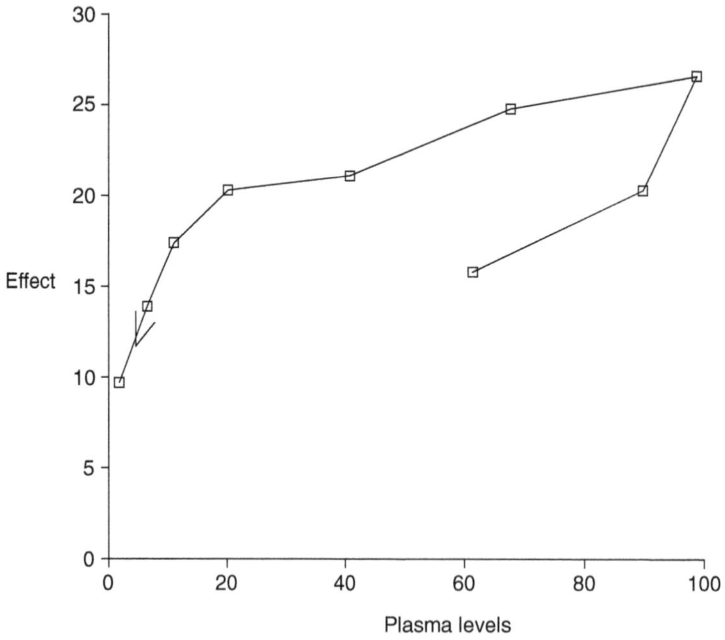

Figure 8.2 *Plot of effect versus plasma concentration showing counter-clockwise hysteresis.*

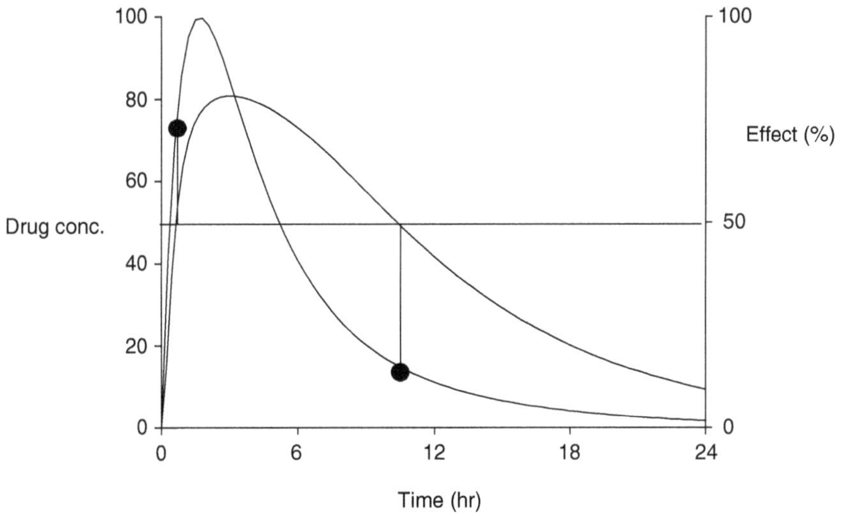

FIGURE 8.3 *Plot of concentration and effect versus time showing the effect lagging behind the plasma concentrations.*

The link model (Holford and Sheiner, 1982) assumes that the delay can be explained by the target receptor being in a separate, non-plasma compartment. Unlike normal PK compartments, this has no volume and hence does not contribute to the mass balance. A first order rate constant, *Keo*, describes the rate of equilibration of this compartment with plasma, and allows a PK/PD model to be constructed that can be used predictively.

The second model is the indirect response model (Jusko, 1990). It assumes that the delay is biochemical. In simple terms, it assumes that the biochemical function under investigation is in a state of equilibrium, with a zero order process producing the function, and a first order process destroying it. A drug can either stimulate or inhibit the production of the function, or stimulate or inhibit the destruction. This is analogous to the steady state infusion situation in PK, where a change in either infusion rate or elimination will change the steady state plasma concentration. As with the link model, the indirect response model can be used predictively with data that shows a delay between plasma concentration and response.

8.4.4 Impact of PK and PD parameters on *in vivo* potency and duration

PK/PD models enable the magnitude and duration of response to be predicted under various scenarios. Whilst the half-life alone does not necessarily reflect the duration of action (the latter is determined by the Hill coefficient, hysteresis and EC_{50} in addition to the half-life), some general rules can be formulated to predict the effect of changing

TABLE 8.1 *Impact of half-life on duration of effect*

Half-life (hours)	Time above 50% effect (hours)
0.5	3
1	6
2	9
4	17
8	30

$E_{max} = 100$, $E_o = 0$, $EC_{50} = 20$, $N = 1$, $Keo = 0.9$, $Co = 270$.

TABLE 8.2 *Impact of dose on duration of effect*

	Time above 50% effect (hours)	
Half-life (hours)	10 mg/kg	20 mg/kg
0.5	3	4
2	9	11

$E_{max} = 100$, $E_o = 0$, $EC_{50} = 20$, $N = 1$, $Keo = 0.9$, $Co = 270$.

half-life, dose and potency on duration. Table 8.1 is an example of a series of compounds with identical PD properties but differing half-lives. This illustrates the point that in general, doubling the half-life doubles the duration of effect.

The effect of doubling the dose (or doubling the potency) is not so dramatic (Table 8.2). That is, in general doubling the dose increases the duration of action by only one half-life. Thus increasing the half-life is a much more efficient means of enhancing the duration of action than is increasing the dose or potency.

8.5 *Summary*

The conventional use of PK only provides information about the disposition of the drug molecule. By joining forces with the pharmacologists the pharmacokineticist can develop PK/PD models that can describe the relationship between plasma concentration and effect. This knowledge allows the likely effect versus time profile in man to be forecast from animal data. It also enables the impact of changing PK parameters on the PD profile to be evaluated. Perhaps most important of all, it assists drug discovery scientists in setting the appropriate PK target during drug candidate selection so that the chance of clinical failure due to inappropriate PK and PD is minimised.

8.6 *References*

Gabrielsson, J. and Weiner, D. (1997) *Pharmacokinetic and Pharmacodynamic Data Analysis*, 2nd edition. Apotekarsocieteten, Stockholm.

Holford, N.H.G. and Sheiner, L. (1982) *Pharmacol. Ther.* 16, p. 143.

Jusko, W.J. (1990) *J. Clin. Pharmacol.* 30, p. 303.

WinNonlin™ Pharsight Cororation, 800 West El Camino Real, Mountain View, California 94040.

CHAPTER 9

Toxicokinetics

Sheila Schwartz

9.1 *Introduction*

In the pharmaceutical industry, the term 'toxicokinetics' is generally used to describe the pharmacokinetics (PK) performed at the dose levels used in the toxicological risk assessment of drugs. The aim of the toxicokinetic evaluation is to define the relationship between systemic exposure to test compound and the administered dose, and to provide information on potential dose- and time-dependencies in the kinetics. Toxicokinetic studies can also aid in determining the effect of age on the PK in animals, provide clearer delineation when there are sex-related differences, determine whether there are any changes in kinetics in pregnancy (during reproductive toxicology studies) and also provide greater detail on inter-species comparisons. However, the overall aim in conducting toxicokinetics during safety studies is to extrapolate the risk assessment from the toxicity test species to humans.

Toxicokinetics is usually monitored as part of the toxicity studies, but is sometimes carried out as a separate study and is always derived from multiple doses. This chapter describes the process for conducting toxicokinetic studies and the application of the data obtained.

9.2 *Study design*

Toxicokinetic study design is well described in the ICH guidelines, note for guidance on toxicokinetics, ICH Harmonised Tripartite Guideline (1994). Multiple dose toxicokinetic studies are usually run concomitantly during the toxicity studies, and may be conducted with serial bleeds or as part of a destructive design, and in individual animals or by using a composite design. Table 9.1 shows an example of a composite design for a small animal toxicokinetic study.

The study should be designed to define the exposure of the drug during a dosing interval, and blood should be collected over a sufficient period of time to estimate the *AUC*. Single time points are not considered suitable for evaluating the toxicokinetics of a compound. There is no requirement to obtain blood samples for 'proof of absorption'. It is not necessary to perform a toxicokinetic assessment if data can be reliably extrapolated from another study.

Relatively large volumes of blood may be demanded from toxicity test animals for toxicokinetic analysis, haematology and clinical chemistry; therefore, it is often necessary to sample blood from a separate ('satellite') group housed under the same conditions (e.g. rats and mice). The blood volume in larger species like dogs is less restrictive, and rather than a satellite group, the test animals themselves are usually used for toxicokinetic bleeds. The collection of blood samples for the derivation of toxicokinetic parameters is dependent on the number of animals and the dosing regimen. For example, a preliminary MRD study (maximum repeatable dose study) may use incremental dosages in one group of animals, and due to haematological or regulatory limitations on blood sampling, it may not always be possible to obtain PK parameters at all dose levels to assess dose proportionality. Monitoring authorities generally accept that maximum blood withdrawal should not exceed 15 per cent of blood volume within a four-week period. For rats and dogs, this represents approximately 1.1–1.3 mL/100 g bodyweight. This has been tested in-house, resulting in an agreement that the haematology parameters may be more seriously affected if removal of 15 per cent blood volume is exceeded.

TABLE 9.1 *Example of a composite design for a small animal toxicokinetic study*

	Animal numbers (n=6)					
	001	**002**	**003**	**004**	**005**	**006**
Bleed times (hours) for each animal (n = 3 bleeds/animal)	1	2	4	8	12	24
	24	1	2	4	8	12
	12	24	1	2	4	8

Resulting in *AUC* of 6 time points with n = 3 samples per time point.

The following sampling scheme is generally recommended for toxicokinetic evaluation:

1 *After intravenous administration*:
Five to six points for the *AUC* with at least two to three time points during the elimination phase.

The sampling may be limited to three time points in subsequent studies in total if the profile proves to be monophasic and dose proportional.

2 *After oral administration*:
Five to six points for the *AUC* with at least:

- one time point during the absorption phase
- one time point at the expected T_{max}
- and two to three time points during the elimination phase.

Pre-dose samples may also be required if the period of drug circulation is longer than the dosing interval (i.e. if drug was still in the blood from the previous day's dose). Alternatively, if a 24-hour time point is selected, the concentration at this time point may be extrapolated as a pre-dose value.

3 *After intravenous infusion*:

- at least one time point during the infusion
- one time point at the end of the infusion
- at least two to three time points during the elimination phase.

The sampling may be limited to one point at steady state during a constant rate infusion.

In formal studies conducted with multiple oral doses, it is often possible to collect concentration–time profiles over a number of time points during the dosing interval, at various occasions throughout the study. These studies should be sampled on the first and last (or close to last) days of the study. In longer-term studies, the kinetics should be monitored with full *AUC* profiles at intervals during the study. For example, blood sampling is strongly recommended during long-term (3–6 months) toxicity studies and over the complete time course of a carcinogenicity study to monitor any changes in the pharmacokinetic as a result of ageing. The toxicokinetics from various studies may be combined to provide a representative picture of the relationships between the kinetics and time/age (i.e. it is not necessary to sample on the same occasions in different studies). During continuous infusion, a number of important pharmacokinetic parameters may be derived from only very few time points. Blood sampling can be minimised by means of a sparse data design resulting in reduced animal numbers with associated ethical and cost benefits.

In general, there is no requirement to evaluate systemic drug levels in animals not receiving test compound; however, this may change in future as more and more often low levels are detected in controls, and the results must be explained. It is important though to bleed control animals to maintain consistency between groups. In these cases, samples from control animals may be stored without analysis and subsequently analysed if the results of the study dictate, or as a standard procedure, only a representative few may be analysed. Exceptions may include dietary and inhalation studies where the likelihood of cross-contamination is increased, in which case all samples should be analysed. Blood sampling is also recommended to monitor the recovery phase of toxicology studies particularly if the elimination half-life of the test compound is relatively long.

Any study done directly in support of a formal safety study must be conducted in compliance with good laboratory practice (GLP). Dosing and bleeding records should be collected and referred to by the kineticist during the toxicokinetic parameter derivation, just in case the doses or bleed times deviated from the nominal protocolled values. Adequate records should be maintained to account for all blood samples taken during a study and their storage conditions. The bioanalytical method is important in underlining the integrity of the toxicokinetic evaluation. The method used to measure test compound should be validated in accordance with the FDA position paper of Shah *et al.* (1992) and a validation report should be available. The validation method should include analyte stability, specificity, precision, accuracy and sensitivity. A calibration line with appropriate limits of quantification should also be defined.

Statistical analysis of toxicokinetic data may overcome uncertainty associated with dose- or time-dependencies in the systemic exposure, or may provide information to optimise study design. A statistical analysis may be appropriate to assess dose proportionality, time-dependence, sex differences or estimate the reliability of *AUC*s obtained from a minimal sampling approach. The kinetics of drugs may become non-linear (supra- or sub-proportional) at higher dose levels. A common method of assessing dose proportionality is to dose-adjust *AUC*s and test for a constant ratio between dose levels. In some studies non-linearity may not be evident because of variability. In this case a non-linear power model may be effective.

The proportionality relationship may be written as a power function:

$$AUC = a \cdot dose^b$$

where, b is the proportionality constant and a the intercept. Linearisation of this relationship gives:

$$\log AUC = \log a + \log \; dose \cdot b$$

The relationship is dose proportional when $b = 1$. Confidence intervals around b can be produced to estimate plausible ranges of true values. This type of model can, therefore, provide a quantitative measure of the deviation from dose proportionality.

Depending on the metabolism of the test compound, it may also be necessary to determine the exposure and kinetics of the metabolites. Optimally, the metabolites in the pre-clinical species should be relevant for humans (i.e. the same metabolites or products of further metabolism). If there were a different metabolite or range of metabolites in humans than in the animals used in the toxicity study, the animal species may not be exposed to the appropriate compound, or desired levels of material, and the risk assessment of the metabolite not adequately evaluated. To support exposure to metabolites, sometimes it is necessary to quantify the levels of the metabolites and perform metabolite toxicokinetics, which ideally should be done in the same assay. Metabolite toxicokinetics is recommended when the test substance is a prodrug, the metabolite(s) are known to be pharmacologically active or toxic, or the toxicity of metabolite is unknown but metabolite levels are high. The toxicokinetics of the metabolite should also be assessed if the test substance undergoes rapid or extensive metabolism, in which case the metabolite may act as a surrogate for exposure to the parent compound. Metabolite toxicokinetics is also useful to help describe the kinetics of the parent drug, particularly if dose- or time-dependent kinetics is seen. However, conducting metabolite kinetics must be carefully assessed on a 'needs basis' prior to such work being conducted.

An approach which is sometimes used in toxicokinetics is that of 'population pharmacokinetics'. This approach takes into account unexplainable inter- and intra-subject effects (random effects) and measured concomitant effects (fixed effects), and such data may be subjected to mixed effect modelling. These methods employ sparse sampling from large study populations, and thus may be suitable for determining the toxicokinetics from oncogenicity studies.

9.3 *PK parameters for toxicokinetic evaluation*

PK parameters have been previously defined in the pharmacokinetics chapter of this book. The most important parameters in toxicokinetic evaluation are those which describe exposure (AUC and C_{max}) and those which may help to assess dose- and time-dependent kinetics ($t_{1/2}$ and CL). Figure 9.1 shows an example of multiple dose concentration–time profile.

As toxicokinetics is concerned with multiple doses (compared to the single dose PK parameters previously described) additional parameters may be described as follows.

9.3.1 Cmaxss, Tmaxss

These are the maximum plasma concentrations at steady state for a multiple dosing profile (C_{maxss}) or a continuous infusion (C_{ss}), or the time at which the steady state

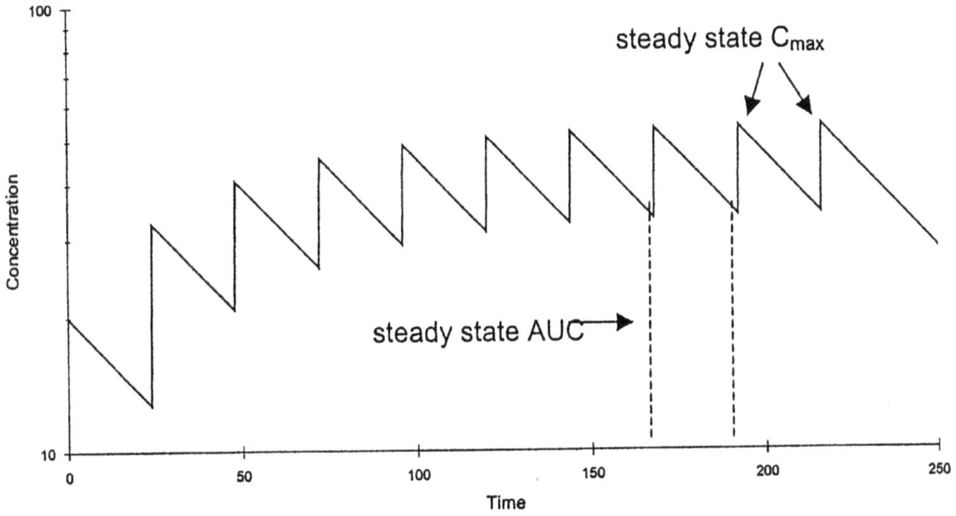

FIGURE 9.1 *Example of a multiple dose concentration–time profile.*

maximum plasma concentration was measured (T_{maxss}). These parameters are obtained directly from the concentration–time data.

9.3.2 AUC_{τ}

The AUC for the dosing interval (AUC_{τ}) after multiple dosing should be calculated using a trapezoidal method (see the pharmacokinetics chapter for more details). The log-linear trapezoidal method is recommended as time points are generally widely spaced in these types of studies, and using the linear trapezoidal rule in these cases (where concentrations have been sampled at intervals greater than the elimination half-life) can overestimate the AUC. Dosing intervals in toxicokinetic studies are usually 24 hours (a dose every day), but may be 12 hours if twice daily dosing is employed. Sometimes the intervals are irregular (e.g. 6 and 18 hours). However, it is common for the AUC for a 24-hour period to be reported, irrespective of the dosing interval.

For a continuous infusion, AUC_{τ} may be estimated from a single sample at steady state:

$$C_{ss} = \frac{AUC_{\tau}}{\tau}$$

It is important to note that AUC for the dosing interval (AUC_{τ}) = AUC at steady state (AUC_{ss}) = AUC extrapolated to infinity for a single dose (AUC_{∞}). This will aid in the interpretation of whether there are any time-dependent changes in the kinetics.

9.3.3 R (ACCUMULATION)

The administration of a drug on a multiple dose regimen will generally result in its accumulation. This type of accumulation is expected and is a function of the half-life of the drug and the dosing interval (τ). Generally when τ is equal to or greater than the half-life of the drug, the extent of accumulation is relatively modest (≤ 2). If τ is much less than the half-life, the extent of accumulation could be substantial. The accumulation factor (R) may be calculated (9.1) or predicted (9.2) as follows:

$$R = \frac{AUC_\tau}{AUC_t} \tag{9.1}$$

$$R = \frac{1}{1 - e^{-\lambda_z \tau}} \tag{9.2}$$

where AUC_τ is the AUC over a dosing interval at steady state, AUC_t the AUC up to time $t = \tau$ after a single dose, and λ_z the terminal elimination phase rate constant. The use of equation 9.2 assumes that each dose is administered in the post-distributive phase of the preceding dose or that the PK is monophasic.

The above equations are useful for predicting what concentrations could be achieved following multiple dosing for different dosing intervals; however, in the toxicology studies, accumulation is generally perceived as a negative factor and is often confused with increased concentrations or exposure resulting from changes in the PK of the drug following multiple dosing. These changes in PK can result in a greater than expected degree of accumulation. Changes in the PK of the drug upon multiple dosing are most easily evaluated by comparing the AUC_∞ following a single dose (e.g. on day 1 of the study) to the AUC over a dosing interval (AUC_τ) at steady state. If the PK of the drug does not change with time, then these two AUCs should not be different. It is this concept/comparison which should be emphasised in the analysis of the multiple dose studies and not the 'R' values.

9.3.4 TIME TO STEADY STATE AND 'EFFECTIVE HALF-LIFE'

After dosing, drug is distributed and eliminated at the same time. When a drug distributes rapidly relative to its elimination, the body acts as one compartment, and it takes 3.3 half-lives to reach 90 per cent steady state. In a more slowly equilibrating pool, the body acts as two compartments, and the elimination half-life of the terminal phase determines the time to steady state. If a lot of drug is eliminated before distribution equilibrium is achieved, the elimination may appear biphasic, but the body acts as a single compartment, and it is the half-life of the initial phase that determines the time to steady state.

A basis for deciding which is the relevant half-life to estimate time to steady state rests on area considerations. The areas associated with the two phases of a biexponential curve are $C1/\lambda_1$ and $C2/\lambda_2$.

The area associated with the terminal portion of the curve is defined as:

$$f_2 = \frac{C2/\lambda_2}{C2/\lambda_1 + C2/\lambda_2}$$

where $f_1 + f_2 = 1$. If $f_2 > f_1$ (which is the normal case), then elimination half-life $= 0.693/\lambda_2$. If $f_1 > f_2$ (>than 0.8), then the terminal half-life is not appropriate to describe time to steady state.

The half-life that controls the time to steady state is the one that is involved with the predominant phase involved in the majority of the area. As a reasonable approximation:

$$\text{'Effective' half-life} = f_1 \frac{0.693}{\lambda_1} + f_2 \frac{0.693}{\lambda_2}$$

When sample time points are limited, as in toxicokinetics studies, the pre-clinical data generally show a monophasic elimination. However, from single dose definitive PK studies, the concentration–time profiles are more rigorously monitored, and often times reveal a biphasic elimination (where the terminal phase of elimination is slower than the initial phase of distribution and elimination). Consideration should be made of the extent that the terminal phase contributes to the total AUC. If not predominant, an 'effective half-life' should be estimated based on the elimination rates in the relative fractions of the AUC, and these used for any allometric scaling, rather than the terminal half-life.

9.4 *Reporting*

Toxicokinetic parameters should be clearly defined in regulatory submissions. The data should take the presentation of tabulated exposure data reflecting the relationship between the exposures (C_{max} and AUC) in animals compared to man (a clinical safety matrix). The AUC should be clearly defined (e.g. AUC_∞ or AUC_T or AUC_t). It is recommended that the toxicokinetics be discussed in the pre-clinical PK section of submission documents and also in the toxicology section. The exposure ratios should be discussed directly in relation to the findings of the toxicity studies in the toxicology section of the document. The method of calculation of the exposure ratios should also be defined (see below). The multiple dose kinetics should be discussed, including any implications these may have on the toxicity findings. Cross referencing of the toxicokinetic data between the PK section and the toxicology section should occur throughout to guide the reviewer to the relevant information.

9.5 Application of toxicokinetic data

The primary use of toxicokinetic data is as a measure of systemic exposure. The safety margin is an assessment of safety in man relative to the toxicological species based on extent of systemic exposure. It is generally expressed as:

$$\frac{AUC \text{ at NOTEL or NOAEL for animals}}{AUC \text{ at therapeutic dose level for man}}$$

where NOTEL is the no-toxic-effect-dose-level and NOAEL is the no-adverse-effect-dose-level (generally related to pharmacological effects). C_{max} may be used instead of AUC, depending on which parameter is considered to be more relevant to the toxicological findings.

Regulatory authorities expect to see this ratio to provide comfort in the assessment of risk (i.e. the animals have been exposed to substantially more drug than in humans), and this data should be constructed into a clinical safety matrix (e.g. a table) in the submission document. There are no common recommended ratios which this comfort factor can be based on. Basically, exposure ratios must be 'suitable' for the proposed clinical trial or for the marketing application. The ratios depend on the therapeutic indication (e.g. treatment of chickenpox in children would likely require a much larger exposure ratio than a curative agent) and dosing regimen (e.g. short-term versus chronic administration). In general, the bigger the exposure ratio the better. Therefore, if exposure at a no-effect-level can be maximised, for example by increasing the mid-dose level, this should be done.

One exception where a ratio has been defined is the ICH proposed 25-fold exposure ratio (on a mg/m^2 basis) as a method for selection of the high dose in rodent carcinogenicity studies (ICH Harmonised Tripartite Guideline, 1994 and 1997). Other acceptable criteria for the selection of the high dose may be dose-limiting PD effects, maximum tolerated dose, saturation of absorption or the maximum feasible dose based on formulation. In the ICH guidelines, the justification for the 25-fold exposure ratio includes the statement 'Those pharmaceuticals tested using a 25 fold or greater AUC ratio for the high dose will have exposure ratios greater than 75 per cent of pharmaceuticals tested previously in carcinogenicity studies performed at the MTD'. This suggests that in 75 per cent of cases, the dose level required to reach a 25-fold AUC ratio will exceed the MTD (maximum tolerated dose), a position which is totally unacceptable. Therefore, the MTD is likely to remain the major criteria for high dose selection in carcinogenicity studies.

The exposure ratio is also applicable to extrapolating animal data to humans to aid in the design of the first human volunteer trials. Suitable doses for trial in humans are often selected by extrapolation of the pre-clinical PK/PD data to man, and then the top dose levels restricted by the exposure ratio of the NOTEL in animals compared to the predicted exposures in man.

Toxicokinetic data plays an important role in determining optimal dose levels. Apart from its direct utility in limiting dose due to supra- or sub-proportional kinetics, toxicokinetic data may also be used to refine the mid-dose, for example, when a higher exposure is desired at a no-toxic-effect level.

Toxicokinetics may also be useful in the species selection process. Typically the rat and dog are chosen for pre-clinical toxicity testing. Using sensitive mass spectrometry techniques, it is possible to compare the metabolite profiles in the species of choice, and this may be done at discovery or early development stage. Furthermore, toxicokinetics may supersede single dose studies in some species (e.g. mouse, rabbit) for the provision of pre-clinical PK data and often provide additional information to ADME studies.

Toxicokinetic data may also be used in allometric scaling to predict PK parameters in humans. This is a method of interpolation and extrapolation based on the anatomical, physiological and biochemical similarities in mammals, and has been described in more detail in the pharmacokinetics chapter of this book. The application of an equation ($y = aW^b$) may permit the extrapolation of animal data to human data and thus predict PK parameters and, together with PK/PD data, therapeutic dose levels in man. However, this author has found that scaling with toxicokinetic data may be misleading due to the limited number of time points from this type of data. The use of single dose PK data for allometric scaling has proven more successful.

9.6 *Toxicokinetic–toxicodynamic relationships*

To achieve maximal application of the toxicokinetic data, it is recommended that the relationships between toxicokinetics and toxicodynamics (TK/TD) are investigated whenever possible. Toxicodynamic parameters include organ and body weight changes, histochemistry and pathology scores. TK–TD relationship is often difficult to assess in general toxicity studies due to limited measurements, and may require a dedicated time-course study.

The TK–TD relationship may aid in the selection of candidate compounds, aid in the selection of the clinical starting dose, characterise active or toxic metabolites, elucidate time-dependent toxicokinetic alterations (e.g. induction, inhibition) and help in the assessment and utilisation of safety margins.

The following considerations should help to achieve useful TK–TD relationships:

1 Selection of the most appropriate toxicokinetic parameter AUC, C_{max}, systemic clearance for intravenous administration, cumulative AUC over complete study period.
2 Protein binding and measurement of unbound drug.

3 Tissue concentration measurements (PET scan, microdialysis).
4 Pooling of plasma concentration data across studies and different species.

Notwithstanding the difficulties associated with establishing a TK/TD model, it is recommended that systemic exposure to test substance is linked in some way to toxicity. In this context, consideration should be given to constructing an exposure–toxicity matrix in the submission, based on the most appropriate indices of systemic exposure (C_{max}, AUC), similar to, or in conjunction with, the clinical safety matrix described previously. The exposure–toxicity relationship should be evaluated across species and any differences assessed in terms of protein binding.

Importantly, toxicokinetic data helps explain unanticipated toxicity. For example, decreases in clearance due to saturation of a metabolic pathway may cause non-linear increases in the exposures and concurrent toxicity. Increases in clearance due to enzyme induction may cause decreases in exposure to the test compound and increases in exposure to a metabolite. In these cases, it may be necessary to quantify the metabolite to provide an exposure ratio to aid in the risk assessment to man. Some real examples follow.

9.7 *Dose- and time-dependencies*

Dose- or time-dependencies in the kinetics of drugs indicate that the kinetics is not linear (Figure 9.2). The term 'non-linear' kinetics most often relates to a dose- or time-dependency which causes a supra-proportional increase in exposure relative to the dose increment and are often related to saturable pathways of elimination. Dose-dependencies which result in sub-proportional increases in the exposure relative to the dose increment are often related to saturable absorption. Time-dependencies resulting in decreases in exposure with time are often related to enzyme induction.

L-N^{G}-monomethylarginine (LNMMA) is eliminated primarily by metabolism and subsequent putative amino acid catabolism (Schwartz *et al.*, 1997). These pathways appear to become saturated, and the exposures to LNMMA increase supra-proportionally with the dose increment in rats and dogs. This results in the kinetics becoming non-linear even at low dose levels. With these types of kinetics, there is also a tendency for the exposures to increase with time due to the saturation of the elimination pathway. Upon multiple dosing, the clearance of LNMMA eventually reaches a new steady state, which may be related to a secondary pathway of elimination (possibly renal excretion). This exemplifies a dose-dependency in the toxicokinetics of LNMMA that results in an increase in exposure with time (Table 9.2).

An example of time-dependent kinetics with opposite connotations is from a 5-lipoxegenase inhibitor programme conducted some years back, prior to the consistent subscription to toxicokinetic assessment. The metabolism of some of these compounds was induced by approximately 50 per cent during multiple dosing for as little as 5–7 days. The candidate series suffered from an inherent potential for renal

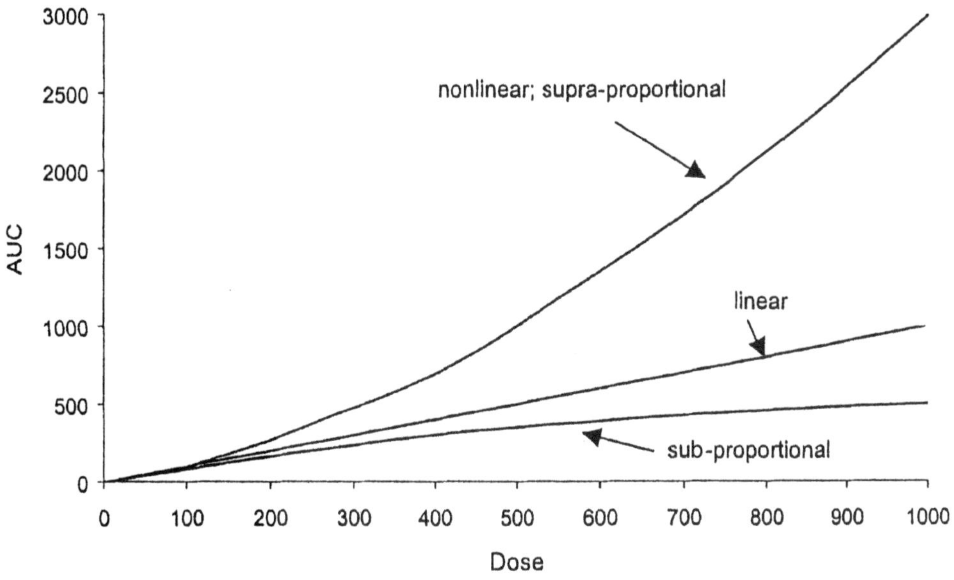

FIGURE 9.2 *Illustration of exposure relationship with dose.*

toxicity, and the successful candidates were selected based on their safety profile. When toxicokinetic data was finally generated, it was clear that the compounds which appeared to produce the best safety profile (minimal or no renal toxicity) were the greatest auto-inducers and thus the compounds which produced the lowest exposures. Indeed, if exposures were increased by incremental dosing following induction, renal toxicity was evident (Figure 9.3). The series was not developed.

Another slightly different example relates to an antiviral compound which was terminated in late phase development. There was renal toxicity associated with this compound also, but it did not manifest itself until the longer-term oncogenicity studies in rats and mice. The exposures to this compound were dose related and remained constant throughout the dosing period. The exposure to the metabolite was sub-proportional with the dose increment (exposures to the metabolite were equal at all doses irrespective of the exposure to the parent compound) during studies of up to approximately three months duration. During longer-term studies, the exposures to

TABLE 9.2 *The toxicokinetics of LNMMA following constant rate infusion; illustrating non-linear kinetics and achievement of steady state clearance*

	0.5 mg/kg/h	1 mg/kg/h	5 mg/kg/h	15 mg/kg/h
C_{ss} (μM)	12	190	630	1190
AUC_{ss} (μM h)	280	4710	15200	28600
CL (mL/h/kg)	230	56	42	67

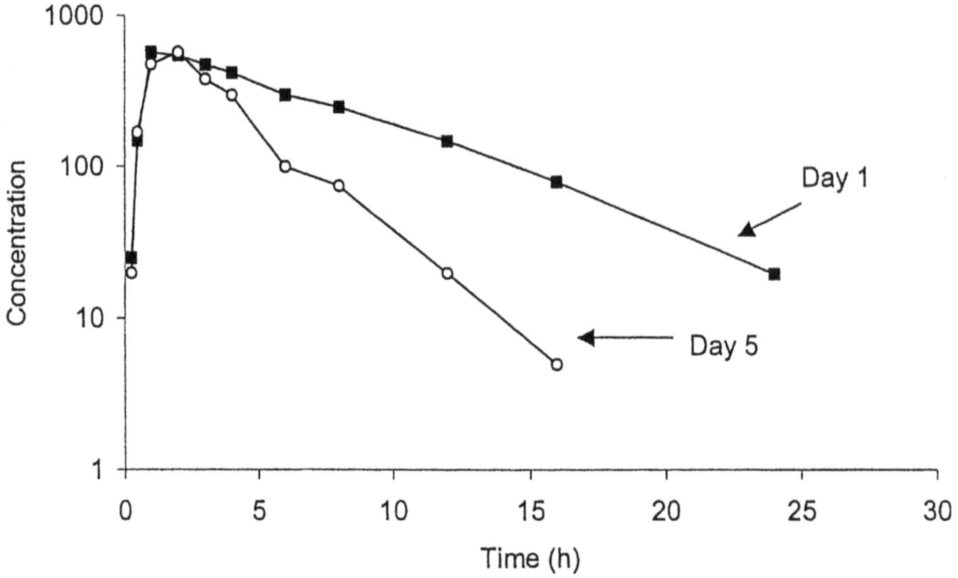

FIGURE 9.3 *Plasma concentration profile of 5-lipoxegenase inhibitor showing enzyme induction in rats.*

the metabolite increased substantially, in a dose-related fashion, without any concomitant decreases in exposure to the parent compound. It was postulated that this was possibly due to an age-related phenomenon (e.g. increased extravascular formation of the metabolite combined with a decrease in clearance of the metabolite). In any case, without the metabolite kinetics, the association between the renal toxicity and the metabolite may never have been drawn (Figures 9.4 and 9.5).

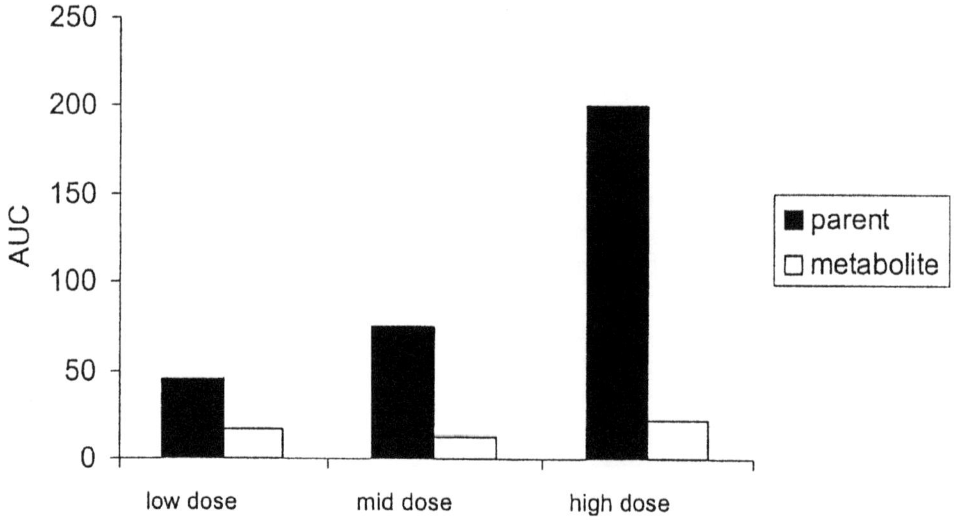

FIGURE 9.4 *Exposure versus dose relationship of an antiviral compound during a 3-month toxicity study in rats; metabolite shows sub-proportional exposure.*

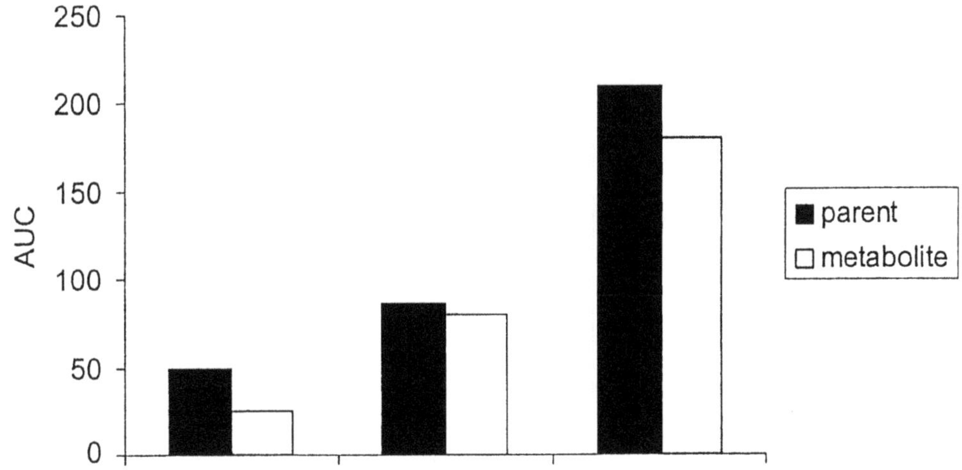

FIGURE 9.5 *Exposure versus dose relationship of an antiviral compound during a 12-month toxicity study in rats; metabolite shows dose-related increase in exposure.*

The reader may find other examples of toxicokinetic applications in the published literature. However, it is often the case that data is not published if there is failure of a developmental project due to toxicity (most often for nothing more than a lack of resource). To truly learn more about how TK and TK–TD may be applicable to the drug development process, scientists should be encouraged to publish more of their successes and failures.

9.8 *References*

ICH Harmonised Tripartite Guideline. Note for guidance on toxicokinetics: the assessment of systemic exposure in toxicity studies (October 1994).

ICH Harmonised Tripartite Guideline. Dose selection for carcinogenicity studies of pharmaceuticals (October 1994) and addendum to 'Dose selection for carcinogenicity studies of pharmaceutical' addition of a limit dose and related notes (July 1997).

Schwartz, S., Clare, R., Devereux, K. and Fook Sheung, C. (1997) Pharmacokinetics, disposition and metabolism of 546C88 (L-N^G-methylarginine hydrochloride) in rat and dog. *Xenobiotica* 27, 1259–1271.

Shah, V., Midha, K., Dighe, S., McGilveray, I., Skelly, J., Yacobi, A., Layloff, T., Viswanathan, C., Cook, C., McDowall, R., Pittman, K. and Spector, S. (1992) Analytical methods validation: bioavailability, bioequivalence, and pharmacokinetic studies. *J. Pharm. Sci.* 81, 309–312.

CHAPTER 10

Protein binding in plasma: a case history of a highly protein-bound drug

Robert J. Barnaby and
Marco Bottacini

10.1 *Introduction*

Protein binding is commonly defined as the reversible association of a drug to the proteins of blood, or more usually plasma. When a drug is administered intravenously or reaches the blood circulation after absorption, it interacts with the available proteins in two different ways: by adsorption on the surface of the proteins or, more rarely, by covalent bonding with active chemical groups of the proteins. When the binding is reversible, there is a dynamic distribution with a transfer between proteins and plasma water. At equilibrium a certain fraction of the total drug amount is bound to plasma proteins. Any factors modifying the nature of the binding interactions (pH change, ionic strength, protein tertiary structure, temperature) and the presence of other competing ligands can modify the extent of binding.

Investigation into the protein binding of new chemical entities is an important activity in the drug development process due to its role in determining clearance and distribution parameters. A summary of the basic concepts with some technical considerations is given, together with a description of a case history of a highly bound drug.

10.2 *The protein binding equilibrium*

The interaction of drugs with proteins can be treated as an equilibrium, obeying the law of mass action kinetics. Therefore it can be described by the reversible equation:

$$[D] + [P] \Leftrightarrow [DP] \qquad (10.1)$$

where [D], [P] and [DP] are the molar concentrations of unbound drug, unoccupied protein binding sites and drug–protein complex, respectively, and k_{on} and k_{off} are the rate constants for the forward (association) and reverse (dissociation) reactions, respectively. The equilibrium *association constant* (K_a, molar^{-1} units) for this reaction is defined as:

$$K_a = \frac{k_{on}}{k_{off}} = \frac{[DP]}{[D][P]} \qquad (10.2)$$

and it provides an index of the affinity between the drug and the binding sites. The total concentration of the binding sites is the sum of unoccupied [P] and occupied binding sites [DP]: this total concentration of sites is referred to as the *capacity constant* (*N*) and has units of sites/L. Since a given protein can have several classes of independent binding sites, the capacity constant represents the product of the 'number of sites/mole of protein' and the molar concentration of protein. Combining all these equations and considering all classes of binding sites, the concentration of bound drug [DP] in a protein solution can be expressed as:

$$[DP] = \sum \frac{Ntot_i[D]}{Kd_i + [D]} \qquad (10.3)$$

where i refers to the number of different classes of binding sites.

10.3 *Determinants of the unbound fraction*

Equation 10.3 can be rearranged so that the *unbound plasma fraction* (*fu*) of drug is represented as:

$$fu = \frac{[D]}{[DP]} = \frac{Kd + [D]}{Ntot + [D] + Kd} \qquad (10.4)$$

Therefore, for a drug that binds to a single class of binding site, the bound drug fraction depends on the equilibrium-free drug concentration, the dissociation constant and the protein concentration. Normally the fraction bound remains constant within a wide concentration range, including the therapeutic range. However, for some drugs (e.g. valproic acid, salicylic acid and several non-steroidal anti-inflammatory drugs), proteins appear to have very limited binding capacity, showing an increase of unbound drug when the total drug concentration is increased (concentration-dependent binding (Lin, 1987; MacKichan, 1992)). Plasma proteins in general have a high capacity for binding and are able to 'extract' certain drug molecules from aqueous solution or suspension. This can be due to a large number of binding sites on each protein molecule and/or high binding affinity. Specific binding sites (high K_a values, low binding capacity) predominate at low drug concentrations, while non-specific binding ones (low K_a values, high binding capacity) predominate at higher concentrations. The possibility of a cooperative binding has also been suggested whereby the affinity of the drug increases as more binding occurs.

10.4 *Principal plasma binding proteins*

Human plasma contains about 100 proteins of which 13 are present at concentrations higher than 1 g/L. Among these latter, six are able to bind drugs: human serum albumin (HSA), α1-acid glycoprotein (AAG), lipoproteins (VLDL, LDL, HDL) and immunoglobulins G (IgG) (Table 10.1). However, albumin is by far the largest contributor to plasma protein binding since it represents 60 per cent of the total plasma proteins. It is principally involved in the binding of most anionic drugs and many endogenous anions. However, many cationic and neutral drugs also bind appreciably to AAG and/or lipoproteins (Table 10.2).

Various disease states can modify the extent of the binding of drugs to plasma proteins (Tillement *et al.*, 1978; MacKichan, 1992). The modification can be due

TABLE 10.1 *Characteristic of the drug binding proteins in plasma*

	Albumin	AAG	Lipoproteins
Molecular weight	66300	40000	200000–1000000
Normal serum conc. (mg/100 mL)	3500–5500	55–140	VLDL: <40 HDL: >35 LDL: 70–205
Half-life (days)	19	5.5	up to 6
Distribution	40% intravascular 60% extravascular		

TABLE 10.2 *Predominant binding proteins of some common drugs bound >70 per cent to plasma proteins*

Albumin	Albumin and AAG	Albumin and lipoproteins	Albumin, AAG, and lipoproteins
Ceftriaxone (A)	Alprenolol (B)	Cyclosporine (N)[b]	Amitriptylline (B)
Clindamycin (A)	Carbamazepine (N)	Probucol (N)[b]	Bupivicaine (B)
Clofibrate (A)	Disopyramide (B)[b]		Chlorpromazine (B)
Dexamethasone (N)	Erythromycin (B)		Diltiazem (B)
Diazepam (B)	Lidocaine (B)		Imipramine (B)
Diazoxide (A)	Meperidine (B)		Nortriptyline (B)
Dicloxacillin (A)	Methadone (B)		Perazine (B)
Digitoxin (N)	Verapamil (B)		Propranolol (B)
Etoposide (N)			Quinidine (B)
Ibuprofen (A)			
Indomethacin (A)			
Nafcillin (A)			
Naproxen (A)			
Oxacillin (A)			
Phenylbutazone (A)			
Phenytoin (A)			
Probenecid (A)			
Salicylic acid (A)			
Sulfisoxazole (A)			
Teniposide (N)			
Thiopental (A)			
Tolbutamide (A)			
Valproic acid (A)			
Warfarin (A)			

[a] A = Acid; B = Base; N = Neutral.
[b] Albumin is minor binding protein.

to a series of both physiological (pregnancy, gender, smoking, obesity, nutritional status, surgery, extremes of age) and pathological conditions (renal and liver disease, infarction, cancer, injuries, diabetes, thyroid diseases, cystic fibrosis, inflammatory arthritis, hyperlipoproteinemia).

10.4.1 Human serum albumin (HSA)

Albumin is a single peptide chain of about 580 amino acid residues. The primary physiological roles of albumin are to maintain colloid osmotic pressure in the vascular system and to transport fatty acid and bilirubin. It is not confined to plasma, but is continuously filtered at a slow rate into interstitial fluid. It is also present in the cerebrospinal fluid (Table 10.3). Albumin-bound drug is therefore found not only in plasma, but also in the interstitial fluid, which contains 60 per cent of the albumin in the body.

Two primary areas of 'high affinity' drug binding sites have been defined on albumin. These have been nominated the *warfarin site* (site I) and the *benzodiazepine site* (site II). Both the sites are in reality shared with other drug and endogenous compounds. Several drugs (e.g. naproxen, tolbutamide, indomethacin) bind to both sites. With the help of fluorescent probes, additional binding sites and their locations have been proposed (Hervé, 1994) (Figure 10.1). Basic drugs can also bind to albumin, but binding of such drugs in plasma is too high to be accounted for by their binding to albumin alone. Albumin tends to show a low affinity and a high capacity for these basic drugs and a variation in albumin concentrations, for example, does not result in marked changes in their plasma protein binding.

10.4.2 α1-Acid glycoprotein (AAG)

AAG (orosomucoid) is a glycoprotein with a lower molecular weight than albumin and is characterised by its high carbohydrate content. It is a monomer of 181 amino acids and 40 per cent of glucid residues. Binding of drugs to AAG appears to involve hydrophobic rather than electrostatic forces. AAG is present in plasma at concentrations which normally are 100 times lower than for albumin. In contrast to the homogeneity of albumin, polymorphic forms of AAG are normally found (Lunde, 1986). These variants may be selective and possess different drug binding capacities. The drug binding sites are believed to be located on the polypeptide chain and may be shared by both acids and bases. Although AAG is known to be a major binding protein for many basic drugs, it also binds some acidic and neutral drugs, but to a lesser extent. Warfarin, for example, can compete with drugs that bind to AAG. In general, AAG is referred to as a 'low capacity, high affinity' protein, while albumin is a 'high capacity, low affinity' one. The plasma concentration of AAG is very much subject to disease and stress state. Elevated levels of AAG are seen in different states of inflammation or injury, therefore an increase in AAG-binding capacity can be observed in these patients compared to healthy volunteers.

TABLE 10.3 *Normal albumin content in various fluids*

	Plasma	Transudates	Pleural fluid	Pericardial fluid	Peritoneal fluid	CSF
Albumin (g/L)	40	20	9	20	9	0.2

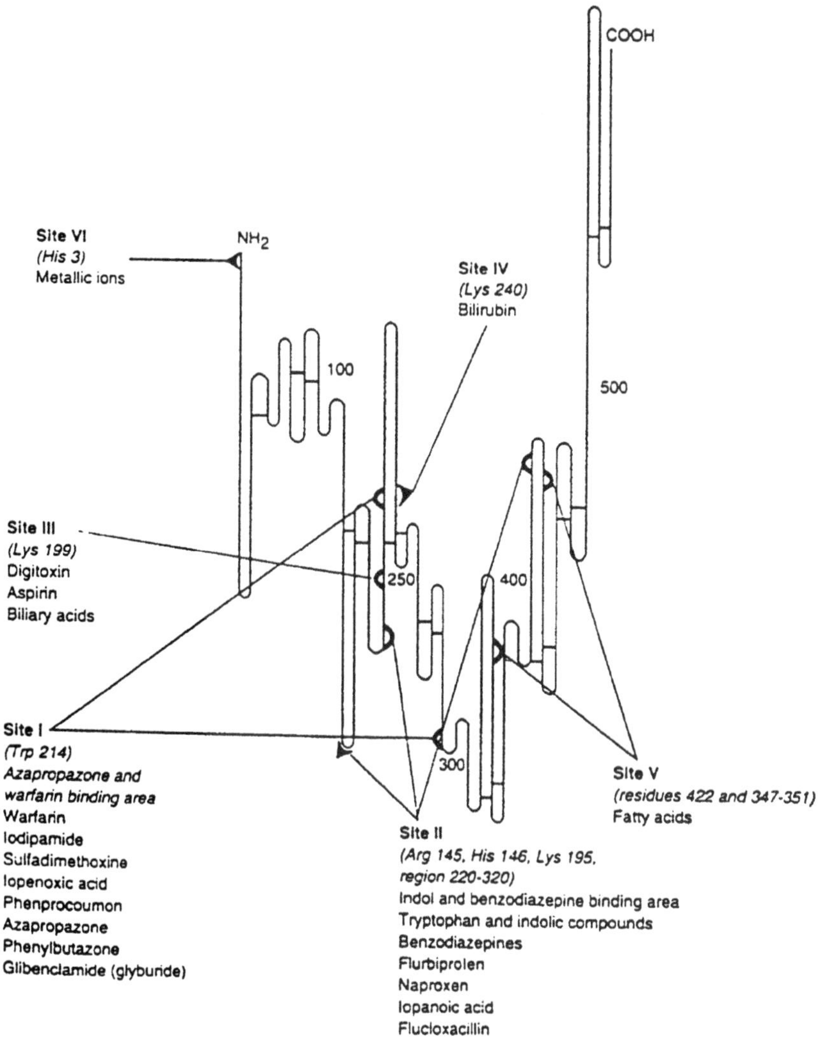

FIGURE 10.1 *Location of binding sites in human serum albumin* (reproduced with permission from Adis International).

10.4.3 LIPOPROTEINS

Lipoproteins are an extremely heterogeneous group of proteins that have a wide range of molecular weights and lipid contents (Zini, 1991). Their tertiary and quaternary structures are not fully elucidated but polar proteins and lipids surround a hydrophobic centre composed of non-polar lipids. The three most important groups are: very low density lipoproteins (VLDL), low density lipoproteins (LDL) and high density lipoproteins (HDL) (Table 10.4). Their concentrations can vary

TABLE 10.4 *Characteristic of plasma lipoproteins*

	VLDL	LDL	HDL
Molecular weight	10^7	3×10^6	3×10^5
Proteins (%)	10	20	50
Cholesterol (%)	20	48	10
Phospholipids (%)	20	24	22
Triglycerides (%)	50	8	18
Fasting conc. (g/L)	1.2	55	32.5
Plasma amount (%)	12.5	55	32.5

extensively in the normal population. They transport fatty acids, triglycerides, phospholipids and cholesterol and may also be responsible for the binding of certain drugs such as chlorpromazine, imipramine, probucol, cyclosporine, tetracyclines and nicardipine. However, nearly all types of drugs are capable of binding to isolated lipoproteins, provided they exhibit a certain degree of lipophilicity. Drugs that 'bind' to lipoproteins are thought to actually be partitioning into the lipid core of the protein instead of associating with a specific site. For this reason competition between drugs for specific sites is not likely to occur and concentration-dependent binding is not expected.

10.5 *The importance of protein binding in drug development*

10.5.1 PHARMACOKINETICS

Plasma protein binding can be important in determining drug distribution, metabolism and elimination. It is widely accepted that only the unbound drug can diffuse across membrane barriers and interact with metabolic enzymes. The interaction of the free drug with the tissues can also affect its distribution. The determinants of binding in tissues exposed to the drug are the same as those for plasma: protein concentration, affinity to the proteins, unbound drug concentration available. However, overall tissue binding in the body (the unbound fraction, fu_t) is difficult to measure, though most recent techniques (i.e. microdialysis) may help.

The PK parameters, which are the determinants of the drug concentration–time plasma profile, are steady-state volume of distribution (V_{ss}), clearance (CL) and elimination half-life ($t_{1/2}$). It is important to understand the influence of protein binding on each of these parameters.

Volume of distribution

The magnitude of drug binding in plasma versus that in tissue is the primary determinant of the apparent volume of distribution of a drug:

$$V_{ss} = V_p + \left(\frac{fu_p}{fu_t}\right) \times V_t \qquad (10.5)$$

where fu_p is the unbound fraction in plasma, fu_t is the unbound fraction of drug in tissue, V_p is plasma volume (approx. 0.07 L/kg in humans), V_t is the tissue volume (0.6 L/kg in humans).

An estimate of overall tissue binding in the body can be made when V_{ss} and fu_p are known and anatomic volumes are assumed.

Many drugs (e.g. amiodarone, many tryciclic antidepressants) have very large distribution volumes (20–70 L/kg) because they are much more highly bound in tissue than to plasma proteins. On the other hand, the small distribution volumes of warfarin, valproic acid, penicillins (0.1–0.5 L/kg) are attributable to high plasma binding relative to tissue binding.

Clearance

The understanding of the relationship between protein binding in plasma and organ clearance is aided by the physiological model of hepatic clearance (Wilkinson and Shand, 1975). According to this model, an organ clearance, and hence the average steady-state concentration C_{ss}, is determined by three physiological variables: organ blood flow (Q), intrinsic organ clearance (CL_{int}) and the unbound fraction of drug in blood (fu_b) as follows:

$$CL = Q \times \frac{CL_{int} \times fu_b}{Q + CL_{int} \times fu_b} \qquad (10.6)$$

The concept of 'restrictive' and 'non-restrictive' clearance needs to be adopted in order to explain how protein binding is involved in the clearance process. A drug is said to undergo restrictive clearance when intrinsic organ clearance is such that:

$$Q \gg CL_{int} \times fu_b$$

Thus, equation 10.6 can be simplified to:

$$CL \approx CL_{int} \times fu_b \qquad (10.7)$$

According to this relationship, the clearance is proportional to the unbound fraction. Displacement of plasma protein binding of one drug by a co-administered drug is possible: however, as long as there is no effect on intrinsic organ clearance (enzyme induction/inhibition), effects of protein-binding displacement will not affect the average free plasma concentration of drugs. Figure 10.2 shows the effect of an increase of unbound fraction (i.e. after displacement) on C_{ss} (unbound), C (bound), CL and fu.

In the case of non-restrictive clearance, protein binding does not appear to protect the drug from elimination. The clearance is determined primarily by organ blood flow, is less influenced by intrinsic clearance and is independent of the unbound fraction. To complicate the situation still further, there is a growing evidence that also the bound fraction, in the form of AAG or lipoprotein complexes, may be taken up into organs by endocytotic mechanisms.

Elimination half-life

The elimination phase is closely related to V_{ss} for most drugs. The half-life of a restrictively cleared drug which has a moderate-to-large V_{ss} value (i.e. >0.4 L/kg) is less influenced by V_p (10.5). It is determined by the simplified equation:

$$t_{1/2} \approx 0.693\left(\frac{V_t}{CLu_{int} \times fu_t}\right) \tag{10.8}$$

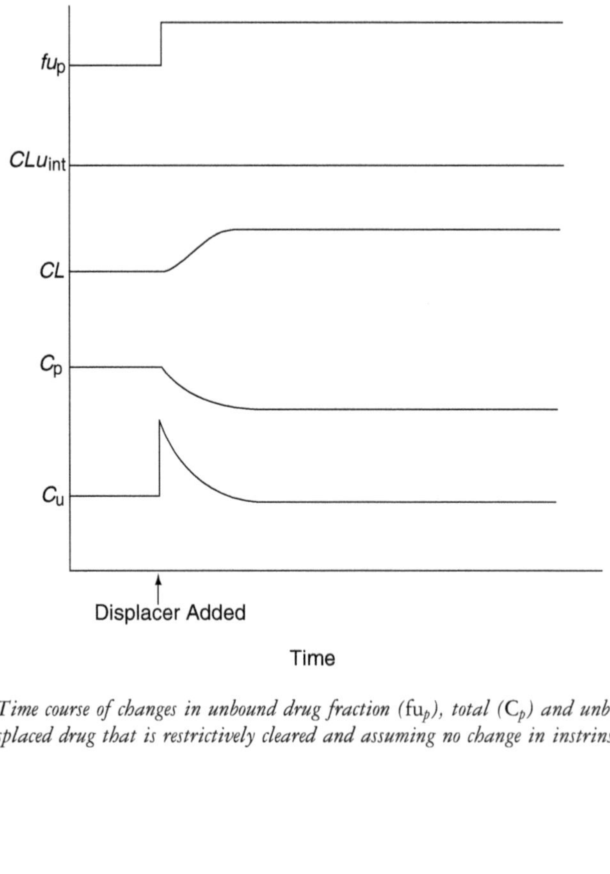

FIGURE 10.2 *Time course of changes in unbound drug fraction (fu$_p$), total (C$_p$) and unbound drug concentrations (Cu$_p$) for a displaced drug that is restrictively cleared and assuming no change in instrinsic clearance.*

So, altered plasma protein binding will have little effect on the half-lives of high distribution volume drugs such as diazepam and phenytoin. When V_{ss} values are less than 0.4 L/kg (warfarin), $t_{1/2}$ is affected by changes in plasma (and tissue) binding according to the simplified equation:

$$t_{1/2} \approx 0.693\left(\frac{V_{\mathrm{p}}}{CLu_{\mathrm{int}} \times fu_{\mathrm{p}}} + \frac{V_{\mathrm{t}}}{CLu_{\mathrm{int}} \times fu_{\mathrm{t}}}\right) \tag{10.9}$$

In the case of non-restrictively cleared drugs, the half-life is influenced by both plasma and tissue binding, according to:

$$t_{1/2} \approx 0.693\left[V_{\mathrm{p}} + \left(\frac{fu_{\mathrm{p}}}{fu_{\mathrm{t}}}\right)V_t\right] \tag{10.10}$$

Decreased binding in plasma will increase the V_{ss} and prolong the half-life, while increased plasma binding will shorten half-life. For drugs with very small volumes of distribution (penicillins), the effects of altered plasma and tissue binding on elimination of half-life will be minimal.

10.5.2 Toxicological cover

Traditionally, in order to predict a potentially toxic dose in man, the exposure of the species to the drug is measured using the plasma area under the time–concentration curve (*AUC*). Ideally, the *AUC* observed at the highest dose in man should not exceed that giving no toxicological effect in animals, and normally it is preferred that there be a reasonable margin to account for potential differences in distribution and elimination of the drug (safety margin). In cases in which the drug shows high restrictive plasma protein binding and/or wide variability in the extent of binding between humans and non-clinical species, it can be more meaningful to determine safety margins on the basis of unbound drug.

10.5.3 Protein-binding displacement

Drug–drug interactions due to alteration of the plasma protein binding of a drug by another drug have been the subject of many debates in the literature. Many of the first examples of clinically significant drug–drug interactions thought to be due to alteration of plasma protein binding were in fact due to metabolic interactions (Rolan, 1994). It was believed by many clinicians that a displacement of protein binding was potentially of critical importance as the free concentration is widely believed to represent the pharmacologically active fraction as only the free concentration is able to pass through membrane barriers. However, a displacement of the protein binding of a drug will only cause a transient increase in free drug concentration, as for most drugs of low to moderate clearance the increase in free concentration will also cause an increase in clearance as well as an increase in volume of distribution. Therefore total concentration will fall until the free concentration reaches previous equilibrium levels (see Figure 10.2). Consequently, the only effect of a protein-binding displacement is to decrease total concentration, increase %unbound but the free concentration remains constant. Therefore, if the pharmacological action depends on the free plasma concentration, no difference in drug activity should occur as long as the transient increase is not relevant. However, this is only partly true as volume of distribution also increases, although not to the same extent as the increase in clearance (MacKichan, 1989; Rolan, 1994; Sansom, 1995).

10.6 *Techniques for measurement: a brief review of the more popular techniques including advantages and disadvantages*

The *in vitro* measurement of drug binding to plasma proteins is used to calculate PK parameters and make predictions on the PK behaviour of the drug. The major concern in this extrapolation from *in vitro* to *in vivo* is the possibility that the binding values could be misleading because of procedure artefacts. The advantages and disadvantages of the three most common methods for plasma protein binding are discussed below. These techniques are useful also in studies where single proteins are used in order to determine the major contributing proteins, kinetics of binding and type of binding sites although this information may have little physiological or clinical relevance. Moreover, some of the listed techniques are also applicable to investigate the binding of the drug to tissue homogenates.

It must be underlined that very often the protein binding values obtained using different techniques can be significantly different due to the different technical aspects. Thus, an overall recommendation is difficult to make as it is important to take into account the final aim of the investigation and the intrinsic characteristics of the drug. The available techniques have been extensively reviewed by Oravcova (1996), Wright (1996) and Zini (1991).

10.6.1 Equilibrium dialysis

Equilibrium dialysis has been by far the more widely used method to study ligand–protein interactions. As a typical example of equilibrium dialysis, the solution of a high molecular weight compound (the protein) containing a ligand (the drug) is separated by a semi-permeable membrane with a known molecular weight cut-off from a buffer solution. After the equilibrium has been reached, the concentration of the free ligand is equal on both sides of the membrane. According to the Fick's law, the rate of diffusion of the ligand depends on the surface area, the thickness of the membrane, the concentration range, the filling volume and the diffusion coefficient. The latter is a function of both the molecular weight, temperature and characteristic of the ligand. To meet the optimal requirements, some dialysing systems (Spectrum® cells, for example) have been specially designed. With these cells, the ratio between the membrane surface and the working volume is optimised. Plasma and buffer are placed in their respective reservoirs separated by the dialysis membrane. The system is then incubated at the desired temperature and allowed to reach equilibrium. Then, the fluid from each reservoir is removed and analysed for drug concentrations. The post-dialysis drug concentration in the buffer reservoir (C_u) will be in equilibrium with the free drug concentration in the plasma reservoir so that the percent of binding will be as follows:

$$\%\text{bound} = \frac{C_t - C_u}{C_t} \times 100 \qquad (10.11)$$

where C_t is the drug concentration in the plasma reservoir after dialysis. There are numerous variables that must be controlled in equilibrium dialysis experiments in order to obtain accurate results: the incubation temperature and time for incubation, the non-specific binding to the apparatus or membrane, the solubility of the drug in the buffer, the radiochemical purity of the drug (Joshi, 1994), the pH at which the incubation is performed, the volume shift due to Gibbs-Donnan equilibrium (Lima, 1983; Bowers, 1984).

10.6.2 Ultrafiltration

This method of separating drug-bound from free drug is extremely popular because of the availability of a large number of commercial easy-to-use filtration devices (Amicon®, Millipore®, BioRad®). Ultrafiltration is mainly used under negative pressure by centrifugation at 1,000–2,000 g for 15–30 minutes. The principle of this separation procedure is that incubation between drug and protein is terminated by putting the incubate through a filtration membrane of known molecular weight, cut-off with the free drug passing through the filter. The free concentration will be constant in ultrafiltrate and retentate. However, the free concentration remains constant during filtration provided that the filtered volume does not exceed 40 per cent of the introduced total volume. The percentage of unbound is calculated by:

$$\%\text{unbound} = \frac{C_u}{C_t} \times 100 \qquad (10.12)$$

where C_u is the drug concentration in the ultrafiltrate (unbound) and C_t is the total concentration before the experiment. As for equilibrium dialysis, non-specific binding may be high with this technique. However, the relative low cost, easiness and speed of assay have contributed to the widespread use of this technique.

10.6.3 Ultracentrifugation

With this technique, the drug–protein complex formed during incubation is determined by pelleting the complex using high speed centrifugation, leaving the free drug in the supernatant. The time and the rate of centrifugation are kept constant as far as the entire sedimentation process is completed. After centrifugation, at typically 100,000 g for some hours, an aliquot of supernatant is taken to measure the free drug concentration.

The percentage of unbound is calculated by:

$$\%\text{unbound} = \frac{C_u}{C_t} \times 100 \tag{10.13}$$

where C_u is the drug concentration in the supernatant (unbound) and C_t is the total concentration before the experiment. The applicability of this technique is limited by a series of factors: costly equipment, low sample throughput, limited volume for free assay, physical phenomena (sedimentation, back diffusion, binding to lipoproteins).

10.7 *GV150526A: a case history of a highly bound drug*

GV150526 is a potent and selective antagonist of the modulatory glycine site of the *N*-methyl-D-aspartate receptor and is in development as a possible therapy to reduce neuronal damage after cerebral ischemia stroke.

The structure of GV150526A (sodium salt) is shown in Figure 10.3. The compound is characterised by a fairly high lipophilicity (log D at pH 7.4 = 1.9) and a fairly acidic carboxylic acid group (pK_a 3.3) and hence it was expected to possess a reasonably high binding to albumin.

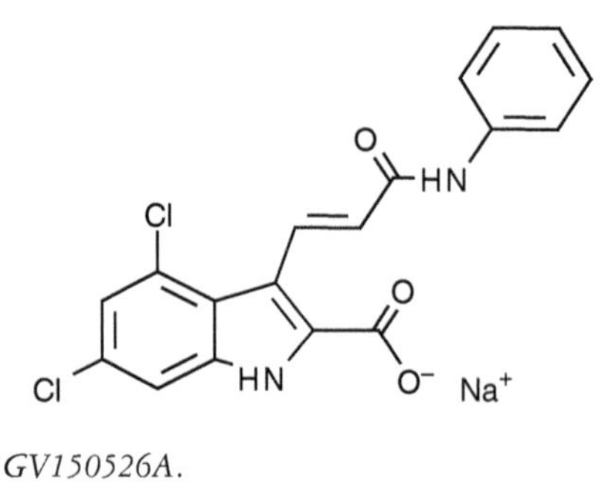

FIGURE 10.3 *Structure of GV150526A.*

Equilibrium dialysis was chosen as the technique of choice because of the high sensitivity required and an already known problem of high non-specific binding.

10.7.1 Non-specific binding

The standards' tests were conducted in order to establish the correct conditions for equilibrium dialysis including estimation of dialysis time to obtain equilibrium, volume shift and non-specific binding to the dialysis material. By dialysing pure solutions of GV150526 in phosphate buffer, evidence was obtained that substantial non-specific binding to the Teflon cells or dialysis membrane was present. However, this factor is not a limitation to performing equilibrium dialysis as long as the degree of non-specific binding or the amount of compound bound non-specifically, is minor compared to the amount in the plasma compartment and enough time is allowed to eventually obtain equilibrium. Plasma protein-bound compound will continually dissociate from its plasma protein binding sites until all non-specific binding sites are saturated and then the true compound bound–unbound equilibrium situation can be measured. In practice, low molecular weight endogenous dialysable material from plasma will also bind to these sites, so in practice equilibrium should be reached relatively quickly. This situation is different to that of ultrafiltration where the unbound fraction is separated from the 'reserve' of bound compound therefore any effect of non-specific binding to the apparatus or filter membrane will produce an underestimate of the free concentration.

10.7.2 Use of radiolabel

Initial attempts to determine the protein binding in plasma were made using a ^{14}C-labelled compound possessing a radiochemical purity of 98 per cent. It was immediately observed that the binding was very high, certainly greater than 99 per cent. However, when the fraction of binding approaches the radiochemical purity the effect of the radiochemical impurities cannot be ignored.

Consequently, care has to be taken when using radiolabelled compounds, without HPLC separation, to measure the binding of highly bound drugs (Honoré, 1987) as any impurity in the radiolabelled compound could have a completely different binding to the parent compound and falsify the result. Analysing the buffer after dialysis by HPLC, in fact, confirmed that the ratio of radioactive impurity (more polar than GV150526) to GV150526 after dialysis was significantly higher than in the starting compound, indicating a much lower binding of the impurity to plasma proteins. Thus the result of binding using the radiolabelled compound without HPLC separation was significantly under-estimated. Therefore all future work was performed using cold compound and HPLC methods.

10.7.3 Identification of principal binding proteins

Studies were performed to determine the main proteins involved in GV150526 binding in human plasma. Albumin, α1-glycoprotein, low and high density lipoproteins and gamma globulin were tested. Albumin was shown to be the most important protein, binding GV150526 to the extent of >99.99 per cent at clinically relevant concentrations. Binding to lipoproteins was in the range 90–94 per cent. Two binding sites to HSA were observed, one with a very high affinity (Kd_1 0.5 μM) and the second with much lower affinity (Kd_2 100 μM).

10.7.4 Linearity of protein binding

The binding of drugs to plasma proteins is usually quoted as a percentage of the total drug that is bound. This value depends on the number of binding sites available which is related to the concentration of protein and the affinity of the drug for the various proteins. The concentration of albumin, the principal binding protein on plasma has a normal concentration of around 40 mg/mL (about 550 μM). When the plasma concentration of drugs with high binding affinity to albumin increases to a level where all the available sites are occupied, then the binding is said to be saturated and the %binding will decrease with increasing plasma concentration. For GV150526 this would be expected in humans when plasma concentrations approach approximately 100 μM (affinity constant Kd_2). The saturation of binding may result in an increased clearance and/or an increased volume of distribution and may result in non-linear kinetics.

In the concentration range studied, the test compound demonstrated non-linear protein binding above certain concentrations (Figure 10.4). These concentrations were different between animals and man and also shown to be different between healthy volunteers and stroke patients. The binding in rat and dog saturated at lower concentrations compared to human volunteers. This causes a complex relationship of %unbound–total concentration between animals and man which was important to understand in the determination of toxicological cover for man (see Section 10.7.5). At lower total concentrations, there is a lower difference between man and animals than at higher concentrations ratio. For example at 75 μg/mL the ratio between rat:dog:human volunteers is 6:16:1 whereas at 150 μg/mL the ratio is 36:50:1. There is a clear difference between healthy volunteer and stroke patients, with, for patients, a lower concentration in which saturation occurs and hence a higher fraction unbound at the higher total concentration studied. This is probably due to a number of factors possibly including lower plasma albumin concentrations due to age factors (Mayersohn, 1992), co-administered medications and altered biochemical parameters due to the disease state. This difference also signifies a different relationship in protein binding between stroke patients and animals. At 75 μg/mL the ratio rat:dog:patients is 4:16:1, whereas at 150 μg/mL the ratio

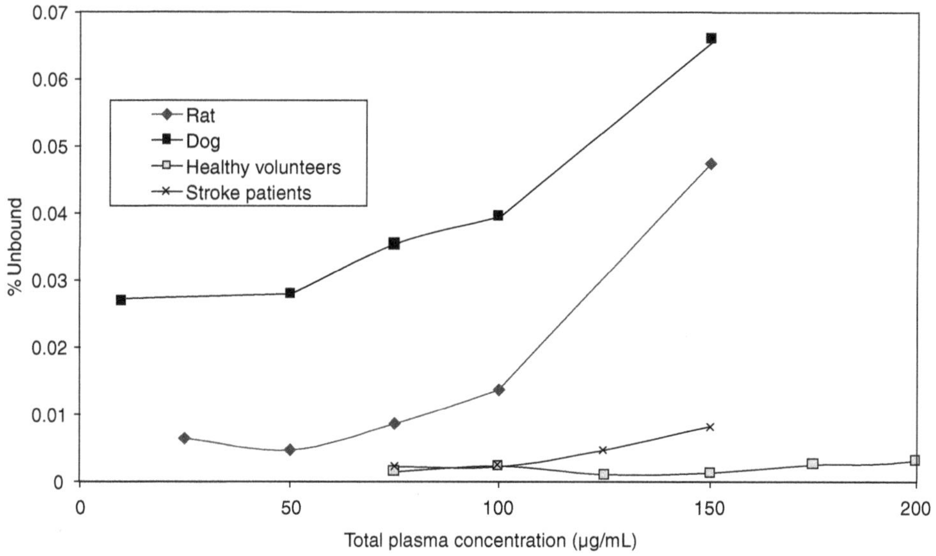

FIGURE 10.4 *Comparison of GV150526 %unbound between rat, dog, human volunteer and stroke patient's plasma.*

becomes 6:8:1, which is considerably less than the ratio between animals and healthy volunteers.

GV150526 is very similar to warfarin in its characteristics as it is a fairly lipophilic acidic compound, which is almost completely eliminated hepatically, and has a very low clearance and volume of distribution in animals and man. Therefore it should be expected that if there are differences in protein binding between animal species, then plasma clearance is also likely to differ. Where binding is very high, as in this case, small changes in %bound can produce large differences in clearance. Figure 10.5 shows the plasma protein binding of GV150526 in mouse, rat, dog, rabbit and man and their correlation with clearance. As can be seen, there is a very close correlation between the fraction unbound and clearance for GV150526, and the inter-species differences in clearance are large. Man has the lowest clearance whilst rat, dog, mouse and rabbit have 15-, 25-, 76- and 200-fold higher clearance, respectively. The inter-species differences in albumin binding may reflect differences in affinity or number of binding sites for GV150526 and are probably caused by the known differences in the amino acid sequence around the principal albumin binding sites between animal species (Lin, 1987).

10.7.5 Toxicological cover

Regarding toxicological cover, two important problems were encountered during the pre-clinical development of GV150526. First, little significant toxicity was

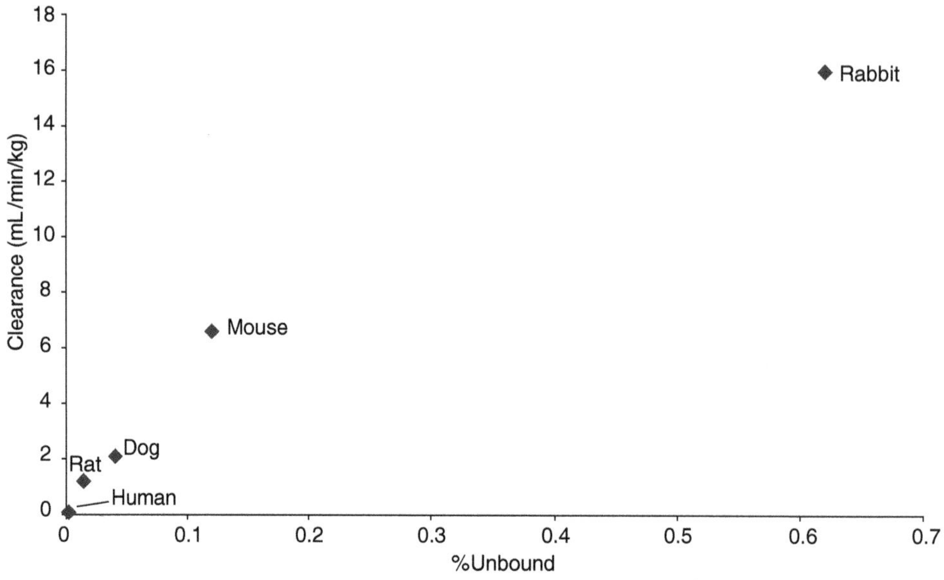

FIGURE 10.5 *Relationship between protein binding (%unbound) in plasma and clearance in toxicological species and man.*

demonstrated at the highest dose administrable in animals. This was in part due to the low intrinsic toxicity of the compound but also due to the fact that chronic testing at very high doses was limited by injection site irritancy. Second, the large differences in protein binding and clearance between the main toxicological species and man made it difficult to obtain standard toxicological cover. As the protein binding in human plasma was higher than all the species tested and consequently clearance was lower, the plasma *AUC* was always much higher in man compared to animals, at a given dose. Therefore these factors made it difficult to administer high enough doses in animals to provide enough toxicological cover for man, based on plasma total concentrations. However in this case the standard approach of using total concentrations to calculate *AUC* is not the most appropriate one. For GV150526, the target organs for toxicity were the eliminating organs, liver and kidney. It is likely that target organ toxicity initiates when a certain critical concentration is exceeded. For drugs with very low clearance and elimination half-life this critical concentration will be exceeded if dose is increased and also if plasma total clearance increases and therefore toxicity should not only be dependent on dose but also on clearance. As, in this case, clearance is highly correlated to the unbound or free fraction in plasma, drug exposure and therefore toxicity of the eliminating organs should be much more closely correlated with the free plasma concentrations rather than total concentrations. Therefore the evaluation of toxicological cover is more correctly based on free concentrations and free *AUC* for this compound. Initially, estimates of free *AUC* were obtained by measuring the free concentration from *in vivo* samples at only the maximum concentration of the time–concentration profile and using the calculated %bound value to determine free *AUC* from the total *AUC* measured. This was done to limit the number of animals used in the study, as the determination of the protein binding of GV150526 with equilibrium dialysis requires 1 mL of plasma, due to the very high analytical sensitivity needed. However, the protein binding of this compound was shown (see Figure 10.4) to be non-linear in rats and dogs at the concentrations observed during the toxicological studies. Therefore, to more accurately estimate free *AUC* in these studies, extensive *in vitro* data on the correlation of %unbound versus total concentration were produced over the entire concentration range encountered. This data was then used to calculate (by linear interpolation) the %unbound at each concentration time point in the profile and so more accurately determine free *AUC* in toxicity studies. This approach was deemed valid as the *in vivo* and *in vitro* %unbound values were very similar, probably due to the fact that the levels of GV150526 metabolites in plasma were generally very low compared to GV150526.

As GV150526 displays restrictive plasma protein binding, it is likely that the fraction unbound will also be related to the degree of brain penetration (Robinson and Rapoport, 1986). To take this into account, the anticipated efficacious dose in man was extrapolated from the principal animal model of activity using free plasma concentrations. An efficacious dose in man was predicted when the free plasma concentration exceeded the maximum free concentration observed after a maximally efficacious dose in the rat pharmacological model. The clinical dosage regimen was then designed so that free concentrations in the clinic were always above this threshold level. Despite the very high restrictive protein binding and the consequent low brain penetration, GV150526 is very efficacious in animal models of stroke due to the high receptor affinity and low toxicity, the latter enabling the administration of very high doses.

10.7.6 Protein-binding displacement

If pharmacological activity depends on distribution into tissues, such as the CNS, a protein-binding displacement due to concomitantly administered medications could potentially cause some change in drug activity.

In the case of GV150526, where the target organs for toxicity were the eliminating organs, kidney and liver, there was much concern over the possibility of abruptly increasing free concentration and so increasing clearance. Renal damage in rats appeared to be related to free concentration. Renal toxicity was more apparent after a bolus administration, where protein binding was saturated at the high plasma concentrations obtained, compared to long infusion and strongly related to the concentration of parent GV150526 in urine. Because of these findings, potential protein-binding displacements in human plasma were studied *in vitro* in order to obtain more information about which type of drugs could potentially alter the plasma protein binding on GV150526 in the clinic and alter toxicity. The real *in vivo* effect of protein-binding displacement by these drugs could then be tested in the clinic. Drugs studied were chosen depending on their likely concommitant administration with GV150526, their binding affinity to albumin and their therapeutic concentrations and on previous knowledge of clinically relevant protein-binding interactions. The drugs studied were warfarin, phenytoin, ibuprofen, phenylbutazone, salicylic acid, heparin and tissue plasminogen activator. Bilirubin was also included. To study a worst case situation, the median peak concentration of GV150526 observed in stroke patients was chosen. The potential displacer was tested at three different concentrations around its normal therapeutic concentration range. The results are summarised in Table 10.5. Phenytoin, ibuprofen, warfarin, heparin and tissue plasminogen activator, at their normal therapeutic concentrations, showed absolutely no displacement. Salicylic acid and phenylbutazone, on the other hand, gave a significant increase in GV150526 free concentration. A slight displacement of GV150526 binding was observed with warfarin at concentrations slightly higher than therapeutic. These results suggest that GV150526 binds to site 1 (Hervé, 1994) of albumin as phenylbutazone and warfarin bind specifically to site I whereas ibuprofen binds with high affinity to site II. The only slight effect by warfarin was probably due to the low concentration of warfarin used. GV150526 was also shown to displace warfarin at normal therapeutic concentrations and this finding caused some concern, as warfarin's action as anti-coagulant has been shown to be related to the free plasma concentration. Therefore a clinical study was performed to study the possible effects of the protein-binding displacement of GV150526 on warfarin. However, no significant effect on anti-coagulant activity was observed.

TABLE 10.5 *The study of the protein-binding displacement of GV150526 in human plasma by possible concomitant drugs, using* in vitro *equilibrium dialysis*

Displacer	Displacer concentration range (μg/mL)	Relative displacement compared to control*
Ibuprofen	20–100	0.5–0.9
Phenylbutazone (ng/mL)	50–300	1.7–12
t-PA (μg/mL)	0.1–4	0.8–1.2
Bilirubin (mM)	10–50 (mM)	0.9–1.0
Phenytoin	3–36	0.8–1.0
Salicylic acid	50–500	1.4–9.0
Warfarin	1–10	1.0–1.2
Heparin	1–100 (units)	1.0–1.1

t-PA = tissue plasminogen activator.

*Calculated from %unbound with displacing drug/%unbound without displacing drug (1.0 = no displacement).

10.8 *References*

Bowers, W.F. (1984) Ultrafiltration vs. equilibrium dialysis for determination of free fraction. *Clin. Pharm.* 9, 49–60.

Hervé, F. (1994) Drug binding in plasma: a summary of recent trends in the study of drug and hormone binding. *Clin. Pharm.*, 26(1), 44–59.

Honoré, B. (1987) Protein binding studies with radiolabelled compounds containing radiochemical impurities. *Anal. Biochem.* 162, 80–88.

Joshi, A.S. (1994) Plasma protein binding of highly bound drug: implications of radiochemical impurities. *J. Pharm. Sci.* 83, 1187–1188.

Lima, J.J. (1983) Influence of volume shifts on drug binding during equilibrium dialysis: correction and attenuation. *J. Pharm. Biopharm.* 11(5), 483–498.

Lin, J.H. (1987) Protein binding as a primary determinant of the clinical pharmacokinetic properties of nonsteroidal anti-inflammatory drugs. *Clin. Pharm.* 12, 402–432.

Lunde, P.K.M. (1986) Inflammation and α1-acid glycoprotein: effect on drug binding. In: *Drug Protein Binding*, edited by Praeger Publisher.

MacKichan, J.J. (1989) Protein binding displacement interactions. Fact or fiction? *Clin. Pharm.* 16, 65–73.

MacKichan, J.J. (1992) Influence of protein binding and use of unbound (free) drug concentrations. In: *Applied Pharmacokinetics. Principle of Therapeutic Drug Monitoring*, edited by Applied Therapeutics Inc.

Mayersohn, M.B. (1992) Special pharmacokinetic considerations in the elderly. In: *Applied Pharmacokinetics. Principle of Therapeutic Drug Monitoring*, edited by Applied Therapeutics Inc.

Oravcova, J. (1996) Drug-protein binding studies: new trends in analytical and experimental methodology. *J. Chrom. Biom. Applic.* 677, 1–28.

Robinson, P.J. and Rapoport, S.I. (1986) Kinetics of protein binding determine rates of uptake of drugs by brain. *Am. J. Physiol.* December; 251 (6 Pt 2), R1212–1220.

Rolan, P.E. (1994) Plasma protein binding displacement interactions – why are they still regarded as clinically important? *Br. J. Clin. Pharmacol.* 37, 125–128.

Sansom, L.N. (1995) What's the true clinical significance of plasma protein binding displacement interactions? *Drug Saf.* 12(4), 227–233.

Tillement, J.P., Lhoste, F. and Giudicelli, J.F. (1978) Disease and drug protein binding. *Clin. Pharm.* 3, 144–154.

Wilkinson, G.R. and Shand, D.G. (1975) A physiological approach to hepatic clearance. *Clin. Pharmacol. Ther.* 18, 377–390.

Wright, J.D. (1996) Measurement and analysis of unbound drug concentrations. *Clin. Pharm.* 30(6), 445–462.

Zini, R. (1991) Methods in drug protein binding analysis. In: *Human Pharmacology*, edited by Elsevier Science Publisher.

CHAPTER 11

Isotope drug studies in man

Graeme Young, John Ayrton and Tony Pateman

11.1 *Radiolabelled studies in man*

11.1.1 Introduction

One of the most important aspects of drug metabolism/pharmacokinetics in drug development is to show that the animals used in toxicology have been exposed to the same chemical species (drug and metabolites) as will your patient. Usually the metabolism and kinetics of the drug are studied in animals with radiolabelled compound and the quickest way of getting the comparative information from man is also to give a radioactive dose.

Ideally the human radiolabel study should be completed as early as possible in a drug's development (before long-term toxicology) if it is going to be useful in the selection of the animal species for toxicology.

To dose the radioactive compound in man you usually need:

1 Basic toxicology data.
2 Basic kinetics and metabolic information in animals.

3 Basic pharmacokinetics of non-radiolabelled compound in man (although assay sensitivity may be insufficient, and the label may be being given to obtain basic pharmacokinetic information).
4 Estimated organ radioactive exposure data from tissue distribution and excretion balance studies.
5 Ethical approval.
6 Administration of Radioactive Substances Advisory Committee (ARSAC) approval.

These studies are not for statistical evaluation. Therefore ethics dictates the use of a limited number of subjects (2–6). Women of child bearing age should not be used.

Normally a single route is used with a radioactive dose of approximately 2 MBq for ^{14}C or 4 MBq for ^{3}H. The exact amount that can be given is determined using ARSAC calculations (see below). Half the amount of radioactivity can be given each time if two routes of administration are used per subject. The dose formulation used should be the one which has the highest bioavailability normally, this will be a solution of the drug. It is often not possible to use a formulation which is equivalent to the proposed clinical formulation (if known) because the method of preparing the clinical formulation may not be practical with the small quantities of radiolabelled drug available. If a solution is not used, the non-radioactive and radioactive material should be dissolved together, crystallised and the resulting homogenous material used.

The choice of isotope should receive a mention here. The counting efficiency of tritium is only about one-third of that of carbon-14. However, the dose constant for tritium is only about one-ninth that of carbon-14, and consequently more Bq of tritium can be administered. The outcome is that the use of tritium affords a 3-fold increase in sensitivity of detection over carbon-14 for a given radiation exposure of a volunteer.

The main objective is to establish the route of elimination of radioactive products and to compare the metabolite pattern in excreta and plasma with those in animals (radio-HPLC/MS). This information can then be used to select/justify the animal species for long-term toxicology. It is not necessary to identify metabolites at this stage although eventually they will have to be identified. As stated above radiolabel can also assist, through the use of radio-HPLC, with conventional pharmacokinetic studies when the properties of the molecules preclude detection by conventional means.

To gain the maximum information:

1 Measure radioactivity in excreta (urine and faeces) and balance with dose. At a stroke this tells us if the biliary excretion seen in animals is replaced by renal excretion in man.
2 Compare metabolites in excreta and plasma with those in animal species used in/intended for toxicology (but what happens if they are different? How far

will a toxicologist go?). This aspect is becoming increasingly important as safety cover based on metabolites as well as parent compound is a developing issue.

3 Measure radioactivity in blood and plasma at different times after dosing. This can give useful information on the distribution in blood and can be supplemented by *ex vivo* protein-binding studies.
4 Measure intact drug in plasma and compare with total radioactivity.
5 If possible, measure a dynamic parameter as well.

If the intravenous route of administration (e.g. IV infusion) is used as well as oral, this can enhance the knowledge of the basic pharmacokinetics of the drug (clearance, volume of distribution, absorption, bioavailability), providing specific measurements of the drug are also included.

11.1.2 ARSAC

Radiolabelled studies in man must first be approved by the ARSAC of the DoH. The guidelines upon which the ARSAC made its decisions, until recently, are to be found in the WHO publication "Use of ionizing radiation and radionuclides on human beings for medical research, training, and non-medical purposes" (1977). There were no specific guidelines for volunteer studies.

The WHO defined three categories of radioisotope work, according to the radiation dose received, these are summarised in Table 11.1.
These exposure limits were recently reviewed on two counts:

1 The data is based on the effects of the bombs in Hiroshima and Nagasaki, and the degree of shielding between the blast and the victims is now considered to have been underestimated.
2 The statistical methods applied to those data are now being questioned.

TABLE 11.1 *Categories of radioisotope work*

	Category		
	I	II	III
Range of effective dose equivalent	<0.5 mSv	0.5–5 mSv	5–50 mSv
Level of risk	within variations of natural background radiation	within dose limits for members of the public	within dose limits for persons occupationally exposed to radiation

This has led to revised calculations which are to be found in ICRP publication 60 (1991).

The ICRP has now modified the WHO exposure categories to take these revisions into account (ICRP, 1992). The following categories have been drawn up specifically to cater for volunteer studies. They are presented in Table 11.2.

Category IIa involves a risk of one in one hundred thousand, and a benefit related to increases in knowledge leading to health benefit. Category IIb is associated with a risk of one in ten thousand, and the benefits will be more directly aimed at the cure or prevention of disease.

In addition to the above, the National Radiological Protection Board (NRPB) advise that the average annual intake over several years should be <15mSv for occupational exposure.

As a general rule, the use of radiolabel should comply with the principles of ALARA (As Low As Reasonably Acceptable), and as such the aim should be to keep volunteers within WHO category IIa or lower. Under these circumstances a volunteer will be exposed to no greater risk than they might be if they were to move from one part of the country to another. The principle of ALARA becomes even more important when we consider that these exposure limits are drawn up from historical data that is constantly being re-appraised.

The purpose of the following sections is to describe the calculations that must be performed on animal data to provide ARSAC with the information they require for a particular study. These calculations can be performed by the pharmaceutical company itself, or by the NRPB. Even if the NRPB route is adopted, a knowledge of the calculations will help to plan the most appropriate animal studies. In addition, it is clearly important to know if a volunteer study that will meet your scientific goals is going to be possible before even submitting the data to NRPB and ARSAC.

It is recommended that for current ARSAC submissions both old and new methods of calculation are performed and the most conservative results used.

The primary calculation required is that of the Committed Effective Dose (1991) or the Committed Effective Dose Equivalent (1977). These calculations are performed on data obtained from quantitative whole body autoradiography studies (Chapter 12) and excretion balance studies.

TABLE 11.2 *Categories for radiolabelled exposure for volunteers*

Level of risk	Risk category	Effective dose range (mSv)	Level of societal benefit
Trivial	I ($\sim<10^{-6}$)	<0.1	Minor
Minor to intermediate	IIa ($\sim10^{-5}$)	0.1–1	Intermediate to moderate
	IIb ($\sim10^{-4}$)	1–10	
Moderate	III ($\sim>10^{-3}$)	>10	Substantial

Both new and old methods of calculation and interpretation will now be covered.

Calculation of committed effective dose (CED); ICRP, 1991

(a) *Which tissues?* ICRP publication 60 specifies the tissues that *must* be taken because of their susceptibility to damage. These are shown in Table 11.3.

(b) *Relative sensitivity of tissues* The dose limits are defined in terms of whole body exposure. However, some organs, such as gonads, are more susceptible to radiation damage than others. Therefore each organ is given a weighting factor (W_T) which takes this into account when calculating total exposure.

The weighting factors take into account the probability of fatal and non-fatal cancer, severe hereditary effects and relative length of life lost.

The weighting factors laid down by the ICRP publication 60 are shown in Table 11.4.

(c) *Transformations per Bq* This is the exposure that an organ receives after administration of 1 Bq to the animal.

For tissues containing radioactivity it is the area under concentration time curve (*AUC*) of label in the organ. This is calculated in the same way as is a plasma level-time *AUC* except that the total radiolabel in the organ is used, and not the concentration.

Melanin binding may be a problem as the half-life may be extremely long and dedicated studies may be required to determine the *AUC*.

(d) Exposure from excreta (urine, bile, intestinal contents) which pass through the body is determined from the percentage dose passing through each route and the

TABLE 11.3 *Tissues specified by ICRP publication 60*

Gonads
Colon (LLI)
Lung
Red bone marrow
Stomach
Bladder
Breast
Liver
Oesophagus
Thyroid
Bone surface
Skin

TABLE 11.4 *Weighting factors*

	W_T
Gonads	0.2
Colon (LLI)	0.12
Lung	0.12
Red bone marrow	0.12
Stomach	0.12
Bladder	0.05
Breast	0.05
Liver	0.05
Oesophagus	0.05
Thyroid	0.05
Bone surface	0.01
Skin	0.01
Remainder	0.05*

* Weighting becomes 0.025.

mean residence time (MRT) in man. An additional factor must also be taken into consideration. Not all the label in, for example, faeces will irradiate the intestinal mucosa, as some radiation will be absorbed by the surrounding excreta. For this reason a 'geometric' factor is used to allow for the reduced exposure.

11.2 *Which isotope?*

The biological effects vary from isotope to isotope. A 'dose constant' is used to provide data for a specific isotope.

11.3 *Calculations*

With the above principles in mind we are now ready to perform the calculations themselves. The guidelines for these are laid down in ICRP publication 60. A number of approaches can be made; the method adopted by the NRPB will be described below.

The following calculations are performed for each organ:

$$H_T = \frac{U\varepsilon\phi A}{m}$$

H_T = equivalent dose to the target organ (S_v).

U = transformation per Bq dose administered, e.g. the AUC of radiolabel in organ (Bq sec).

m = mass of the source organ in man (Kg) obtained from ICRP publication 23.

ε = dose constant for radioisotope in use

$$= 9.12 \times 10^{-16}\,\text{kg Gy Bq}^{-1}\,\text{s}^{-1} \text{ for } {}^{3}\text{H}$$

$$= 79.4 \times 10^{-16}\,\text{kg Gy Bq}^{-1}\,\text{s}^{-1} \text{ for for } {}^{14}\text{C}.$$

It is the mean energy of radiation per nuclear transformation. That is, a measure of how damaging a given isotope will be.

ϕ = Fraction of radioactive emissions absorbed ('geometric factor'). It is 1.0 (label in tissue) or 0.5 (label in excreta).

A = amount of radiolabelled drug administered (Bq).

The effective equivalent dose is the whole body dose which would produce the same risk as a non-uniformly distributed absorbed dose. It is calculated for each organ from the equivalent dose using the formula:

$$\text{Weighting factor} = H_T \times W_T$$

The effective equivalent dose of the remainder is a mass weighted mean of the equivalent doses of the contributing tissues.

$$\text{Effective equivalent dose} = \frac{\text{mean of } (H_T \times \text{mass})}{\text{mean of mass}}$$

The effective equivalent doses for all the organs are then summed to produce the 'committed effective dose'. It is this value that must be below 1.0 mSv to fall within a risk category IIa.

11.3.1 SOURCE OF DATA

All the information required for the above calculations is available from tables except for the value of U, and it is this that must be determined experimentally from quantitative tissue distribution, QTD (or quantitative whole body autoradiography, QWBA; see Chapter 12) and excretion balance studies.

The exact amount of data required is unclear, and it probably varies from compound to compound. At one end of the spectrum would be QTD in a rodent and dog, using perhaps nine or ten time points in the rodent and two in the dog. At the other end of the spectrum, it may be possible to use the rodent only and use quantitative WBA at only three or four time points. In both cases an excretion balance study in both species would also be required. If the latter course is adopted the only work involved is encompassed by the normal ADME package.

Quantitative WBA has now gained wide acceptance and clearly offers a great saving in labour over the conventional QTD. Standard organ weights must be used to convert concentrations to organ contents.

Whichever approach is adopted, the organs can be divided into 'tissues' for which QTD or QWBA provides the data, and 'excreta' for which excretion balance studies are the source data.

(a) *Tissues*
A common approach is to take four time points. One point would be the expected peak level, and the other three would be chosen to characterise the elimination. Depending on the compound, the last point may be 24 hours, 48 hours, or even as long as a week or two after dosing.

The value of U is readily obtained by the trapezoidal rule. Integration may also be used. The value of A_0 in the formula A_0/λ would be either the peak amount of label in the organ or the value extrapolated to time zero, whichever is the greater. λ is the half-life of the biological elimination of radioactivity in the organ.

In either case, the exposure must be extrapolated beyond the end of the experiment by assuming that any label remaining has a half-life of 100 days. That is,

$$U = \frac{A_0}{\lambda} + \frac{A_Z \times (100 \times 24 \times 60 \times 60)}{0.693}$$

The value of U is normalised to a dose of 1.0 Bq.

(b) *Melanin*
Binding to ocular melanin may have a half-life in excess of 100 days. For this reason melanin binding must be treated as a special case, should it occur, and detailed pharmacokinetics should be obtained.

(c) *Excreta*
Because this has a finite residence time in the body, and therefore exposure to radiation is linked to bodily function as opposed to metabolite pharmacokinetics, a different approach is used.

$$U = F \times MRT \text{ (remember SI units)}$$

F is the fraction of the dose that passes through a particular excretion route (i.e. a fraction of the 1.0 Bq nominal dose).
MRT is the mean residence time for that route in man (Table 11.5)

NB If significant label resides in the walls of the intestines, bladder, etc. this must be calculated separately and added to the exposure from the excreta. It should be remembered that the GI tract is considered as four organs and that biliary excretion in rat might be replaced by urinary excretion in man.

TABLE 11.5 *MRT is the mean residence time for that route in man*

Tissue	MRT (hours)
Stomach	1
Small intestine	4
Upper large intestine	13
Lower large intestine	24
Urine	10
Bile	2.53

Typical calculations supplied by the NRPB are:

Thyroid

Mass of thyroid = 0.02 kg

Transformations per Bq = 4.5

$\phi = 1$

Equivalent dose = 7.57×10^{-7} Sv

Effective equivalent dose = 2.27×10^{-8} Sv

Small intestine (from contents)

Mass of contents = 0.4 kg

Fraction activity = 1.0 (p.o dose)

$MRT = 4$ hours

Transformations per Bq = 14,400

$\phi = 0.5$

Equivalent dose = 6.02×10^{-5} Sv

Effective equivalent dose = 3.61×10^{-6} Sv

The sum of all the effective equivalent doses gives us the CED, which must be <1mSv for a category IIa study.

11.3.2 Calculation of committed effective dose equivalent (CEDE); ICRP 1977

The calculation of the CEDE is similar to that of the CED. The major difference is that a different set of tissues is mandatory and the weighting factors are consequently different.

ICRP publication 26 specifies six tissues that *must* be taken because of their susceptibility to damage. These are:

Gonads
Breast
Bone marrow) usually combined, and assume all activity in marrow
Bone surface)
Lung
Thyroid

In addition, five other tissues must be selected. These should be the ones receiving most exposure.

The weighting factors, laid down by the WHO report number 611 are shown in Table 11.6.

The effective dose equivalents for the ten organs are then summed to produce the 'committed effective dose equivalent'. It is this value that must be below 0.5 mSv to comply with a WHO category I experiment.

The sum of all the effective equivalent doses (dose equivalents) gives us the committed effective dose (or committed effective dose equivalent) to a human volunteer for a given dose. For example, if a CED of 550 μSv is arrived at based on the administration of 1.0 MBq, then a maximum of 1.8 MBq could be administered to be within the 1 mSv limit of a WHO category IIa experiment. If the calculated CEDE is higher than the CED, the amount of radioactivity that could be administered would be reduced as this would be the more conservative estimate. Also, it should be remembered that the category IIa upper limit is twice that of the old category 1, and that exposure of greater than 0.5 mSv would need to be very carefully considered. Above all, remember ALARA!

The term ALARA may take on a whole new meaning when we consider the use of the technique of accelerated mass spectrometry in support of radiolabelled studies in man.

TABLE 11.6 *Weighting factors laid down by the WHO report number 611*

	W_T
Gonads	0.25
Breast	0.15
Red bone marrow	0.12
Bone	0.03
Lung	0.12
Thyroid	0.03
Five other organs	0.06 × 5
	1.00

11.4 Accelerator mass spectrometry

As indicated in the section above, in the United Kingdom, it is a pre-requisite for human radiolabelled studies to gain approval from the ARSAC. This can be a lengthy process and the conditions placed on the design of the study are very stringent. An exception to gaining this approval can be made by using an extremely low dosage of radioactivity which results in an ionising radiation exposure to the subject of $<1\,\mu$Sv. To ensure that the expected exposure to radiation will be $<1\,\mu$Sv, the calculations outlined above will still have to be performed. The analytical tool known as accelerator mass spectrometry (AMS) can make the use of such a low radioactive dose, a viable alternative. AMS is an established technology, which allows the measurement of extremely small quantities of rare and radioactive isotopes, such as radiocarbon (^{14}C), with high precision (Scott *et al.*, 1990; Vogel *et al.*, 1995). AMS is mainly used in the geochemical and archeological areas, such as in radiocarbon dating, but following use of AMS for biomedical applications by the Lawrence Livermore National Laboratory (LLNL), California, USA, the technique is being used more widely in this area of science. A facility known as the Centre for Biomedical Accelerator Mass Spectrometry (CBAMS) Ltd dedicated to the use of AMS for biomedical applications is now operational, near York, England. AMS can detect ^{14}C at concentrations 10^3–10^6 lower than the techniques currently used in drug metabolism studies, such as liquid scintillation counting. AMS differs from conventional radioisotope counting since it is a nuclear detection technique, rather than a decay counting technique.

With increased focus on the safety aspects of using humans in drug trials, AMS offers the advantage of lowering the amount of radiolabelled material administered from typically 2 MBq to circa 4 kBq and thus greatly reducing the exposure to ionising radiation.

Since the levels of exposure to radiation can be lowered to such a degree, it opens the way for carrying out experiments that are more difficult to arrange for ARSAC studies such as administration of both intravenous and oral administration to the same subject, i.e. it is possible to administer radiolabelled drug by two routes in an ARSAC study but the dosage on each administration would be half of the approved dosage.

The current AMS instruments are very large (see photograph of an instrument in Figure 11.1) and can cost in the region of £2million. AMS is currently limited in its application by the complexity of the sample preparation involved. Sample throughput is fairly low, being in the region of 100 samples that can be prepared per technician/day. Advances in automating the process, possibly by radical change, may be required in the future to enhance throughput.

The sensitivity of the instrument is such that ^{14}C contamination from areas where higher levels have been handled is a very real obstacle to obtaining meaningful results. There is therefore a need for controlled access to and use of facilities, to attempt to limit the cross-contamination potential.

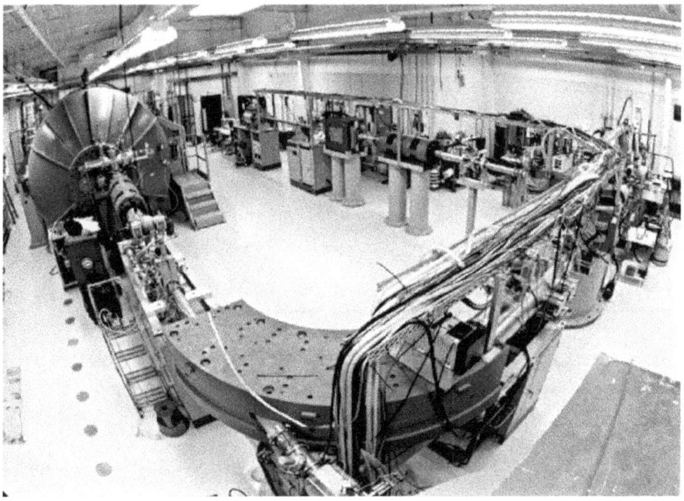

FIGURE 11.1 *Wide angle view of the 10 MV FN tandem accelerator and mass spectrometer located in the Center for Accelerator Mass Spectrometry (CAMS) at the Lawrence Livermore National Laboratory in Livermore, California, USA.* At the NIH NCRR National Resource for Biomedical Accelerator Mass Spectrometry the 10 MV AMS is used for the analysis of biomedical samples.

11.4.1 SAMPLE PREPARATION FOR AMS

The schematic representation in Figure 11.2 shows part of the process of sample preparation which involves sample combustion and reduction to graphite, prior to analysis by AMS.

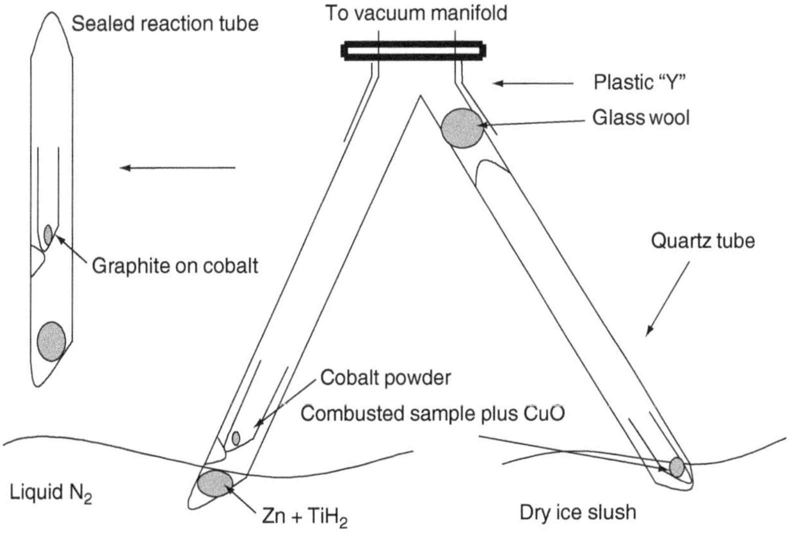

FIGURE 11.2 *Graphite production from biological samples.*

The carbon from the sample, typically 50μL of plasma for example, is isolated as CO_2 by oxidation for 2 hours at 6,500 ℃ in the presence of copper oxide (CuO). The CO_2 is isolated cryogenically from other oxidation products and reduced to graphite with H_2 and Zn on a cobalt catalyst by heating to 5,500 °C for 4 hours. The carbon/cobalt sample is then transferred into a sample holder which is introduced into the AMS via a sample wheel.

11.4.2 Instrumental details of AMS

Figure 11.3 shows a schematic representation of the nuclear physics involved in the technique of AMS. The graphite sample is bombarded by a caesium–sputter ion source which results in production of negatively charged nuclear and molecular isobars of carbon (e.g. $^{14}C^-$, $^{12}CH_2^-$). The carbon ions are then selected using a mass spectrometer and accelerated along a tandem electrostatic accelerator where charge conversion occurs to produce positively charged ions. The ion beam is then deflected through a second mass spectrometer resulting in further 'purification' of the ion beam and for a few milliseconds every second, the ^{13}C content is determined by means of a Faraday cup. The ion beam is then focussed towards a final ionisation detector

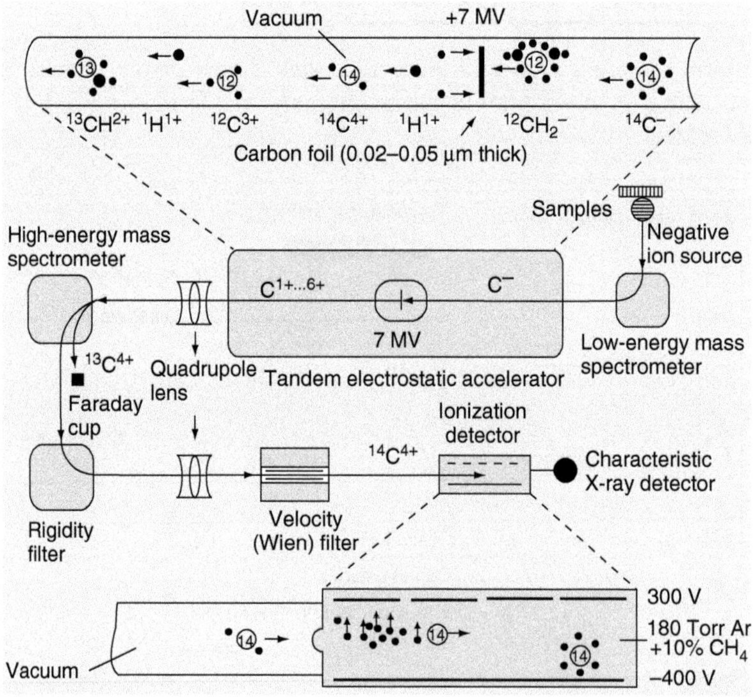

FIGURE 11.3 *Instrumental operation* (reproduced with permission from John S. Vogel and Lawrence Livermore National Laboratory).

where the ^{14}C content is measured. The ratio of ^{13}C to ^{14}C can be used to determine the amount of ^{14}C in the sample above the background level, which in turn allows determination of analyte concentration, i.e. drug and/or metabolite(s) of interest in the initial sample. In order to ensure that the AMS is operating correctly, an international standard of known ^{13}C:^{14}C is measured with each set of samples. There are a number of such standards in use, including the commonly used Australian National University sucrose standard.

The sensitivity advantage of AMS relative to decay counting is shown by the equation:

$$dN/dt = -(1/\tau) \times N$$

where (dN/dt) = the activity or the rate of decay, τ = the mean half-life of the isotope, and N = the total number of isotope nuclei present. Decay counting techniques such as liquid scintillation counting, indirectly predict N by measuring dN/dt, which is a very small percentage of N for all but the shortest lived isotopes. AMS counts N directly, independent of the mean life, resulting in sensitivity of detection increases relative to scintillation counting of 10^3 for ^3H and 10^6 for ^{14}C.

Elemental analysis of any samples submitted for AMS analysis is required in order to determine the %carbon content of the samples. Quantitation of ^{14}C content of samples relies on knowledge of the full carbon inventory of the samples i.e. the sources of carbon in the samples. If there is insufficient carbon in the samples to allow sufficient graphite to be prepared then addition of a carrier of known ^{14}C content, e.g. tributyrin, is required.

The technique of AMS could not only allow reduction of exposure of human subjects to radioactivity in drug development studies, but also make many experiments possible which are currently impossible. Examples of these are the monitoring of systemic exposures following administration of very small quantities of drug, e.g. when administered by the inhaled, intranasal or topical routes. Microsampling of tissues following administration at conventional doses may also be possible.

11.5 *Future of AMS*

A potential application for AMS may be to include the administration of radiolabelled material in Phase I human studies for all new chemical entities. This would increase greatly the amount of metabolism and pharmacokinetic information made available early in drug development, thereby enhancing the potential of the investigators to make good development decisions on the new chemical entity (NCE).

AMS may also be of use in the future in research experiments with extremely low dosages where there is little need for toxicology safety cover. There will however, always be the additional concerns of possible non-specific adsorption problems and lack of linearity to therapeutic dosages. Advances in sample preparation and/or introduction will be very important if AMS costs are to be reduced and sample throughput increased. Both of these factors are likely to have great influence on the development and use of the technique in the future.

11.6 *Stable isotope studies*

Stable isotope labelling of the drug under development can be a useful alternative to studies using the radiolabelled isotopes or indeed stable and radioactive isotopes can be used in combination. Commonly carbon-13 or deuterium is used to produce stable labelled drug. The isotope pattern produced is very distinctive when samples from a study are analysed by mass spectrometry and this makes identification of metabolites facile. The disadvantage of using solely stable isotope labelling as opposed to radioactive labelling tends to be one of sensitivity, i.e. since the background levels of stable isotopes tend to be much higher than radioactive isotopes, it is a less sensitive technique to use.

All of the techniques and approaches mentioned in this chapter have both advantages and disadvantages. AMS offers an exciting new approach to the conduct of isotope studies in the future but there may still be a place for conventional radiolabel studies where AMS cannot supply all of the information required.

11.7 *Acknowledgements*

Lawrence Livermore National Laboratory, California.

11.8 *References*

ICRP (1991) *1990 Recommendations of the International Commission on Radiological Protection.* ICRP publication 60, *Ann. ICRP*, 21(1–3), Pergamon Press, Oxford.

ICRP publication 62 (1992) Radiological Protection in Biomedical Research.

ICRP publication 23 (1975) *Reference Man: Anatomical, Physiological and Metabolic Characteristics*, edited by ICRP, 0–08–017024–2, EUR 122, USD 12.

ICRP (1977) *Recommendations of the International Commission on Radiological Protection.* ICRP publication 26, *Ann. ICRP*, 1(3).

Report of a WHO Expert Committee. Technical Report Series 611, WHO, Geneva, 1977.

Scott, E.M., Long, A. and Kra, R. (1990) Radiocarbon, 32.

Vogel, J.S., Turteltaub, K.W., Finkel, R. and Nelson, D.E. (1995) *Anal. Chem.* 67, 353A–359A.

CHAPTER 12

Whole body autoradiography

Lee Crossman, Kenneth Brouwer and Jeanne Jarrett

12.1 *Introduction*

The technique of whole body autoradiography (WBA) was introduced in 1954 by Sven Ullberg, in Upsala, Sweden. WBA involves the cryosectioning of whole animals such as mice, rats, rabbits and monkeys and was developed to study the distribution of compounds in the intact animal's body. In the early days, cryosectioning was performed by technicians dressed in fur coats in a cold room maintained at −15 °C using a hand-driven sledge microtome (Ullberg, 1954, 1958). Today, the technique has been refined substantially, and highly specialised equipment has been designed for all aspects of WBA techniques. WBA was developed in part to overcome the technical problems encountered in traditional methods of studying compound distribution. Many compounds are soluble in water or other liquids used in the histological preparation of tissue specimens and may therefore be extracted from the specimen during processing. WBA allows for the fixation of the compound in the intact animal by freezing, thereby preventing any tissue preservation liquids from coming into contact with the test compound. As such, the localisation of the compound is preserved (Ullberg, 1977). WBA has many applications, but its most frequent use is to generate comprehensive information about the distribution pattern of new drug candidates. For this application, WBA data are used to support histopathology data from toxicity testing, and to generate radiolabelled dose estimates for human studies. The technique may also be used for a variety of other applications, including the identification of target tissues for a test compound, receptor identification, to investigate blood–brain barrier or placental permeability, or to generate samples for micro-autoradiographic studies.

Although we have attempted to cover as many of the applications of WBA as possible, our experience is limited to use of this technique within the pharmaceutical industry, and as such the information contained within this chapter is from that perspective. The methods presented are intended to serve as general guidelines for the design of WBA studies.

12.2 *Historical background*

The published observation of Niepe de St Victor (1867) of the autoradiographic (ARG) phenomenon pre-dated the discovery of radioactivity per se and assisted in the discovery and awareness of radioactive principles by Henri Bequerel (1896) and Pierre and Marie Curie (1898). The first macro ARG was thought to have been produced by London (1904). The first systematic use of the ARG phenomenon was by Lacassagne and Lattes (1924). Advances in biology, chemistry and physics during and after the 1940s gave scientists access to ever increasing numbers of radioisotopes. These were used to study biological distribution of both endogenous and exogenous substances. Prior to 1954, most macroscopic ARG studies were performed using either Lamholt (1930) or Libby's (1947) method. Lamholt method was only suitable for preparing individual organs, whilst Libby was cutting 5 mm thick whole body sections using a bandsaw. Both methods involved impregnating the sectioned tissue with liquid paraffin, which made it unsuitable for working with soluble compounds. In 1954 Ullberg's method was published, and most autoradiographers today work to a variation of this method for studying the distribution of radiolabelled compounds *in vivo*.

12.3 *Methodology*

For a typical WBA study, a radiolabelled compound is administered to an experimental animal, and the compound is allowed to distribute for various periods of time. At each time point, each animal is euthanised, immediately frozen in a bath of solvent (usually hexane or heptane) and dry ice and the frozen animal embedded in a chilled solution of carboxymethylcellulose. Using this process, a frozen block is formed on a large microtome stage and the block is mounted in a large cryomicrotome. Sagittal sections are taken, collected onto tape and freeze-dried. The dried sections are then exposed to X-ray film or storage phosphor film, and the latent or digital image generated is quantified using densitometry software. In general, the darkest areas indicate the highest radioactivity concentrations. It is important to note that WBA allows for the detection of radioactivity, which may correlate with parent compound, metabolites or impurities.

12.4 *Study design*

12.4.1 Animal selection

In general, for WBA studies performed to generate tissue distribution data for a test compound, animals are chosen to correlate with the rodent species used in the toxicity testing of the compound under investigation, which supports the interpretation of toxicity data. Usually, the toxicological species is an albino rodent strain. Another consideration in the selection of animals is the evaluation of the potential for melanin binding. If a compound is found to bind to melanin, this may limit the radiolabelled dose in a human study. It is therefore recommended to include pigmented animals in the study design. Consideration of the current regulatory requirements of each country where the drug is to be marketed must also be considered; for example, the Japanese authorities require data from albino animals only and do not investigate melanin binding.

12.4.2 Dose selection

For WBA studies performed to generate tissue distribution data for a regulatory submission, the dose is often chosen to correlate as closely as possible with the low dose used in toxicity testing and the effective clinical dose. This practice ensures that the WBA data can be used with more confidence to support toxicity data and to generate human radiolabelled dose estimates. The dose vehicle should also reflect that used in toxicity testing and in clinical studies. It is critical to use the purest radiochemical possible (>98 per cent), because an impurity could bind preferentially to a particular tissue, resulting in misleading data. Since WBA allows for the study of the tissue distribution of radioactivity, if a radiolabelled impurity were to bind exclusively to a particular tissue, this could be interpreted as the distribution of the parent compound.

12.4.3 Time point selection

In the selection of time points for a WBA study, the compound T_{max}, half-life and pharmacokinetic profile in the rodent species in which WBA will be performed should be considered. Time points chosen for studies should provide adequate data to allow for the calculation of tissue half-lives, which will be used to calculate the radioactivity exposure for each tissue. Time points chosen for the study should also illustrate that the compound of interest has entered the body and is subsequently excreted. A reasonable course of action is for the early time point to coincide with the T_{max} of the compound in blood. The final time point should be based on the period of time in which it is expected that little or no compound will remain in the body, and unless the compound half-life is very long, or very short, a reasonable choice is seven days post-dosing. Additional time points are chosen based on the pharmacokinetic profile. Different laboratories study different numbers of time points; however, it is generally agreed that five time points are sufficient to provide comprehensive data on the distribution pattern of the compound, while allowing for the calculation of tissue half-life data for most tissues.

12.5 *Obtaining whole body sections*

12.5.1 Freezing and embedding

To prepare animals for WBA, the freezing mixture (usually dry ice added to hexane or heptane) and the embedding agent (2 per cent w/v carboxymethyl cellulose) should be prepared in advance. Animals should be frozen immediately after euthanasia to minimise the diffusion of test compound between tissues. The body should be straightened and positioned to facilitate sectioning, tissue identification and to obtain a pleasing image. The animal should be placed within a freezing frame, and chilled CMC solution poured around the carcass and worked into the fur and crevices before the embedded animal is re-frozen. A 250–300 g rat should be entirely frozen in the freezing mix for a minimum of 20–30 minutes to ensure that ice crystals, which are detrimental to the imaging process, do not form. Once the animal has been frozen, the tail and limbs are trimmed away.

12.5.2 Sectioning

The frozen animal embedded in a solid CMC block is mounted on a cryomicrotome (Figure 12.1), and the animal is trimmed until a level of interest appears. When tissues or organs of interest have been identified, a strip of transparent tape is adhered to the surface of the block. A section is obtained as the microtome knife cuts swiftly under the tape, and the section is lifted away from the block. The thickness of the section is an important factor in the accurate quantification of radioactivity within tissues. It is suggested that 40 μm is the optimum section thickness as there are adequate amounts of radioactivity within the section, but

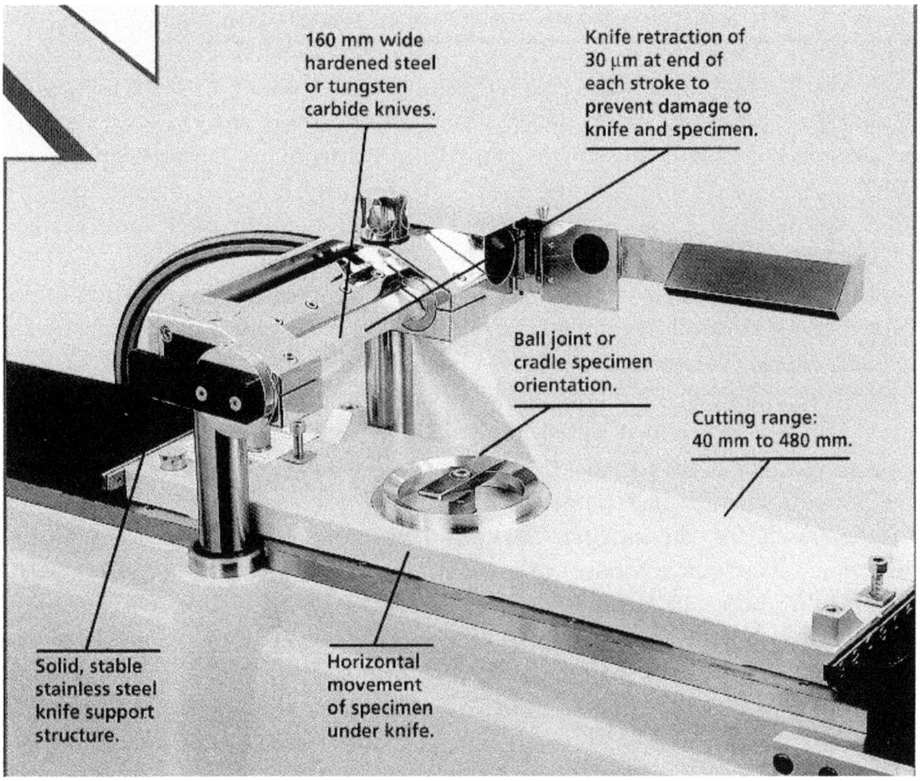

FIGURE 12.1 *Microtome.*

tissue self absorption is minimised and resolution maximised. In this fashion, sections are obtained which contain tissue samples from all tissues of interest for the particular study. After the sections are obtained, they are freeze dried by sublimation at −20 °C in the microtome. Freeze-drying for four days minimises density differences between the tissues, which occur as a result of tissue water content. A light dusting of talc can be applied to the edges of each section prior to exposure, to prevent the tape from adhering to the imaging media.

12.6 *Imaging*

The sections are exposed to the surface of X-ray film or a phosphorimaging plate along with standards. In general, sections are exposed for 4–10 days, depending on the radioisotope, specific activity and time point. Studies show, that after ten days of exposure to a ^{14}C phosphorimaging plate, the signal to noise ratio begins to decrease, so there is no value in exposure times of longer than ten days.

12.6.1 Principle of imaging plate methodology

In the late 1960s, X-ray photography was the only available means for medical imaging diagnostics (Miyahara, 1989). The development of imaging plate technology was made in the 1970s by the Fuji Film company of Japan. Commercially available instruments were introduced in 1981, exclusively for the medical industry, and it was not until the 1990s that analytical phosphorimagers were available globally.

Phosphors are powdered substances that emit light when exposed to radiation, UV rays or an electron beam, or when heated, mechanically hit or stimulated by chemical reaction (Miyahara, 1989). A phosphor emits light when stimulated, for example, by radiation. The light disappears instantaneously when the stimulation ceases. This phenomenon is called 'fluorescence'. Some of the phosphors continue to emit light for a time after the stimulation has stopped, this is 'phosphorescence'. 'Luminescence' incorporates both of these light emission phenomena. The phosphor used for the imaging plate utilises 'photostimulable luminescence' (PSL) which is neither fluorescence nor phosphorescence, but involves a substance that emits light again upon the second stimulation by light having a longer wavelength than the luminescence wavelength of the first stimulation, e.g. radiation.

The imaging plate (IP) is a flexible image sensor in which groups of very small crystals of photostimulable phosphors of barium fluorobromide, containing a trace amount of bivalent europium as a luminescence centre are uniformly coated 150–300 μm thick on a polyester support film (Motoji *et al.*, 1995).

Exposure of samples to the IP is performed in a manner similar to that of X-ray film (Gahan, 1972; Shindo, 1979). The exposed IP is scanned with a He–Ne laser beam of red light (633 nm) whilst the plate is conveyed with high accuracy through a phosphor reader. Resolution and reading density are dependent upon the specification of the machine, and with current technology are 25–100 pixels/mm^2. The reading sensitivity and sensitivity range can also be selected based on the objective. A bluish purple (400 nm) PSL released upon laser excitation is collected via the light collecting guide and passed through the photo multiplier tube (PMT) where it is converted to an analogue signal and then to a digital image. The higher the radioactivity within the sample, the higher the PSL value. This shows up with increased tissue density in the image displayed on the screen.

12.7 *Quantitative whole body autoradiography*

Once the image has been obtained, visual analysis of the image can give qualitative information of the distribution, retention and excretion of radiolabelled material. However, prior to administering the test compound to humans it is important to be able to obtain quantitative information on the concentrations of drug that each tissue will be exposed to. To perform quantitative WBA, standards of known radiological activity are exposed to the IP along with the sections. Commercially available polymer standards, or blood standards prepared in the laboratory can be used for quantitative WBA. It is essential that the calibration standards are of the same thickness as the sections, or suitably calibrated, because direct comparison of the two on the same imaging plate is central to the quantitative process.

A standard curve is prepared which plots the PSL values against the known concentration of radioactivity. The PSL of each area of interest within the sample can be measured and when plotted against the standard curve, enables the radioactive content of the tissue to be calculated. By knowing the specific activity of the source and the amount administered, the radio-concentration of a tissue can be equated to the concentration of drug that has accumulated in that tissue. The information obtained from QWBA studies can be used to calculate a safe dose of radiolabelled compound for administration to human volunteers.

12.8 *Applications of quantitative whole body autoradiography*

WBA studies provide a rapid way to provide preliminary information on the ADME properties of radiolabelled compounds. WBA is the only method available that can allow the scientist to evaluate the tissue distribution of a drug without having to make prior assumptions regarding the tissue distribution of the compound under evaluation. Although limited to detecting total radioactivity, WBA can none-the-less provide valuable information in many areas relevant to preclinical drug development. In all of the following images, darker areas of the image represent higher levels of radioactivity.

12.8.1 Absorption/distribution

WBA studies provide a rapid method to determine the extent to which a compound is absorbed, and where it distributes within the body. Figure 12.2 is an autoradiogram following an oral dose of a drug candidate at 24 hours post-dose. The compound was well absorbed and distributed into all tissues. Significant distribution into the brain tissue is evident, along with fairly high levels of radioactive drug-related material in the liver, salivary gland and adrenal gland. Non-absorbed or excreted radiolabelled material is also seen clearly in the faecal pellets found in the colon. Note the small structures in the brain (pineal body) where distribution can be visualised and quantified.

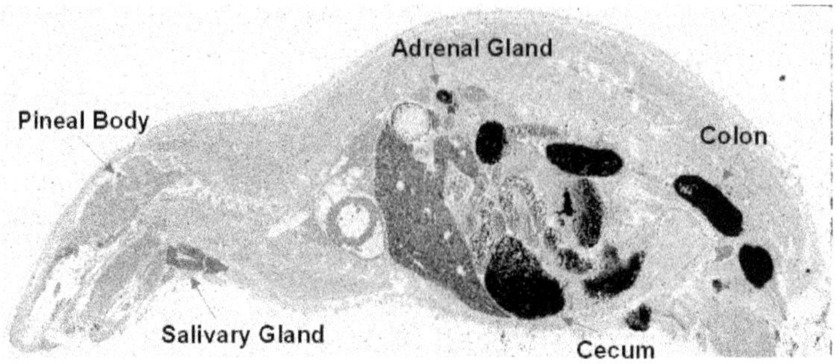

FIGURE 12.2 *Distribution of a ^{3}H-drug candidate in the male albino rat, 24 hours after oral administration.*

12.8.2 Excretion

During pre-clinical development, it is important to determine the various routes of elimination for the compound under evaluation. Pre-clinical metabolic excretion balance studies often require the investigator to account for the majority (90 per cent or greater) of the administered dose. Information from WBA studies can identify unsuspected routes of elimination (i.e. skin, bile, saliva, CO_2) which may increase the potential for complete recovery in the metabolic studies. WBA studies can also provide information on retention of radiolabelled material in the tissues or organ systems.

Figure 12.3 is an image following intravenous administration of a drug candidate to a rat, even at 15 minutes post-dose, extensive uptake by the liver is observed with some distribution in the lung and kidney. Distribution into the other tissues of the body, with the exception of the skin is minimal. The presence of radiolabelled material in the stomach suggests that the drug candidate may be directly secreted into the stomach, even at this early time point.

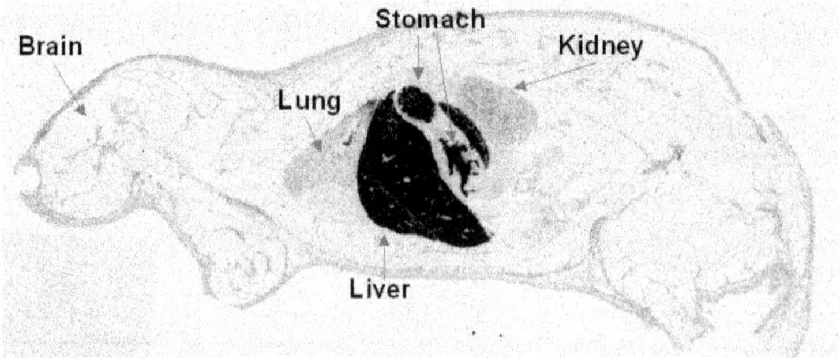

FIGURE 12.3 *Distribution of a ^{14}C-drug candidate in the male albino rat, 15 minutes after intravenous administration.*

12.8.3 SITES OF METABOLISM

High concentrations of radioactivity in a specific organ system (e.g. liver, kidney or lung) may suggest a possible site of metabolism that could be confirmed using *in vitro* tests. If radiolabelled metabolites are available, the distribution of parent and metabolite(s) can be evaluated. Figure 12.4 depicts a drug candidate with high amounts of drug-related material present in the liver at 24 hours post-dose. In this case the presence of the radioactivity correlated with liver toxicity. Subsequent extraction of liver tissue and identification of the radiolabelled material suggested a toxic metabolite.

WBA can also differentiate between the distribution of a metabolite generated *in vivo* following administration of the parent, or when it is administered as a separate entity. Plate A in Figure 12.5 represents the distribution of a ^{14}C drug candidate at 24 hours following IV administration to a male albino rat. Renal toxicity was associated with this compound in the rat species. Pre-clinical studies demonstrated that this compound was rapidly and extensively metabolised to a single metabolite, eliminated in the urine. Other species used in the toxicology studies did not produce this metabolite, and did not demonstrate renal toxicity. A study of the distribution of the metabolite in the rat was performed (Plate B, Figure 12.5) and demonstrated that the distribution of the radioactivity 24 hours post-dose was dramatically different. Subsequent toxicology studies indicated that no renal toxicity was observed when the metabolite was administered.

12.8.4 RESIDUES AND TOXICITY

WBA studies provide a method for correlating the distribution and/or retention of radiolabelled material with observed or potential toxicity. The potential for WBA studies to evaluate unanticipated sites of distribution and/or retention is one of the most appealing aspects of this technique. An example of this is a study where radiolabelled drug was administered to male albino rats by both the intravenous (IV) and oral (PO) routes. The distribution of total radioactivity to various organ

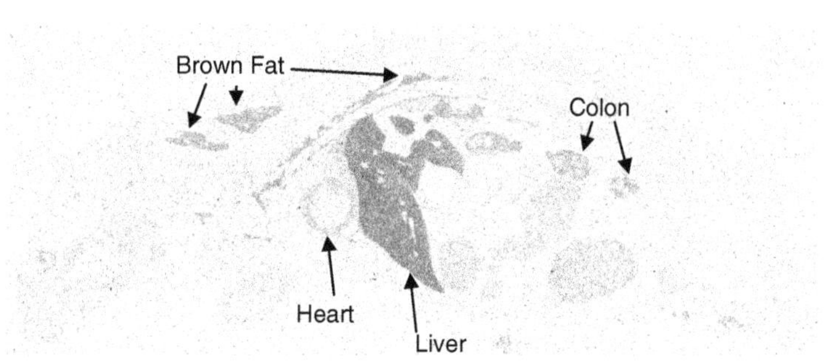

FIGURE 12.4 *Distribution of a ^{14}C-drug candidate in the male albino rat, 24 hours after intravenous administration.*

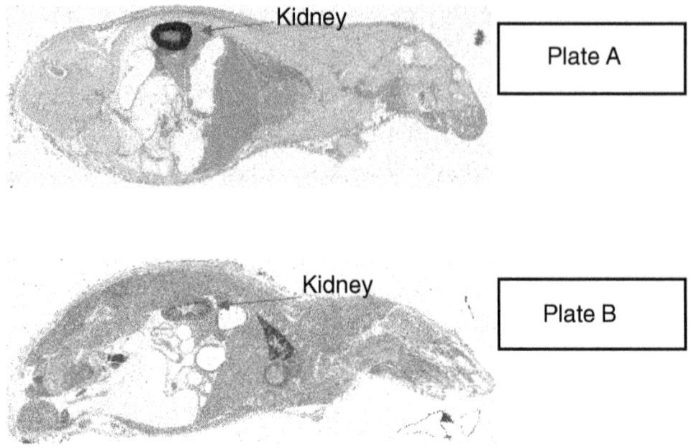

FIGURE 12.5 *Differentiation distribution of parent and metabolite following intravenous administration in the male rat. Plate A – ^{14}C parent drug candidate, Plate B – ^{14}C metabolite.*

systems was monitored for up to 96 hours after dosing. The data was then used to support the micronucleus test by indicating that there was continuous and increased exposure (relative to blood) of the bone marrow to the test material and its metabolites. In this case, the quantitative WBA data also demonstrated that there were no differences between the IV and PO routes in bone marrow exposure.

This information would also be critical in the design of the human radioactivity studies, since it suggested that drug-derived material may accumulate in the bone marrow, and this could limit the amount of radioactivity which could be administered.

Figure 12.6 provides an excellent example of how visualisation and quantification of radiolabelled material can impact upon the development of a drug candidate. During the development of this drug, QWBA studies were performed in albino animals. In the toxicology studies in dogs, histopathology work suggested

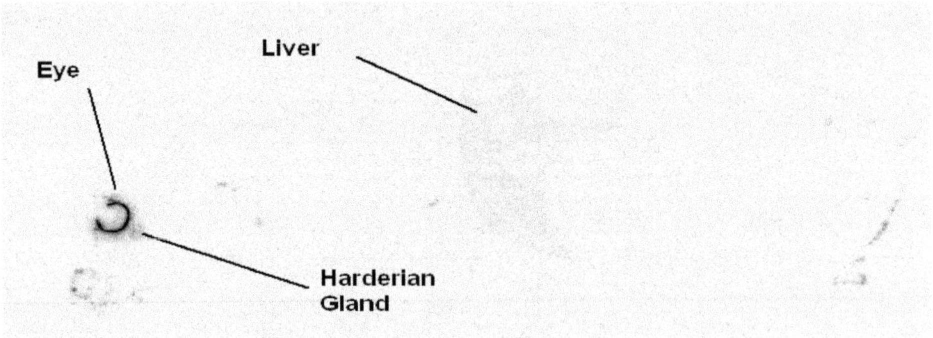

FIGURE 12.6 *Distribution of a ^{14}C-drug candidate in the male pigmented mouse, 13 days after oral administration.*

a potential structural alteration in the eye. QWBA studies in albino rats did not give any evidence for distribution into the eyes of these animals. However, when QWBA studies were performed in pigmented animals a different picture emerged. Pigmented rats demonstrated a significant amount of distribution and accumulation in the uveal tract (retina) of ^{14}C drug-related material. This observation resulted in further efforts to evaluate the time course of elimination from this site and the nature of the binding. These efforts cumulated in the identification of the metabolite responsible for the binding, and impacted the clinical program by the inclusion of ophthalmologic evaluations during the initial clinical studies.

12.8.5 Therapeutic activity

Quantitative WBA can also be used to support the potential of therapeutic activity for development compounds. Often during a drug's development the question is raised as to whether the drug is or can distribute to the site of action. QWBA provides a method to answer this question and quantitative information on the time course of the drug. Figure 12.7 demonstrates the tumour penetration and retention in mice of an agent designed to enhance the effect of anti-cancer drugs. In addition to demonstrating good tumour penetration, the agent appears to be retained in the tumour longer than in the rest of the tissues, especially blood. This could translate into a sustained effect of the compound, which can often be beneficial when developing compounds of this type.

CNS penetration of new chemical entities is also readily and rapidly evaluated using WBA. In this example, WBA was used to demonstrate a change in distribution due to the interaction of two compounds. A *p*-glycoprotein inhibitor, was administered to two groups of male mice once a day for four days prior to administration of a protease inhibitor. Following a single ^{14}C-labelled dose of protease inhibitor to each group of animals, the autoradiograms obtained at 2 hours

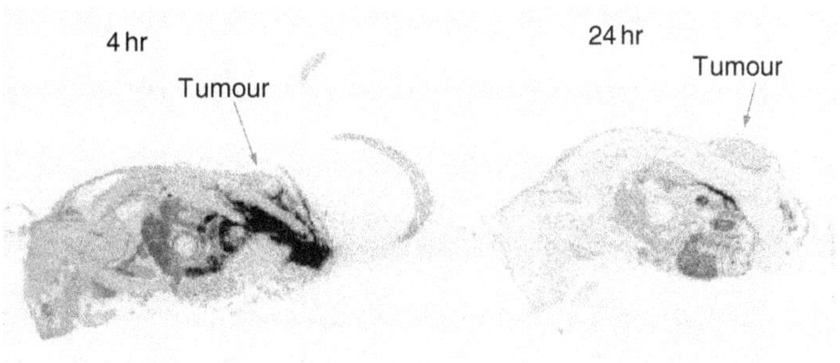

Figure 12.7 *Tumour penetration and retention following a single oral dose of ^{14}C candidate to male SCID mice.*

post-dose are shown in Figure 12.8. This time point was chosen because metabolism studies in mice indicated that the majority of the ^{14}C-labelled material circulating at this time was parent compound. Plate A is the control animal, and Plate B is a section from one of the animals that was pre-treated with the *p*-glycoprotein inhibitor. Quantification of these images revealed that there was an approximately 8-fold increase in the brain:blood ratio in the presence of the protease inhibitor, and a 2-fold increase in the CSF:blood ratio. The studies readily demonstrated the ability of *p*-gp inhibitors to dramatically alter the distribution *p*-gp substrates. It was also noted that blood levels were not substantially different between the two groups, suggesting that the absorption/elimination was not affected to any great extent (Polli *et al.*, 1999).

In the second example (Figure 12.9), WBA was used to demonstrate the lack of CNS distribution for a neuromuscular blocker under pre-clinical development. In this set of studies, the ^{14}C-labelled neuromuscular blocker was administered by continuous IV infusion to male cynomolgus monkeys (*Macaca fascicularis*) for 30 minutes. The animals were anaesthetised and ventilated during the infusion period. Quantification of the processed samples demonstrated that only very low levels of radioactivity (just above the limit of detection) were observed in brain tissue, while the meninges and cerebro-spinal fluid had slightly higher levels of radioactivity, suggesting that the compound and its metabolites have very limited penetration across the blood–brain barrier.

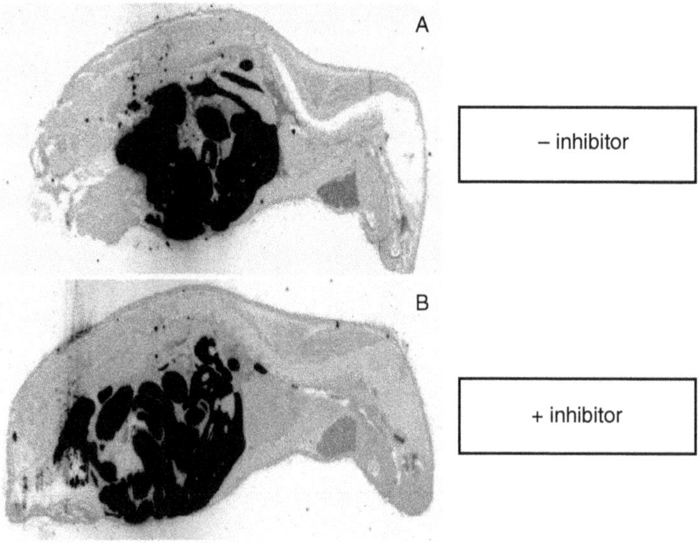

FIGURE 12.8 *Distribution of ^{14}C-p-gp substrate in male CD-1 mice pretreated with a p-gp inhibitor.*

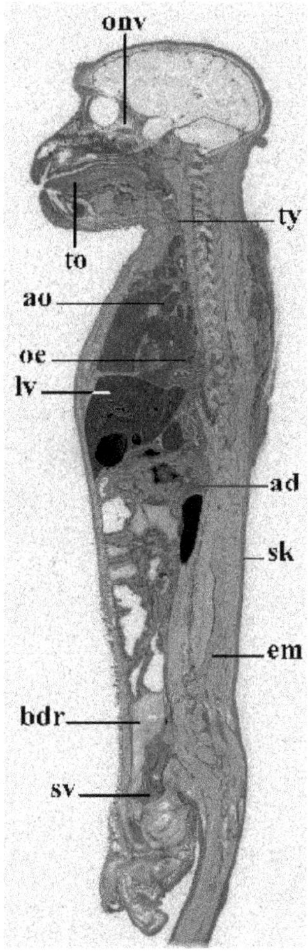

FIGURE 12.9 *Autoradiogram of a ^{14}C neuromuscular blocker in the male cynomolgus monkey following a single 30 minute intravenous infusion. ONV = optical nerve, TO = tongue, TY = trachea, OE = oesophagus, AO = Aorta, LV = liver, AD = adrenal, SK = skin, EM = epimysium, BDR = bladder, SV = Seminal vesicle.*

12.8.6 Reproductive toxicology studies

QWBA studies can also be used to provide information to support reproductive toxicology studies, by indicating the potential for accumulation in relevant target tissues, including the placenta and developing foetus. Figure 12.10 demonstrates the distribution of a ^{14}C-drug candidate following oral administration to a pregnant rat. The foetal unit (fs), uterus (ut) and placenta (pl) can be readily identified, allowing the distribution of radiolabelled drug-related material to be quantified and the drug exposure estimated.

Figure 12.11 is an enlargement of Figure 12.10 providing further information on the distribution of the radiolabelled material within the foetal unit. At this higher

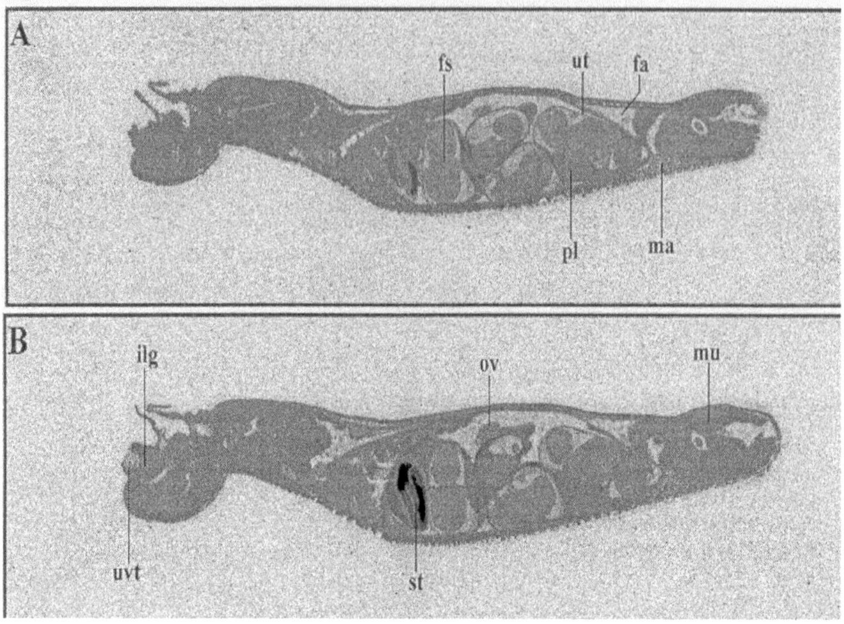

FIGURE 12.10 *Whole-body autoradiograms of a pregnant albino rat 1 hour following a single oral administration of ^{14}C-drug candidate. FS = foetus, UT = uterus, ILG = intraorbital lachrymal gland, UVT = Uveal tract, OV = ovary, ST = stomach, MU = muscle, PL = placenta, MA = mesenteric artery, FA = (white) fat.*

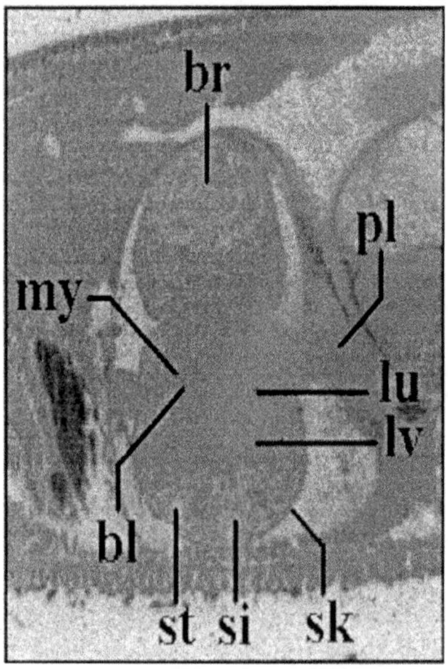

FIGURE 12.11 *Enlargement of Figure 12.10 to show additional foetal distribution detail. BR = brain, BL = blood, MY = myocardium, ST = stomach, SI = small intestine, SK = skin, LV = liver, LU = lung, PL = placenta.*

resolution, additional organs such as the brain (br), myocardium (my), blood (bl), lung (lu) and liver (lv) can be identified and ^{14}C levels quantified. Information such as this can serve to support the reproductive toxicology tests by demonstrating foetal exposure to ^{14}C-labelled drug material.

12.8.7 Human dosimetry studies

QWBA studies are often used to estimate the quantity of radiolabelled material that can be administered to humans. The amount of radioactivity is quantified in individual organs or tissues at various time points to account for the disposition and elimination of the radiolabelled material. This quantitative information is then used to estimate the exposure of the organ or tissue to the radioactivity in the animal model. This exposure in the animal model is then scaled to humans using physiologic modelling on various computer software packages such as MIRDOSE 3.0. Figure 12.12 provides an example where a compound exhibits extensive binding to melanin following oral administration in the rat. Although binding was extensive in the rat, retention was minimal, and the persistence did not adversely affect the amount of radioactivity that could safely be administered to humans.

Figure 12.6 (residues and toxicity section) gave an example of where the retention of radiolabelled material would affect the administration of radiolabelled material to humans. The extent of binding in all melanin-containing tissues and the persistence over time in the eye impact on the amount of radioactivity that could be administered in the human study. Additional WBA studies at later time points suggested that the elimination half-life in the retina of the eye was greater than 1,000 days.

Over the past ten years, QWBA has increasingly replaced traditional tissue dissection experiments undertaken to investigate the tissue distribution and retent-

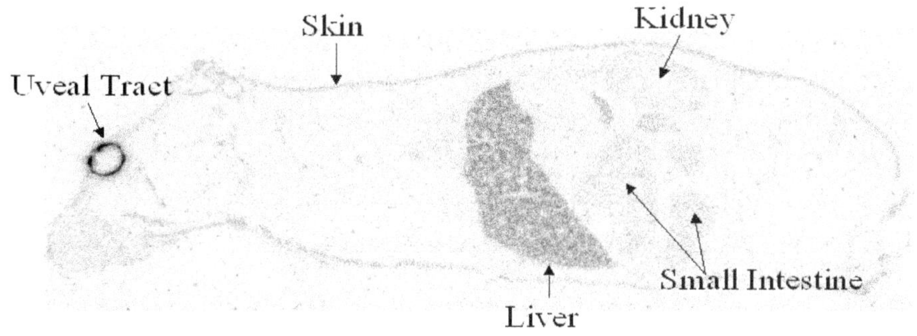

FIGURE 12.12 *Retention of ^{14}C-labelled material 7 days after an oral dose.*

ion and/or elimination of radiolabelled test materials. WBA offers several advantages over tissue dissection studies, including:

- Preservation of drug candidate localisation within the animal.
- Determination of the distribution in all organs utilising relatively few animals.
- Permitting the observation of unforeseen localisation and retention locations.
- Allowing for determination of the differential distribution within an organ system.
- Providing quantitative and qualitative information.

The primary disadvantages in the technique are that it allows for visualisation and quantification of only radiolabelled material and it is difficult to estimate the actual percent of dose within a specific organ.

However, future advances may remove some of these disadvantages. Recent experiments (Troendle *et al.*, 1999) suggested that by using a quadrupole ion trap mass spectrometer laser microprobe instrument and matrix-assisted laser desorption/ionisation (MALDI) detection, pharmaceutical compounds can be detected in intact tissue. In these studies, MALDI MS–MS was used to detect physiological relevant concentrations of paclitaxel in a human ovarian tumour. Further development of this technology may offer the ability to image the distribution of parent and metabolites of all tissues.

12.9 *References*

Becquerel, H. (1896) Sur les radiations invisibles emises per les corps phosphorescents. C.r. hebd. Séanc. *Acad. Sci.* Paris, 122, 420–421.

Curie, P. and Curie, M. (1898) Discovery of radium, anon.

Gahan, P.B. (1972) *Autoradiography for Biologists*, 1st edition. London, Academic Press.

Lacassagne, A. and Lattes, J. (1924) Repartition du polonium (injecte sous la peau) clans l'organisme du rats porteus de greffes cancereuses. C.r. Seonc. *Soc. Biol.* 90, 352–353.

Lamholt, S. (1930) Investigation into the distribution of lead in the organism on the basis of a photographic (radiochemical) method. *J. Pharmac. Exp. Ther.* 40, 235–245.

Libby, R.L. (1947) Anon. Trans. N.Y. *Acad. Sci.* 9, 249.

London, E.S. (1904) Etudes sur la valeur physiologique de l'emanation du radium. *Arch. Elec. Med.* 12, 363–372.

MIRDOSE 3.0 – Radiation Internal Dose Information Center, Oak Ridge Institute for Science and Education. Oak Ridge, TN 37831.

Miyahara, J. (1989) Visualising things never seen before. The image plate: a new radiation image sensor. *Chemistry Today*, 223, 29–36.

Motoji, N., Hayama, E. and Shigematsu, A. (1995) Studies on the quantitative. 1. Radioluminography for quantitative autoradiography of ^{14}C. *Biol. Pharm. Bull.* 18(1), 89–93.

Niepe de St Victor (1867) Sur une nouvelle action de la lumiere. C.r. hebd. Séanc. *Acad. Sci.*, Paris 65, 505.

Polli, J.W., Jarrett, J.L., Studenberg, S.D., Humphreys, J.E., Dennis, S.W., Brouwer, K.R. and Woolley, J.L. (1999) Role of *P*-glycoprotein on the CNS disposition of amprenavir (141W94), an HIV protease inhibitor. *Pharm. Res.* Vol. 16, No. 8.

Shindo (1979) Autoradiography for visual to ultramicro objectives, 1st edition. Tokyo city and medical dental press.

Troendle, F.J., Reddick, C.D. and Yost, R.A. (1999) Detection of pharmaceutical compounds in tissue by matrix-assisted laser desorption/ionization and laser desorption/chemical ionization tandem mass spectrometry with a quadrupole ion trap. *J. Am. Soc. Mass Spectrom.* 10, 1315–1321.

Ullberg, S. (1954) Studies on the distribution and fate of ^{35}S-labelled benzylpenicillin in the body. *Acta Radiol.* (Suppl. 118), 1–110.

Ullberg, S. (1958) Autoradiographic studies on the distribution of labelled drugs in the body. *Proc. Second UN Int. Conf. Peaceful Uses of Atomic Energy, Geneva, 1958*, 24, 248–254.

Ullberg, S. (1977) The technique of whole body autoradiography, cryosectioning of large specimens, *Science Tools, The LKB Instrument Journal, Special Issue.*

CHAPTER 13

Phase I metabolism

Peter Eddershaw and Maurice Dickins

13.1 *Introduction*

The overriding aim of an organism when exposed to a potential toxicant is to remove it from the body as quickly as possible. Whilst this is a sensible strategy from the point of view of survival of the organism, it represents a major barrier to the scientist seeking to produce an effective medicine. In higher mammals, myriad systems have evolved to facilitate the efficient removal of xenobiotics (i.e. foreign chemicals such as drugs, pesticides, food additives, etc.) of which the drug metabolising enzymes are a major part. The term drug metabolism enzymes may be something of an over simplification since they are often involved primarily in the metabolism of endogenous compounds. Moreover, interference with these endogenous pathways by drug molecules can result in unwanted side-effects which may not have been readily predicted from the primary pharmacology of the molecule. Therefore, a good understanding of the nature of the enzymes involved in drug metabolism can be vital in achieving a balance between efficacy and safety during the optimisation of potential new medicines.

Drug metabolism can be conveniently divided into two areas, Phase I and Phase II. Phase I metabolism, and in particular, the cytochrome P450 system, has traditionally attracted the greatest attention from the drug metabolism community and the purpose of this chapter is to provide a concise introduction to this area.

TABLE 13.1 *Reaction types catalysed by Phase I enzymes*

Enzyme	Reaction
Cytochrome P450s (CYPs)	oxidation, reduction
Monoamine oxidases (MAO)	oxidation
Flavin-containing monooxygenases (FMO)	oxidation
Alcohol dehydrogenase	oxidation
Aldehyde dehydrogenase	oxidation (reduction)
Xanthine oxidases	oxidation
Epoxide hydrolase	hydrolysis
Carboxylesterase and peptidases	hydrolysis
Carbonyl reductases	reduction

However, it is important to stress that Phase II enzymes also play a vital role in both the detoxification and elimination of drugs and that it is the combination of the two phases that helps to produce such an effective barrier to xenobiotics. Phase 2 enzymes are discussed in detail in Chapter 14. Phase I metabolism includes a range of activities such as oxidation, hydrolysis, reduction and hydration. These are often termed functionalisation reactions since they generally lead to the introduction or uncovering of key functional groups (e.g. OH, COOH, NH_2, SH, etc.) which may facilitate removal from the body, either directly, or via conjugation with the polar co-factors of Phase II metabolising systems. Table 13.1 lists the major classes of Phase I enzymes involved in drug metabolism which are described in more detail in the following sections.

13.2 *Cytochrome P450s*

The cytochrome P450s (CYPs) are a superfamily of haem-thiolate containing enzymes which play a major role in the metabolism of many drugs and other xenobiotics. A number of carcinogens are also metabolised by CYPs and it is often these metabolites which are the ultimate carcinogenic species. It has been estimated that over 50 per cent of the most commonly prescribed drugs are cleared primarily by CYPs. In addition to their role in drug metabolism, CYPs have important endogenous functions such as the synthesis and regulation of steroid hormones, eicosanoids and bile acids. Because of this, CYPs are almost ubiquitous in the human body, although the major site of drug metabolism is the liver. CYPs involved in drug metabolism are predominantly membrane bound within the endoplasmic reticulum of cells, together with the flavoprotein NADPH-cytochrome P450 reductase which is involved in the transfer of electrons from NADPH to CYPs.

In contrast to most enzymes, the CYPs involved in xenobiotic metabolism have evolved a broad substrate specificity which enables them to metabolise a very wide range of compounds to which an organism may be exposed. Despite differences in the active site architecture between CYPs, the catalytic mechanism is essentially constant across isoforms. CYPs catalyse the oxidation of bound substrates through the redox action of the haem moiety and the activation of molecular oxygen (Figure 13.1). By this mechanism, CYPs are able to carry out a variety of hydroxylations, dealkylations and heteroatom oxidations as shown in Figure 13.2. The nature of the resultant product(s) is governed by the steric interactions between enzyme and substrate, which determine the regions of a molecule that are accessible to the oxidising species, and thermodynamic factors, which can influence the relative rates of competing pathways.

A systematic nomenclature has been developed to classify the CYP superfamily. This is based on the amino acid sequence of each isoform rather than a particular reaction or substrate of individual CYPs. Isoforms with greater than 40 per cent sequence homology are assigned to the same gene family (e.g. CYP1, CYP2, CYP3, etc.). Isoforms with greater than approximately 60 per cent homology are further classified as belonging to the same subfamily (e.g. CYP2A, CYP2B, etc.). Each member of a subfamily is then given a number to denote the individual isoform (e.g. CYP2A1, CYP2A2, etc. (Table 13.2). This system does not specify in which species a given isoform is found, or provide information on the function of the enzymes. For instance, the metabolic profiles of many substrates in rat mirror those seen in human, although the P450 isoforms involved may differ. This is exemplified by the CYP3A/2C 'cross-talk' between rat and human. Thus, mephenytoin is hydroxylated predominantly by CYP2C in human but by CYP3A in rat; and

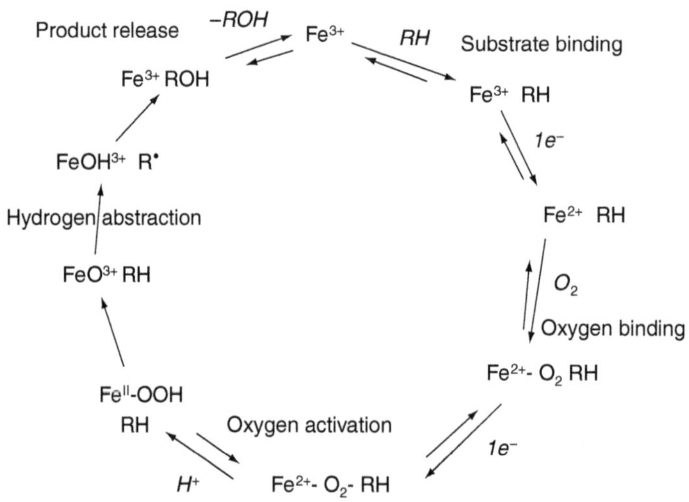

FIGURE 13.1 *Catalytic cycle of cytochrome P450s.*

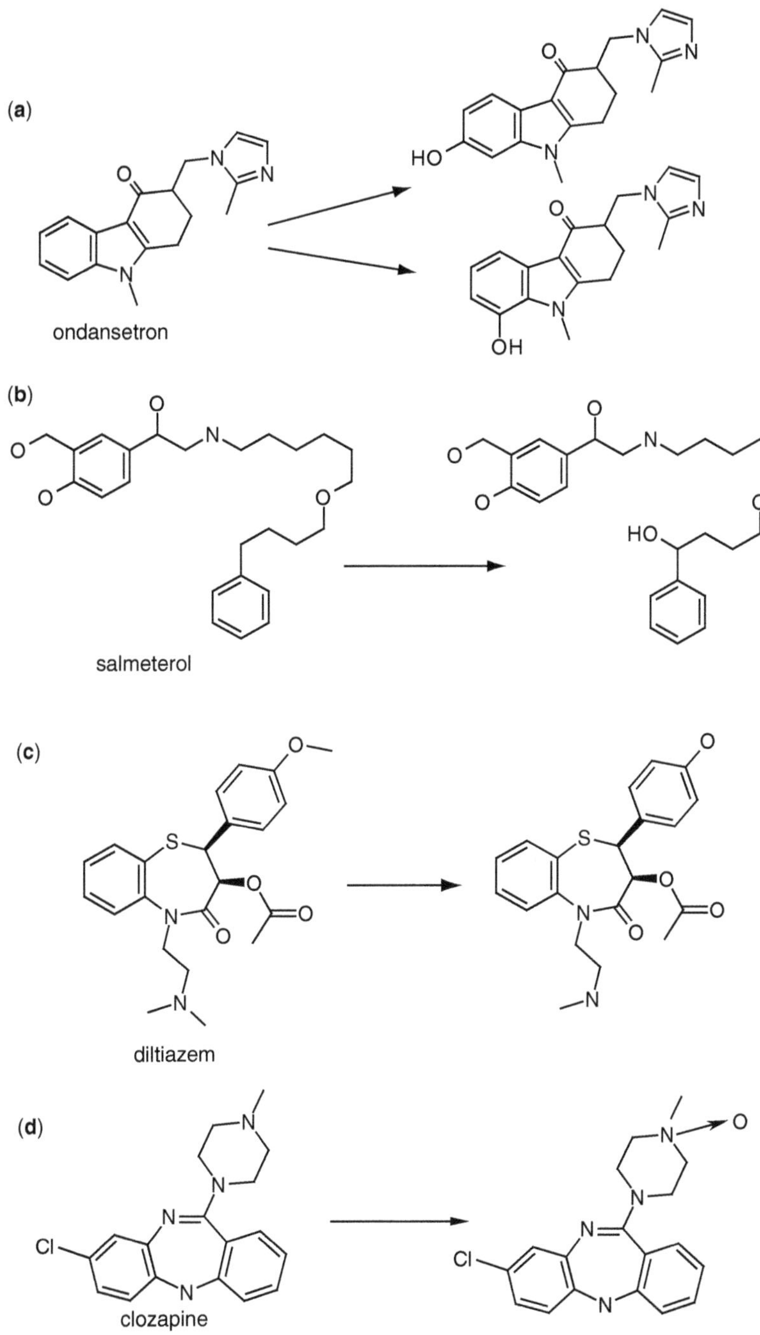

FIGURE 13.2 *Examples of reactions catalysed by CYP: (a) aromatic hydroxylation; (b) aliphatic hydroxylation; (c) N-, O-dealkylation; (d) N-oxidation.*

TABLE 13.2 *Major CYP forms*

CYP	Tissue	Inducibility	Total P450 (%)
HUMAN			
1A1	Extra hepatic	Inducible	
1A2	Liver	Constitutive/inducible	13
2A6	Liver		4
2B6	Liver	Constitutive	0.2
2C9/19	Liver	Constitutive	20
2D6	Liver	Constitutive	2
2E1	Liver	Constitutive/inducible	7
3A4	Liver/others	Constitutive/inducible	30
RAT			
1A1	All tissues	Inducible	<1
1A2	Liver	Constitutive	2
	All tissues	Inducible	
2A1	Liver	Constitutive	7–30
	Liver	Inducible	(varies according to strain/induced state, etc.)
2B1/2	Lung, testis	Constitutive	5
	All tissues	Inducible	
2C11	Liver	Constitutive	54
2D1	Liver/kidney	Constitutive	
	Inducible		
2E1	Liver/kidney	Constitutive	
	Liver/lung	Inducible	
3A1	Liver/intestine	Constitutive/inducible	17
DOG			
1A	Hepatic	Inducible	similar to human
2B11	Liver	Constitutive	high levels c.f. human
2C21	Liver	Constitutive	minor form
2D	Liver	Constitutive	lower levels c.f. human
3A12	Liver/others	Constitutive	similar to human levels 3A; higher catalytic efficiency

lidocaine and nifedipine are classic CYP3A substrates in human but are preferentially metabolised by CYP2C in rat.

The number of identified CYPs is increasing on a seemingly daily basis. Fortunately, the group of isoforms involved in the majority of human drug metabolism is currently limited to only five or six: CYP1A2, 2C9, 2C19, 2D6 and 3A4/5 (Figure 13.3). Despite the relatively small number of CYPs involved, marked intra- and inter-individual variability exists in both the genotype and phenotype of the

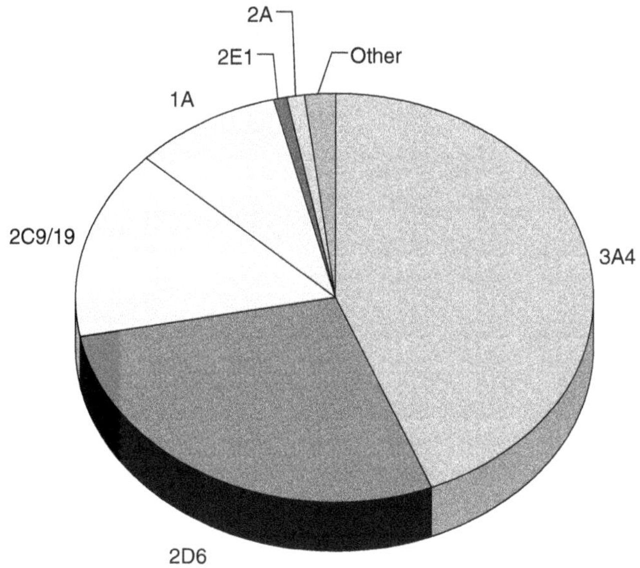

FIGURE 13.3 *Percentage of commonly prescribed drugs metabolised by each CYP isoform.*

human population, which can often be a major cause of the variability in efficacy and/or toxicity of many prescribed medicines observed in patients.

In addition to the effects of age and gender, the range and extent of CYP activity are influenced by both genetic and environmental factors. Inherited mutations in the coding and/or regulatory regions of CYP genes may prevent synthesis of a particular CYP or result in a protein that has reduced catalytic activity. The impact of polymorphism amongst CYPs on human drug metabolism has been most clearly demonstrated for CYP2D6, CYP2C9 and CYP2C19. These isoforms are an important part of the human complement of drug-metabolising enzymes and thus deficiencies in their activities can have important consequences for the disposition of compounds which are dependent on them for clearance. Significant proportions of various ethnic populations have been identified as poor metabolisers of drugs such as debrisoquine (a substrate for CYP2D6) and *S*-mephenytoin (CYP2C19) (Table 13.3) and many other examples have been observed. From a clinical perspective, the appearance of a poor metaboliser phenotype for a given drug is dependent largely on the fraction of the administered dose that is cleared via the affected isoform and the availability of alternative or competing clearance mechanisms. For example, the 5-HT_3 receptor antagonists, ondansetron and tropisetron can both be metabolised *in vitro* by the polymorphic CYP2D6. However, whilst this is the major pathway for tropisetron, metabolism by CYP3A4 is the predominant route of clearance for ondansetron. Thus, in patients who are deficient in CYP2D6, the plasma concentration half-life of tropisetron increases from approximately 9 to 30 hours whereas no change in the half-life of ondansetron is observed. Whether the existence of polymorphism in drug clearance

TABLE 13.3 *Distribution of polymorphic CYPs in human populations*

			Allele frequency (%)		
Enzyme	**Variant allele**	**Enzyme function**	**Caucasian**	**Asian**	**Black African**
CYP2A6	CYP2A6 × 2	Inactive	1–3	0	–
	CYP2A6del	Enzyme absent	1	15	–
CYP2C9	CYP2C9 × 2	Reduced affinity for reductase	8–13	0	–
	CYP2C9 × 3	Altered substrate specificity	6–9	2–3	–
CYP2C19	CYP2C19 × 2	Inactive	13	23–32	13
	CYP2C19 × 3	Inactive	0	6–10	–
CYP2D6	CYP2D6 × 2 × n	Increased activity	1–5	0–2	2
	CYP2D6 × 4	Inactive	12–21	1	2
	CYP2D6 × 5	Enzyme absent	2–7	6	4
	CYP2D6 × 10	Unstable enzyme	1–2	51	6
	CYPD6 × 17	Reduced	0	–	34

has any adverse clinical consequences is in turn dependent on the therapeutic margin of the drug and any impact its elevated concentrations may have on co-administered medications.

Environmental agents such as drugs, other xenobiotics or disease can also cause a (usually) more transient attenuation of CYP activity, either through the prevention of gene expression or by inhibition of the subsequently expressed protein. Inhibition of CYP activity by drug molecules is an area of intense interest for drug metabolism scientists. The occurrence of adverse drug–drug interactions and/or the disruption of endogenous biochemical pathways as a result of CYP inhibition can severely compromise or even preclude the clinical viability of a drug candidate. Several well-documented examples of this exist, including the interaction between the antihistamine, terfenadine, and the antifungal, ketoconazole, in which potent inhibition of the CYP3A4-mediated metabolism of terfenadine by ketoconazole resulted in cardiac toxicity and, in some cases, death, in patients taking both agents concurrently. Despite the increased awareness of the occurrence of CYP inhibition and the development of an array of *in vivo* and *in vitro* methodologies to investigate potential interactions, the recent withdrawal of mibefradil (Posicor^{TM}) from the market, due to a plethora of unforeseen drug–drug interactions, shows that this can still be a serious problem in drug development.

Conversely, increases in CYP activity can also lead to variability in the disposition of drugs. The presence of multiple copies of a CYP gene can give rise to higher constitutive levels of active enzyme than in individuals possessing only a single copy of the gene. More commonly, certain CYP levels can be induced by exposure to a variety of xenobiotics, typically as drugs, dietary components or cigarette smoke (Table 13.4).

TABLE 13.4 *Inducers of human liver CYPs*

CYP1A2	CYP2C9	CYP2C19	CYP2E1	CYP3A4
Cruciferous	Rifampicin	Rifampicin	Ethanol	Rifampacin
Vegetables			Isoniazid	Dexamethasone
β-Naphthoflavone				Carbamazepine
Omeprazole				Phenobarbital
Tobacco smoke				Phenytoin
3-methyl				Troleandomycin
Cholanthrene				Troglitazone

The exact mechanisms by which CYP induction occurs are in some cases only partially understood at present. The role of receptors such as the aryl hydrocarbon (Ah), pregnane X (PXR) and constitutive androstane (CAR) receptors has been characterised in the induction of CYP1A, CYP3A and CYP2B, respectively. However, given the importance of the CYP system in so many biochemical processes within the body, it is likely that the regulation of these enzymes is under a complex control system with multiple inputs which are yet to be identified. Induction of CYPs is generally triggered by a degree of prolonged exposure to a given chemical, either through multiple dosing of a drug or the persistence of a longer-lived acute therapy. Induction of a specific CYP isoform may manifest itself clinically through a reduction in the systemic exposure of the inducing agent itself on repeat administration ('autoinduction') and/or that of co-administered drugs and thus result in a significant decrease in the efficacy of drug treatment. For instance, induction of CYP3A4 by the antibiotic, rifampacin, causes a decrease in the systemic exposure of synthetic steroids such as ethynyloestradiol which are metabolised by this isoform, with subsequent loss of contraceptive activity.

13.3 *Monoamine oxidases (MAO)*

MAO enzymes are present in humans as two forms, MAO-A and MAO-B. The enzymes are located in the mitochondria and are present in a range of tissues such as liver, kidney, intestine and brain. MAO-A preferentially oxidises serotonin (5-hydroxytryptamine) whereas MAO-B substrates include arylalkylamines such as phenylethylamine and benzylamine. Substrates of MAO undergo oxidative deamination but, unlike CYPs, the oxygen incorporated into the metabolite is derived from water rather than molecular oxygen. The initial step of the reaction appears to be abstraction of hydrogen from the α-carbon adjacent to the nitrogen atom.

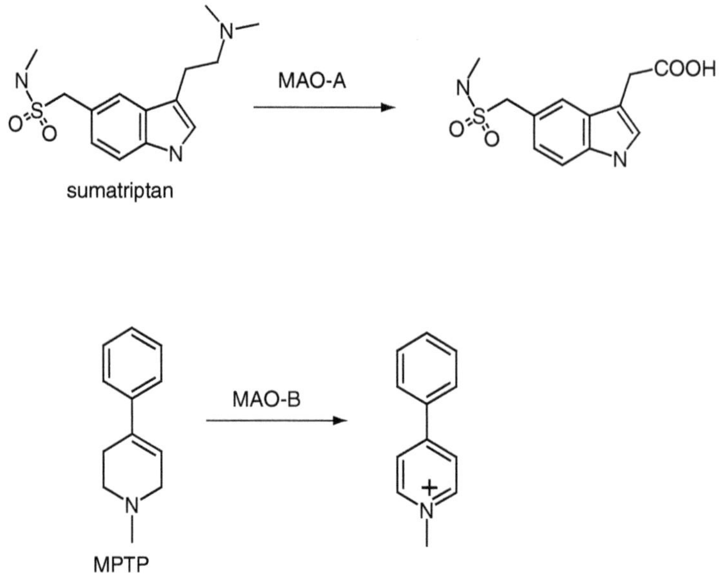

FIGURE 13.4 *The metabolism of sumatriptan and MPTP (1-methyl-4-phenyl-1,2,5,6-tetrahydropyridine) by MAO-A and MAO-B.*

Pharmaceutical agents such as the anti-migraine drugs (5-$HT_{1B/1D}$ receptor agonists) sumatriptan and zolmitriptan are known to be metabolised by MAO-A (Figure 13.4). More recent compounds of this class are substituted at the α-carbon atom, making them resistant to metabolic attack by MAO-A.

An example of an MAO-B substrate is the experimental compound MPTP (1-methyl-4-phenyl-1,2,5,6-tetrahydropyridine) which causes symptoms of Parkinson's disease in primates. The ultimate metabolite MPP^+ is a neurotoxin which selectively degrades cells in the substantia nigra region of the brain which generates the neurotransmitter dopamine.

13.4 *Flavin monooxygenases (FMO)*

The FMO are a family of microsomal enzymes which complement the CYPs in that they typically carry out oxidation by nucleophilic attack at heteroatoms such as N-, S- and P-CYP substrates are metabolised by electrophilic attack, more usually at carbon atoms. However, both CYPs and FMOs have the same cofactor requirements, NADPH and molecular oxygen, although the mechanism of the reaction is very different. For FMO, the reaction involves formation of a peroxide intermediate which then oxygenates the substrate (Figure 13.5). The activation of the enzyme/

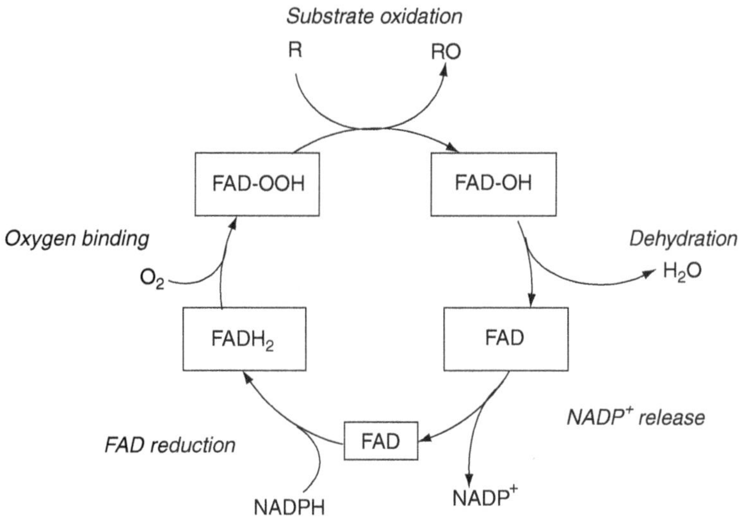

FIGURE 13.5 *Catalytic cycle of FMO.*

cofactor complex prior to interaction with a substrate has led FMOs to be likened to a loaded gun awaiting a target!

As for CYPs, the FMOs are an enzyme superfamily which consists of isoforms FMO1–FMO5. There are also species differences in the occurrence of these isoforms – for example, FMO1 is prevalent in the liver of rat, pig and rabbit but FMO3 is the major human hepatic isoform.

Substrates for FMO3 include nicotine and the H_2-antagonist ranitidine (Figure 13.6).

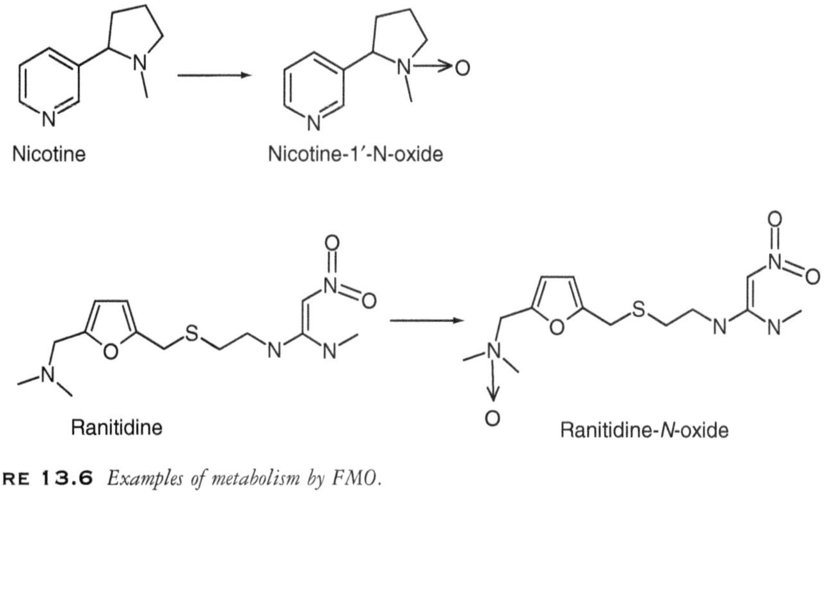

FIGURE 13.6 *Examples of metabolism by FMO.*

13.5 *Alcohol dehydrogenases (ADH) and aldehyde dehydrogenases (ALDH)*

ADH and ALDH are cytosolic enzymes which convert alcohols to aldehydes (by the action of ADH), and the aldehyde products are subsequently metabolised to carboxylic acids by ALDH enzymes. Both ADHs and ALDHs are found mainly in the liver but are also found in the kidney, lung and gastrointestinal tract and require NAD^+ as cofactor. One form of an atypical ADH is prevalent in Japanese (85 per cent of the population) which results in unusually rapid conversion of ethanol to acetaldehyde. However, the ALDH enzyme responsible for the further oxidation of acetaldehyde to acetic acid is atypical in that about 50 per cent of Japanese are poor metabolisers of acetaldehyde. Thus the unwanted effects of acetaldehyde (flushing, nausea) explain why the Japanese are notoriously intolerant to alcohol.

ADH and ALDH are not widely involved in the metabolism of drugs although the antiviral agent abacavir is an example of a compound which is metabolised by the enzymes.

13.6 *Molybdenum hydroxylases*

13.6.1 Xanthine oxidase (XO)

XO catalyses the sequential oxidation of hypoxanthine to xanthine and uric acid. Monomethylated xanthines can also be oxidised to the corresponding derivatives of uric acid, but dimethylxanthines (theophylline, theobromine) and 1,3,7-trimethylxanthine (caffeine) are oxidised to these types of metabolite by CYP. A classic inhibitor of xanthine oxidase is allopurinol, a drug used to treat gout, a condition due to the over production of uric acid which results in crystal deposits of the poorly soluble acid in the joints.

The prodrug, 6-deoxyaciclovir, is efficiently converted to the anti-viral agent acyclovir by the action of xanthine oxidase (Figure 13.7).

13.6.2 Aldehyde oxidase (AO)

Like XO, AO is a cytosolic molybdenum containing oxidase which functions as a true oxidase, that is the enzyme is first reduced and then re-oxidised by molecular oxygen. However, the oxygen atom incorporated in the metabolite is from water and not molecular oxygen.

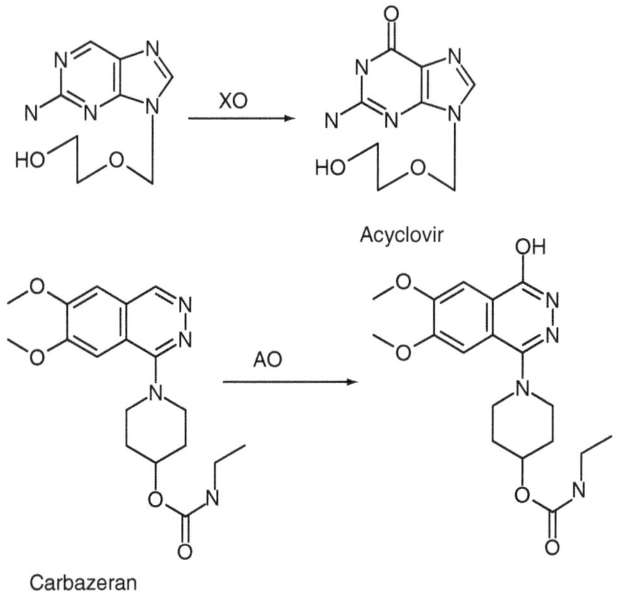

FIGURE 13.7 *Examples of reactions catalysed by xanthine oxidase and aldehyde oxidase.*

The substrates for these enzymes are typically aromatic azaheterocycles such as pyrimidines and purines. Oxidation takes place at a carbon which is electron deficient, typically adjacent to the N heteroatom (which renders the carbon electron deficient). A number of drugs are substrates for aldehyde oxidase including the antiviral prodrug molecule famciclovir which undergoes C-6 oxidation and ester hydrolysis to generate the active antiviral molecule, penciclovir. Phthalazines such as carbazeran are also oxidised by aldehyde oxidase (Figure 13.7).

13.6.3 EPOXIDE HYDROLASE

Epoxide hydrolase (EH) catalyses the conversion of epoxides and arene oxides to diols through the addition of water. These potentially toxic electrophilic epoxides are often formed as the result of oxidation of alkenes and aromatic hydrocarbons by CYP. The importance of this role is reflected in the widespread distribution of EH throughout the body in a manner which closely parallels that of the CYPs. Similarly, many known inducers of CYP are also able to induce EH.

Hydrolysis of epoxides by EH is effected by abstraction of a proton from a water molecule to form a nucleophilic hydroxide ion which then attacks one of the carbon atoms of the epoxide. This attack usually occurs at the less-hindered carbon atom, with the subsequent protonation of the alkoxide ion intermediate preferentially occurring on the opposite side of the molecule to give the *trans* configuration. Substrates for EH include the epoxide metabolites of carbamazepine and several

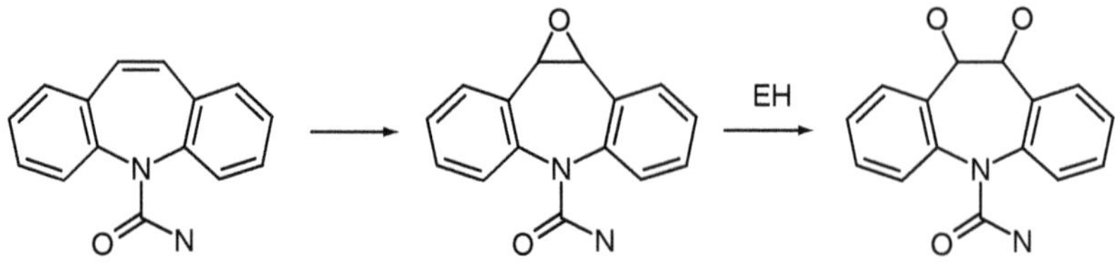

FIGURE 13.8 *Metabolism of carbazepine by epoxide hydrolase.*

polycyclic aromatic hydrocarbons. Metabolism of carbazepine by epoxide hydrolase is illustrated in Figure 13.8.

13.6.4 Carboxylesterases and peptidases

The carboxylesterases comprise a family of enzymes that are able to hydrolyse various drugs and other xenobiotics containing acid, amide or thioester functions. Some carboxylesterases play an important role in the detoxification of organophosphate pesticides (OPs) and it is this activity which is commonly used to classify the enzymes; A-esterases are able to hydrolyse OPs, B-esterases are inhibited by OPs and C-esterases do not interact with OPs. Many A-esterases contain a cysteine residue in the active site whilst the majority of B-esterases contain a serine atom which may explain the difference in behaviour towards OPs of the two groups.

The peptidases are a related group of enzymes found extensively in the blood, liver and other tissues where they are responsible for the hydrolysis of peptides and peptide-mimetics through nucleophilic attack on the carbonyl function of a peptide bond.

13.6.5 Carbonyl reductases

Carbonyl reductases are enzymes which reduce aldehydes and ketones to primary and secondary alcohols. These enzymes require NADPH as cofactor in contrast to ADH and ALDH. Typical drug substrates are ketones rather than aldehydes since very few therapeutic agents contain an aldehyde function due to its reactive nature. A number of therapeutic agents such as haloperidol, daunorubicin, warfarin and nafimidone undergo metabolism by these enzymes. The smoking cessation drug buproprion is reduced to 494U73 by this class of enzyme (Figure 13.9).

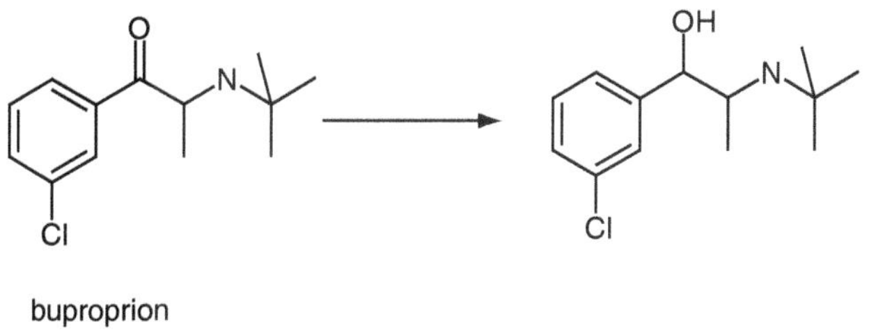

FIGURE 13.9 *Metabolism of bupropion by carbonyl reductases.*

13.7 *Conclusions*

It is clear from even the brief overview presented here that Phase I metabolising enzymes represent a formidable challenge for drug discovery scientists. It has become increasingly clear that the successful development of safe and effective medicines requires a detailed understanding of the way in which drug molecules interact with the drug-metabolising enzymes. This is true not only in terms of achieving optimal pharmacokinetics for a drug candidate itself but also in ensuring that the impact on other co-administered therapies is negligible. To this end, considerable effort continues to be directed towards characterising all aspects of the structure, function and regulation of the major Phase I enzyme systems. Of particular note in this regard is the impact of computational modelling and data analysis methods on improving our ability to rationalise and, ultimately, predict the metabolic disposition of drug molecules in humans. This increase in knowledge of the fundamental principles underlying Phase I metabolism will contribute greatly to a more rational, hollistic approach to drug design.

CHAPTER 14

Phase II enzymes

Gary Manchee, Maurice Dickins and Elizabeth Pickup

14.1 *Introduction*

Phase II enzymes are becoming increasingly important in drug discovery and drug development. Although Phase I oxidations are recognised as providing the major rate-limiting processes to metabolic clearance, there are a number of pharmaceutical agents which are primarily cleared metabolically by Phase II enzymes, for example, NSAIDs, tricyclic anti-depressants, β_2-agonists and some anti-HIV drugs (Miners and Mackenzie, 1991). The recognition of this fact is driving the need for more detailed and comprehensive information on the nature of the individual Phase II enzymes and their catalytic properties. This knowledge lags behind that available for CYPs, but it is important to identify specific isoforms within enzyme families that are involved in the Phase II metabolism of new chemical entities (NCEs), particularly with a view to their use in multidrug therapies in patient populations.

There are a variety of Phase II conjugating enzyme systems that attack at functional groups such as –OH, –COOH, $–NH_2$, –SH, which are either present naturally on the target molecules or which have been generated by Phase I oxidative metabolism. Whilst Phase II metabolic reactions usually generate hydrophilic metabolites which are readily excreted in urine or bile, it should be noted that such metabolism may also give rise to reactive, potentially toxic metabolites which may bind covalently to tissue macromolecules.

When considering the scope of Phase II enzymes, it is also of importance to remember their role in the metabolism of endogenous substrates. Whereas a number of CYPs carry out highly selective, specific reactions (e.g. CYPs involved in cholesterol biosynthesis), the same Phase II enzymes involved in xenobiotic metabolism frequently metabolise a number of endogenous substrates such as bilirubin, steroids and biogenic amines. Hence it is feasible to envisage situations in which xenobiotics and endogenous compounds may compete for the same Phase II metabolic pathway.

This chapter will describe Phase II reactions, nomenclature and the emerging information, which concentrates on the use and nomenclature of Phase II enzyme systems, and focuses on some issues which may be relevant in the development of new medicines such as polymorphisms, induction and drug–drug interactions.

14.2 *Phase II enzyme reactions*

Xenobiotic and endogenous compounds undergo metabolism by Phase I (functionalisation) and Phase II (conjugation) enzymes. For some compounds, Phase I metabolism occurs before a Phase II reaction is possible, and in some cases Phase II products undergo further Phase I metabolism (sulphated steroids). Table 14.1 details the Phase II enzymes. Phase II reactions generally result in the generation of more polar, more easily excretable compounds which are largely devoid of significant pharmacological or toxicological activity.

TABLE 14.1 *Phase II enzymes and their reaction with functional groups*

Enzyme	Reaction	Functional group
UDP-glucuronosyltransferase	Glucuronidation	–OH, –COOH, –NH, –NOH, $–NH_2$, –SH, ring N
UDP-glycosyltransferase	Glycosidation	–OH, –COOH, –SH
Sulphotransferase	Sulphation	–OH, –NH, –NOH, $–NH_2$,
Methyltransferase	Methylation	–OH, $–NH_2$
Acetyltransferase	Acetylation	–OH, $–NH_2$, $–SO_2NH_2$
Amino acid conjugation		–COOH
Glutathione-S-transferase	Glutathione conjugation	Epoxide, organic halide
Fatty acid conjugation		–OH

Adapted from Gibson and Skett, 1994.

14.2.1 Glucuronidation

Glucuronidation is a major pathway of Phase II metabolism and involves the transfer of the sugar acid, D-glucuronic acid with the acceptor substrate. Such conjugation reactions are catalysed by a family of enzymes called uridine diphosphate (UDP)-glucuronosyltransferases or UGTs (Tephly and Burchell, 1990). For glucuronidation the cosubstrate UDP-glucuronic acid (UDPGA) is required and this is synthesised from glucose-1-phosphate and UTP in a two-stage reaction (Figure 14.1). The product of the initial reaction is UDP-glucose (UDPG) which is then oxidised by the UDPG dehydrogenase enzyme to produce UDPGA (Dutton, 1966).

The UDP-glucuronosyltransferases are membrane-bound proteins located on the inside of the endoplasmic reticulum (ER) and nuclear membrane of cells. They are found in highest concentration in the liver but are also present in many other tissues including small intestine, kidney, lung and skin. Most UGTs are capable of glucuronidating a wide range of xenobiotics but show a greater specificity for endogenous compounds (e.g. estrogens, androgens, bilirubin) which generally react with one specific form of UDPGT (Tephly and Burchell, 1990). Some examples of the glucuronidation of xenobiotic compounds are shown in Figure 14.2.

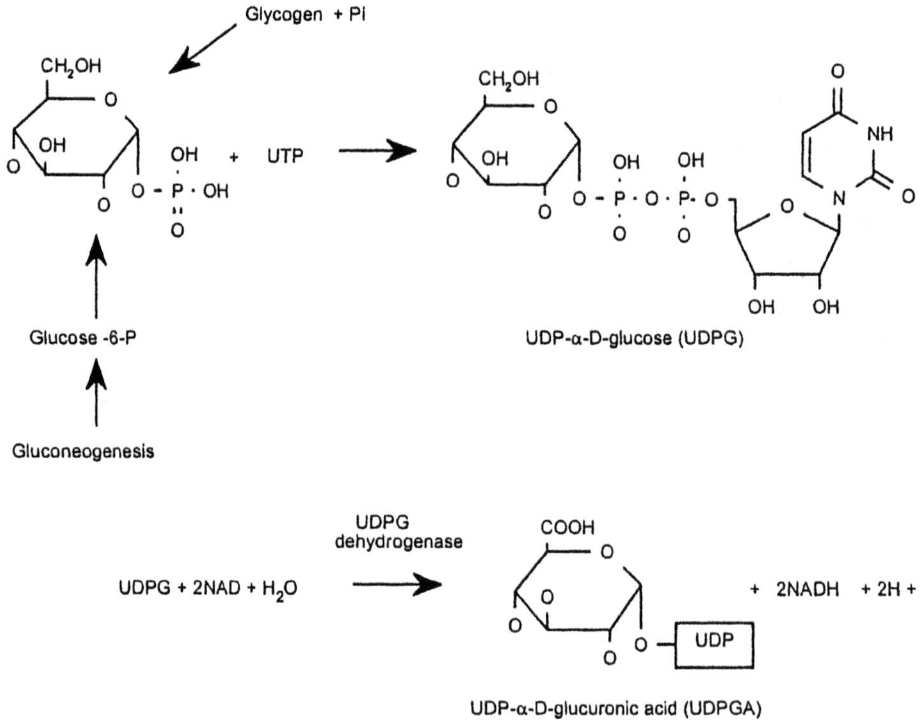

FIGURE 14.1 *Synthesis of UDPGA.*

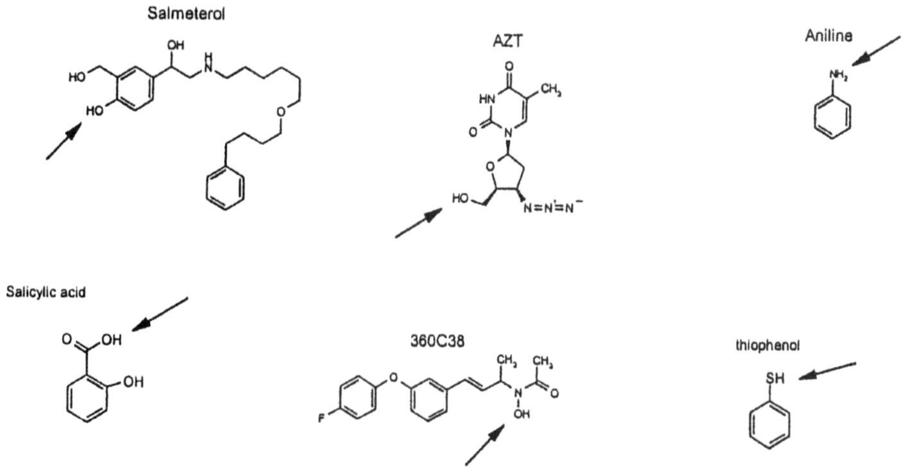

FIGURE 14.2 *Glucuronidation of some xenobiotic compounds.*

There is a wide variation in data obtained from microsomal UGT assays due to latency of the membrane-bound enzyme (Burchell and Coughtrie, 1989). Detergents such as Lubrol PX cause the release of this latent UDPGT activity by disrupting the membrane structure (Vanstapel and Blanckaert, 1988). Following on from this, a model has been proposed in which transport of UDPGA is rate limiting for glucuronidation in intact microsomes, but perturbation of the ER membrane by detergents allows free access of UDPGA and releases the latent UGT enzyme activity. However, substrate access to the enzyme may actually be more rate limiting than UDPGA access (Burchell and Coughtrie, 1989). Studies of the topology of UGTs have revealed a small C-terminal region on the cytoplasmic side of the membrane, linked by a transmembrane-spanning domain to the majority of the protein which is located in the lumen of the ER (Tephly and Burchell, 1990).

14.2.2 SULPHATION

Sulphation is a major pathway of Phase II drug metabolism and is carried out by a family of enzymes called the sulfotransferases (STs). These enzymes play a fundamental role in the metabolism and excretion of both endogenous compounds and xenobiotics. They exhibit a broad range of substrate specificities encompassing endogenous compounds, such as steroid hormones, bile acids, iodothyronines, monoamine neurotransmitters, sugar residues of glycoproteins and glycosaminoglycans, and tyrosine residues in proteins and peptides, as well as detoxifying xenobiotics including drugs, environmental pollutants and food additives (Falany *et al.*, 1993).

Two types of ST enzymes exist in man, which are distinguished by their subcellular localisation and functions. The first type is located in a membrane-bound state in the Golgi apparatus (Falany, 1991). These STs are responsible for the sulphation of endogenous proteins, peptides and glycans, often on tyrosine residues to produce post-translational modifications. The second type of STs is cytosolic enzymes involved in the detoxification and metabolism of endogenous and exogenous compounds (Weinshilboum and Otterness, 1994). Sulphation, like glucuronidation, also occurs in many mammalian tissues with generally greatest activity in the liver and small intestine (Wong and Yeo, 1982; Pacifici *et al.*, 1988). Sulphation of steroids occurs in most tissues, although the highest activity is found in adrenal, kidney, brain, etc. (Falany *et al.*, 1993). The cytosolic ST enzymes will be discussed in detail in this chapter. It is important to note that STs often form a low-capacity–high-affinity partner to the UGTs, which are typically high-capacity–low-affinity enzymes for xenobiotics.

The enzymes catalyse the transfer of a charged sulphonate group from the cofactor PAPS by electrophilic attack at the oxygen and nitrogen atoms of –C–OH, –N–OH and –NH groups. The cofactor PAPS is synthesised from ATP and inorganic sulfate by the sequential action of two enzymes (Figure 14.3), ATP sulphurylase and adenosine 5′-phosphosulphate kinase. Some examples of the sulphation of xenobiotic compounds are shown in Figure 14.4.

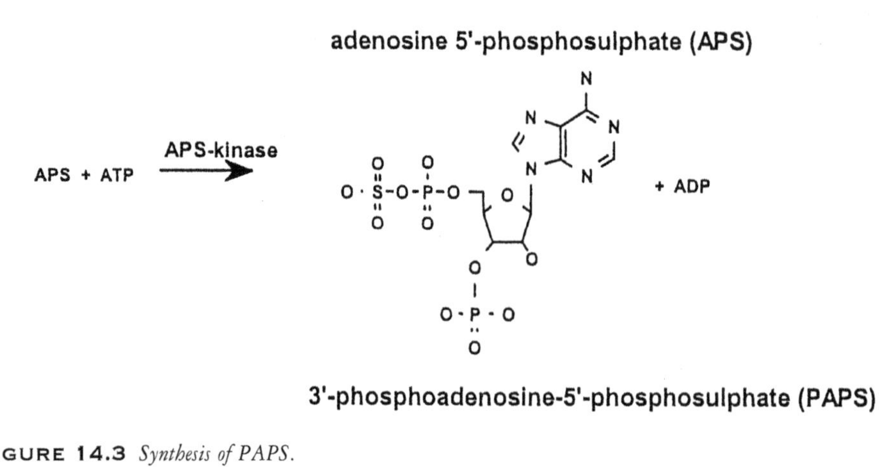

FIGURE 14.3 *Synthesis of PAPS.*

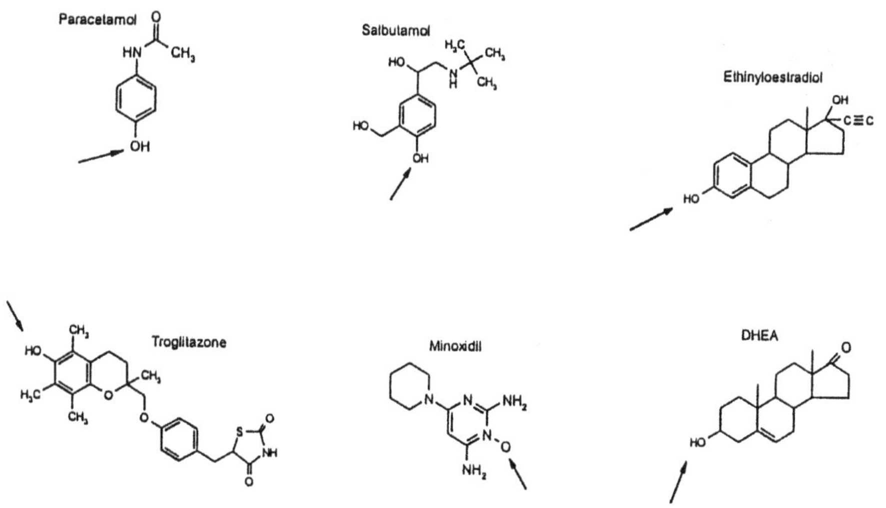

FIGURE 14.4 *Sulphation of some xenobiotic compounds.*

14.2.3 Methylation

Methylation is a minor pathway for xenobiotic metabolism although it is an essential step for some endogenous compounds such as catechols, catecholamines, histamine and *N*-acetylserotonin. Methylation differs from other Phase II reactions because it usually results in a decrease in the water solubility of xenobiotics. This is not always the case since N-methylation of pyridine groups, e.g. nicotine can produce quaternary ammonium ions that are very water soluble.

The cofactor for methylation is *S*-adenosylmethionine (SAM). The synthesis of SAM is shown in Figure 14.5. The methyl group bound to the sulphonium ion in SAM is transferred to acceptor substrates by nucleophilic attack from an electron-rich heteroatom (*0*, *N* or *S*).

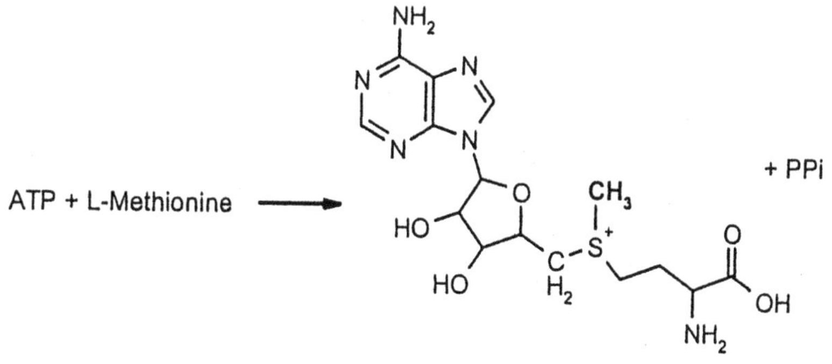

FIGURE 14.5 *Synthesis of SAM.*

Methylation of phenols and catechols is catalysed by two different enzymes known as phenol *O*-methyltransferase (POMT) and catechol *O*-methyltransferase (COMT) (Weinshilboum, 1989, 1992). POMT is a microsomal enzyme that methylates phenols but not catechols, and COMT is a cytosolic enzyme with the converse substrate specificity. COMT has a more important role in the metabolism of catechols than POMT has in the metabolism of phenols. COMT is present in most tissues with the highest concentrations in the liver and kidney. Substrates for COMT include neurotransmitters like adrenaline, noradrenaline and dopamine and catechol drugs like L-dopa, isoprenaline and isoetharine. In humans, COMT is encoded by a single gene with alleles for a low- and high-activity forms (Weinshilboum, 1989, 1992). In Caucasians, these allelic variants are expressed with equal frequency whereas in African Americans the higher activity form is more prevalent.

Two *N*-methyltransferases have been described in humans, one is known as histamine *N*-methyltransferase which methylates the imidazole ring of histamine and related compounds. The other enzyme is known as nicotinamide *N*-methyltransferase which methylates compounds containing a pyridine ring, like nicotine or an indole ring like serotonin. Classification of human *N*-methyltransferases may not be applicable to other species. S-methylation is also an important pathway in the metabolism of some xenobiotics such as captopril, D-penicillamine and 6-mercaptopurine. In humans, S-methylation is catalysed by two enzymes, thiopurine methyltransferase (TPMT) and thiol methyltransferase (TMT). TPMT is a cytoplasmic enzyme with preference for aromatic and heterocyclic compounds like 6-mercaptopurine and azathioprine. TMT is a microsomal enzyme with preference for aliphatic sulph-hydryl compounds like captopril. TPMT is encoded by a single gene with alleles for low- and high-activity forms. The gene frequency of TPMT, low (6 per cent) and high (94 per cent), activity forms produces a trimodal distribution of TPMT activity expressed in 0.3, 11.1 and 88.6 per cent of the population, respectively. Low TPMT activity in cancer patients can lead to toxicity, whereas high TPMT activity may result in poor exposure to the drug. Some examples of the methylation of xenobiotic compounds are shown in Figure 14.6.

14.2.4 Acetylation

Acetylation is a major route of metabolism for xenobiotics containing an aromatic amine ($R–NH_2$) or a hydrazine group ($R–NH–NH_2$), which are converted to

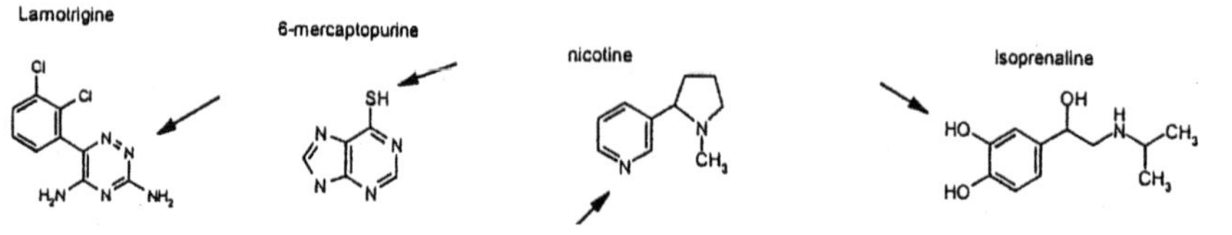

FIGURE 14.6 *Methylation of some xenobiotic compounds.*

aromatic amides (R–NH–$COCH_3$) and hydrazides (R–NH–NH–$COCH_3$), respectively. The acetylation of xenobiotics requires the cofactor acetyl-coenzyme A. The acetyl group of acetyl-CoA is transferred to the enzyme with the release of CoA. The acetyl group is then transferred to the amino group of the substrate.

Xenobiotics containing primary aliphatic amines are not a common substrate for N-acetylation, although cysteine conjugates, which are formed from glutathione conjugates, are converted to mercapturic acids by N-acetylation in the kidney. N-acetylation often causes a reduction in water solubility of the parent molecule via addition of a non-ionisable group.

N-acetylation of xenobiotics is catalysed by the cytoplasmic enzyme *N*-acetyltransferases (NAT) which is present in the liver (Kupffer cells) and other tissues of mammalian species, with the notable exception being the dog. There are only 2–3 enzymes present in any one species and in humans they are called NAT1 and NAT2. NAT1 is expressed in most tissues, whereas NAT2 is expressed in the liver and gut. There are no specific substrates although *p*-aminosalicylic acid, sulphamethoxazole and sulphanilamide are preferentially acetylated by NAT1 while isoniazid, procainamide dapsone and hydralazine are preferentially acetylated by NAT2. The carcinogenic amine, 2-aminofluorine is acetylated equally well by NAT1 and NAT2. Some examples of the acetylation of xenobiotic compounds are shown in Figure 14.7.

14.2.5 Amino acid conjugation

There are two mechanisms for the conjugation of xenobiotics with amino acids. Xenobiotics with a carboxylic acid group can react via the amino group of amino acids such as glycine and taurine. This biotransformation step first requires the activation of the xenobiotic with CoA by acyl-CoA synthase, which produces an acyl-CoA thioester. The second step, catalysed by acyl-CoA: amino acid *N*-acyltransferase, involves the transfer of the acyl group of the xenobiotic to the amino group of the amino acid (Figure 14.8). Substrates for amino acid conjugation are limited to certain aliphatic, aromatic, heteroaromatic, cinnamic and arylacetic acids. Xenobiotics with aromatic hydroxylamine groups can react with a carboxylic acid of amino acids

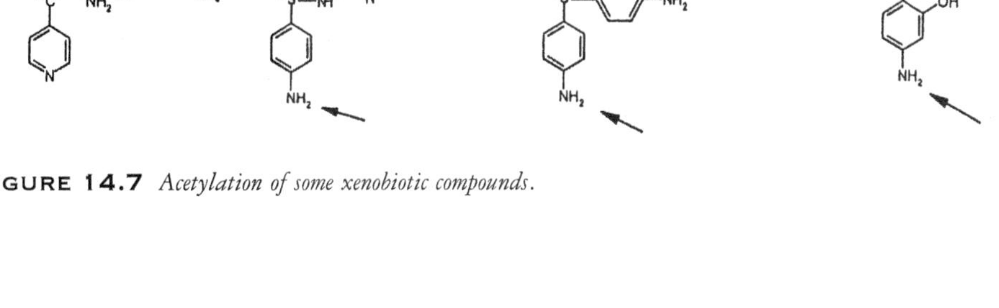

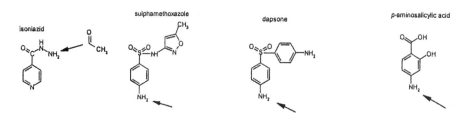

FIGURE 14.7 *Acetylation of some xenobiotic compounds.*

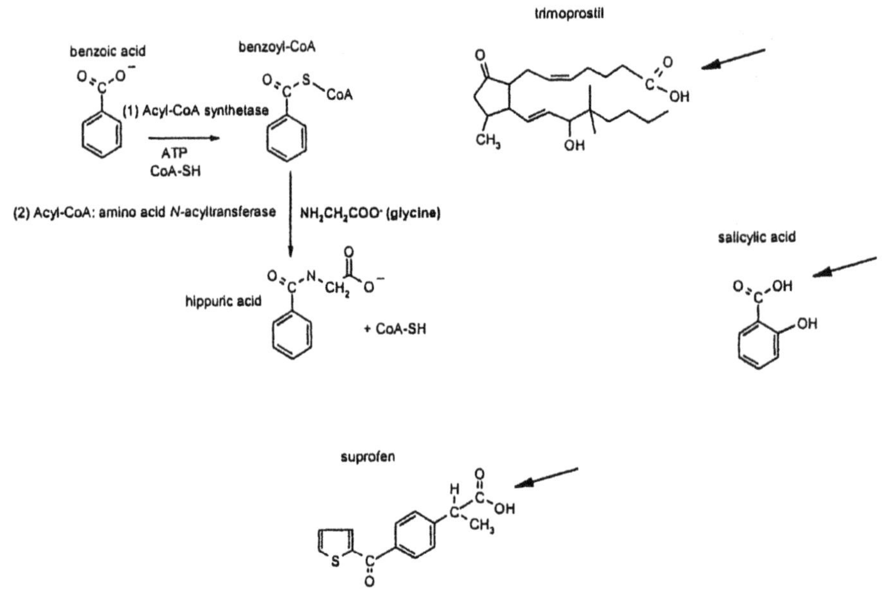

FIGURE 14.8 *Amino acid conjugation of some xenobiotic compounds.*

like proline or serine to produce *N*-esters that can degrade to form reactive electrophilic nitrenium and carbonium ions.

Amino acid conjugation of xenobiotics depends on steric hindrance and substitution on aromatic rings or aliphatic side-chains. In rats, ferrets and monkeys, phenylacetic acid undergoes amino acid conjugation whereas diphenylacetic acid undergoes glucuronidation in these species. Bile acids are endogenous substrates for taurine and glycine conjugation with activation to an acyl-CoA thioester via the microsomal enzyme cholyl-CoA synthetase. Conjugation with glycine and taurine is catalysed by a single cytosolic enzyme, bile acid-CoA:amino acid *N*-acyltransferase (Falany, 1991). In contrast, xenobiotic activation occurs mostly in mitochondria which contain a number of acyl-CoA synthetases. Subsequent xenobiotic conjugation occurs via cytosolic and/or mitochondrial *N*-acyltransferases. Two types of *N*-acyltransferases have been isolated from hepatic mitochondria, one preferring benzoyl-CoA, the other arylacetyl-CoA. The acceptor amino acid is both species and xenobiotic-dependent. For benzoic, heterocyclic and cinnamic acids the acceptor amino acid is usually glycine. Aryl acetic acids are also conjugated with glycine except in primates which use glutamine. In mammals, taurine is also used.

14.2.6 Glutathione conjugation

Glutathione *S*-transferases (GSTs) are a family of mainly cytosolic enzymes which are present in most tissues, with high concentrations in liver, intestine, kidney adrenal and lung. Glutathione is a tripeptide which is comprised of glycine, cysteine and glutamic acid – the latter is linked to the cysteine via the γ-carboxyl group rather than the more usual α-carboxyl function (Figure 14.9). Glutathione conjugation occurs with a wide variety of electrophilic compounds or compounds that can be transformed into electrophiles. The mechanism of the reaction is one of nucleophilic attack of glutathione thiolate anion (GS^-) with an electrophilic carbon, oxygen, nitrogen or sulphur atoms in the molecule concerned. Substrates for GSTs have three common features, they are hydrophobic, contain an electrophilic atom and

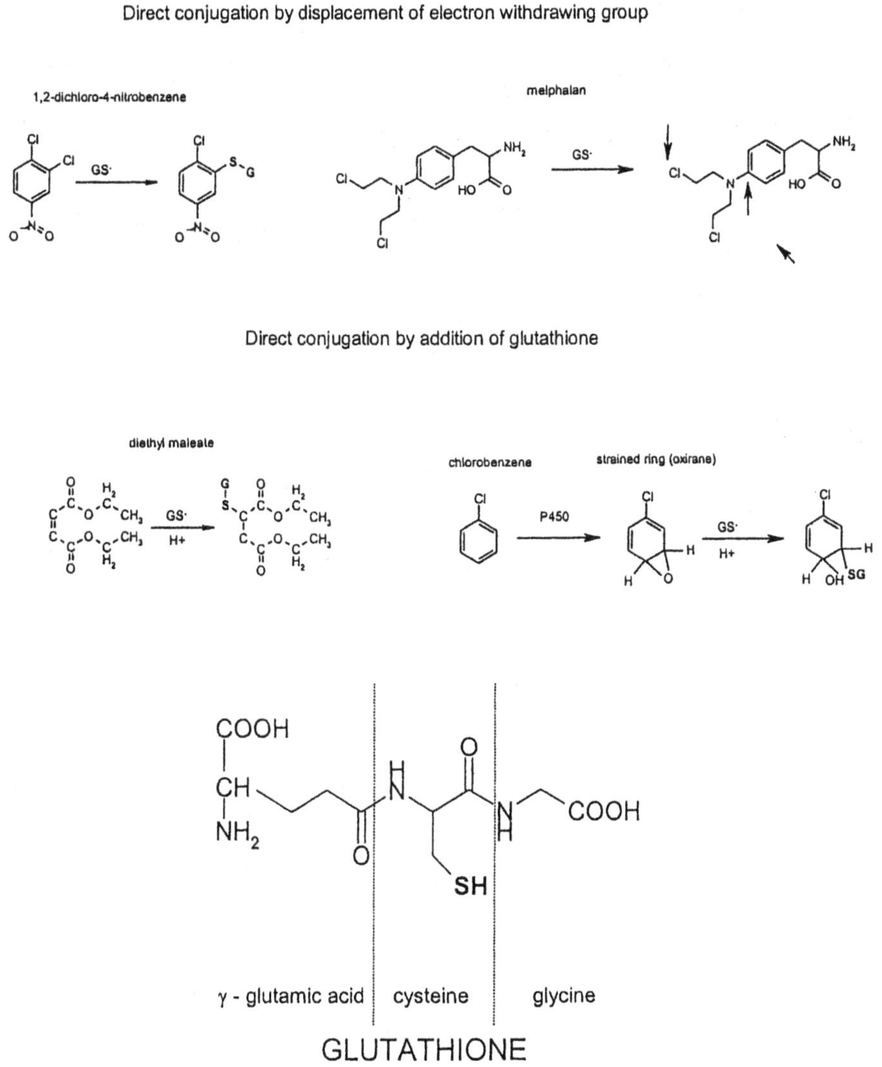

FIGURE 14.9 *Glutathione conjugation with an electrophilic carbon atom.*

react chemically with glutathione to some degree (e.g. paracetamol, nitrosurea). Substrates for GSTs can be classified into two groups, those that are sufficiently electrophilic for direct conjugation and those which undergo biotransformation to an electrophilic metabolite prior to conjugation. The conjugation reactions can be divided into two types, addition and displacement reactions (Figure 14.9).

Glutathione can also conjugate xenobiotics with electrophilic heteroatoms (*O*, *N*, and *S*). An example of this is trinitroglycerine (Figure 14.10). In many cases, the initial conjugate formed between glutathione and the heteroatom is cleaved by a second molecule of glutathione to form oxidised glutathione. The second step is usually non-enzymatic in nature.

Glutathione conjugates can be excreted intact in bile or they can be transformed to mercapturic acids in the kidney and excreted in urine. The process for the generation of mercapturic acids involves the sequential cleavage of the glutamic acid and glycine residues, followed by N-acetylation of the remaining cysteine conjugate. The glutathione conjugate, leukotriene C_4, undergoes metabolism to leukotriene D_4 and then leukotriene E_4 via sequential loss of amino acids. Similarly, the glutathione conjugate of naphthalene undergoes sequential degradation to 1-naphthylmercapturic acid. Also, cysteine conjugates can be degraded by kidney β-lyase which leads to the generation of thiol metabolites which can then undergo further metabolism via methylation or oxidation at the sulphur atom.

14.3 *Nomenclature of phase II enzymes*

The nomenclature systems used for each of the four major Phase II enzyme families are discussed below, accompanied by a table of the major enzymes in humans for each family.

14.3.1 UDP-GLUCURONOSYLTRANSFERASE (UGT) NOMENCLATURE

A nomenclature system, based on evolutionary divergence, has been adopted for *UGT* genes (Burchell *et al.*, 1991; Mackenzie *et al.*, 1997). Each UGT encoding

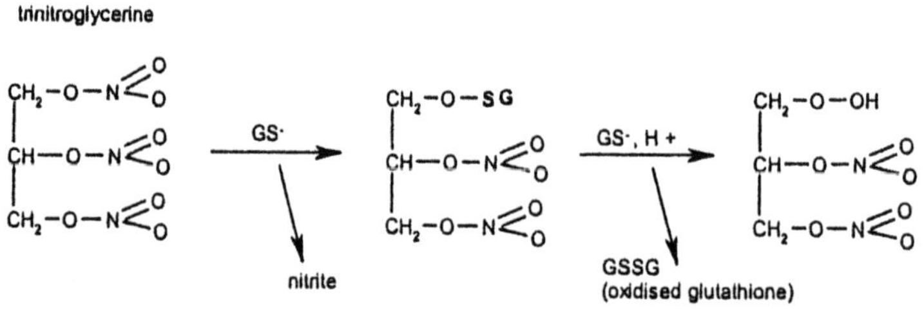

FIGURE 14.10 *Glutathione conjugation of trinitroglycerine.*

gene, *UGT*, is followed by an arabic numeral for the family it belongs to, a letter to denote the subfamily, and finally another arabic numeral for each individual gene (Burchell *et al.*, 1991). A UGT protein sequence from one gene family must have at least 45 per cent sequence identity with another member of that family, whilst subfamilies have greater than 60 per cent sequence identity.

In mammals at least 47 cDNAs and genes have been described which belong to three families, namely *UGT1*, *UGT2* and *UGT8*. The *UGT1* family comprises two subfamilies named *UGT1A* and *UGT1B*, whilst the *UGT2* family contains three subfamilies designated *A*, *B* and *C*, respectively. To date no subfamilies have been identified for the *UGT8* family. This is summarised in Table 14.2.

At least 15 human UGTs have been identified. The *UGT1* gene is unusual in that it is a single gene locus which can generate a number of different UGT isozymes. The *UGT1* gene consists of four common exons (exons 2–5) and a variable exon 1. The presence of a unique exon 1 for each UGT1 isozyme (produced by alternative splicing of exon 1) means that UGT1A1, UGT1A3, UGT1A4, etc. are all transcripts of the *UGT1* gene. In contrast, the *UGT2* genes each generate an individual UGT2 isoform (UGT2B7, UGT2B8, etc.).

14.3.2 Sulphotransferase (SULT) nomenclature

As a result of advances in the cDNA cloning of SULT enzymes in recent years, the nomenclature in this field has become increasingly difficult to understand. Indeed at recent meetings, prizes should have been awarded to those actually able to

Table 14.2 *Human UDP-glucuronosyltransferase enzyme nomenclature*

UGT1 family	UGT2 family	UGT8 family
UGT1A1	UGT2B4	UGT8
UGT1A2P	UGT2B7	
UGT1A3	UGT2B10	
UGT1A4	UGT2B15	
UGT1A5	UGT2B17	
UGT1A6		
UGT1A7		
UGT1A8		
UGT1A9		
UGT1A10		
UGT1A11P		
UGT1A12P		

This table includes all UDPGT enzymes for which a human cDNA sequence has been elucidated. Adapted from Mackenzie *et al.* (1997) *Pharmacogenetics* 7, 225–269.

identify the SULTs being discussed in posters! In an attempt to clarify the situation and devise a universal nomenclature system, the SULT nomenclature committee has proposed some guidelines.

The abbreviation SULT will be used to refer to all cytosolic sulfotransferase enzymes and will be in italics when referring to a gene rather than the enzyme protein or mRNA. For enzymes isolated from mice only the first letter will be in capitals, e.g. Sult.

A family of sulfotransferase enzymes will include proteins with 45 per cent or greater amino acid sequence identity, whilst subfamilies will have 60 per cent or greater identity. Families will be assigned arabic numerals, subfamilies capital letters, and individual gene products another arabic numeral e.g. SULT1A1. Orthologues across different species will have the same designation but will be followed by a three-letter species suffix in lower case (Table 14.3).

At least 11 human SULTs have been identified. In addition to the individual isoforms such as SULT1A1, SULT1A2, etc. major variant alleles have also been described which differ by single amino acids e.g. SULT1A1*1 (Arg213) and SULT1A1*2 (His213).

14.3.3 *N*-ACETYLTRANSFERASE (NAT) NOMENCLATURE

N-acetyltransferase enzyme activity was one of the first drug-metabolising activities shown to exhibit polymorphic variation (Meyer, 1993), which results in inter-individual variation such that individuals can be separated into slow or rapid acetylators.

Three *NAT** loci (*NAT1**, *NAT2** and *NAT3**) have been found in vertebrates. Advances in DNA technology have been responsible for a vast expansion in the acetylation field, allowing the identification and characterisation of numerous allelic variants at these *NAT** loci.

A nomenclature system has been adopted (Vatsis *et al.*, 1995) based upon nucleotide changes observed in cDNA and genomic clones, or within PCR-generated fragments of *NAT* genes. A nomenclature system based on evolutionary divergence

TABLE 14.3 *Human sulphotransferase enzyme nomenclature*

Phenol STs		Estrogen STs		Hydroxysteroid STs	
New name	**Current name**	**New name**	**Current name**	**New name**	**Current name**
SULT1A1	HTSPST1 or PPST1	SULT1E1	hEST	SULT2A1	hDHEAST
SULT1A2	HTSPST2 or PPST2				
SULT1A3	HTLPST MPST				

This table includes the proposed new nomenclature and the current (old) name for all SULT enzymes for which a human cDNA sequence has been elucidated.

is not possible due to insufficient structural information on *NAT** loci. The *N*-acetyltransferases are assigned the root symbol *NAT*, which is followed by an arabic numeral denoting the gene family and an asterisk which indicates that this is a gene. Individual alleles are then assigned a combination of up to three arabic numerals and latin letters (e.g. NAT2*2, NAT2*5A, NAT1*10, etc.) in chronological order irrespective of the species they were derived from (Table 14.4).

14.3.4 Glutathione-*S*-transferase (GST) nomenclature

Molecular cloning of GSTs in mouse, rat and human has allowed the identification of four classes of enzyme. Within each class, GSTs possess greater than 40 per cent identity whilst those with less than 30 per cent are assigned to a different class (Hayes and Pulford, 1995). The elucidation of gene structures and chromosomal localisation for a wide range of rat and human *GST* genes supports the hypothesis that each class does indeed represent a separate GST family (Rushmore and Pickett, 1993).

The classes of GST enzymes have been designated alpha, mu, pi and theta. The diversity of GST enzymes found in mammals is achieved by the dimeric nature in which subunits come together to form GST enzymes. A novel nomenclature system designates the alpha, mu and pi enzymes as GSTA, GSTM and GSTP, respectively.

TABLE 14.4 *Human* N*-acetyltransferase alleles and their corresponding proteins*

NAT1* locus		**NAT2* locus**		**NATP locus**	
Allele	**Protein**	**Allele**	**Protein**	**Allele**	**Protein**
*NAT1*3*	NAT1 3	NAT2*4	NAT2 4	*NATP1*	None
*NAT1*4*	NAT1 4	*NAT2*5A*	NAT2 5A		
*NAT1*5*	NAT1 5	*NAT2*5B*	NAT2 5B		
*NAT1*10*	NAT1 10	*NAT2*5C*	NAT2 5C		
*NAT1*11*	NAT1 11	*NAT2*6A*	NAT2 6A		
		*NAT2*6B*	NAT2 6B		
		*NAT2*7A*	NAT2 7A		
		*NAT2*7B*	NAT2 7B		
		*NAT2*12A*	NAT2 12A		
		*NAT2*12B*	NAT2 12B		
		*NAT2*13*	NAT2 13		
		*NAT2*14A*	NAT2 14A		
		*NAT2*14B*	NAT2 14B		
		*NAT2*17*	NAT2 17		
		*NAT2*18*	NAT2 18		

In the case of NATP there is no corresponding protein as this is a psuedogene in humans. Adapted from Vatsis *et al.* (1995).

This is followed by arabic numerals which denote the subunits present in the dimeric enzyme e.g. GSTA1-1. Allelic variants can also be indicated by lower case letters e.g. GSTM1b-1b which is a homodimeric Mu class enzyme composed of the 1b allelic variant (Table 14.5).

14.4 *Phase II enzymes and drug development*

14.4.1 Toxicity of conjugated metabolites

As eluded to in the introduction, the conjugated metabolites produced by Phase II conjugation reactions do not always result in a reduction in activity. Situations in which conjugates, particularly glucuronides and sulphates give rise to reactive, potentially toxic metabolites are described below.

Glucuronides

A number of compounds which contain a carboxylic acid grouping are susceptible to conjugation catalysed by UGTs, leading to the formation of acyl glucuronides (reviewed in Spahn-Langguth and Benet, 1992). A number of these acyl glucuronides have been shown to bind irreversibly to proteins and exert toxic effects. In addition, acyl glucuronides undergo a reaction known as acyl migration where the aglycone can move from the 1′-hydroxyl group to other hydroxyl groups on the glucuronic acid sugar residue. Such changes in the molecule render the conjugate resistant to β-glucuronidase, and the protein-bound adducts formed may pre-dispose individuals to immunologic problems. Typical substrates which are metabolised to acyl glucuronide conjugates include the non-steroidal anti-inflammatory drugs (NSAIDs, such as the profens), and these compounds have been associated with toxic responses.

TABLE 14.5 *Human glutathione-S-transferase enzyme nomenclature for gene locus and corresponding protein*

Alpha class		**Mu class**		**Pi class**	
Gene locus	**Protein**	**Gene locus**	**Protein**	**Gene locus**	**Protein**
GSTA1	GSTA1-1	*GSTM1*	GSTM1a-1a	*GSTP1*	GSTP1-1
GSTA2	GSTA2-2	*GSTM1*	GSTM1b-1b		
		GSTM2	GSTM2-2		
		GSTM3	GSTM3-3		

Adapted from Mannervik *et al.* (1992) *Biochem. J.* 282, 305–308.

Sulphates

It has been known for a number of years that sulphation is traditionally associated with inactivation and detoxication of xenobiotics (reviewed in Glatt, 1997). However, the sulphate group is electron withdrawing and can act as a good leaving group, thus generating reactive, potentially toxic metabolites. Typical substrates which generate toxic metabolites via this mechanism include heterocyclic aromatic hydroxylamines, formed as a result of N-hydroxylation of the primary amine group. The hydroxyl group introduced into the molecule (typically by CYP1A2) is then available for conjugation with sulphate catalysed by SULT enzymes. Chemical degradation of the sulphate conjugate occurs, generating a reactive, electrophilic species which can bind covalently to nucleophiles such as DNA and protein. Metabolites generated in this way via CYP and SULT pathways have been shown to be potent mutagens *in vitro* and thus provide a mechanism for the genotoxic and carcinogenic properties of heterocyclic amines and polycyclic aromatic hydrocarbons containing benzylic groups.

14.4.2 Stereoselectivity in metabolism by Phase II enzymes

A number of UGT substrates have shown various degrees of selectivity in relation to the glucuronidation of chiral compounds. Glucuronidation of NSAIDs with chiral centres has shown this route of metabolism for several compounds (e.g. naproxen, ketoprofen) to be stereoselective. The enantiomers of a series of reverse hydroxamic acids (e.g. BW360C) (Figure 14.11) which possessed a single chiral centre showed marked differences in their metabolism by human liver microsomal UGTs. In such cases, the *R*-enantiomers were preferentially and extensively metabolised by human UGTs whereas the corresponding *S*-enantiomers were almost resistant to glucuronidation. In contrast, a series of close structural analogues of the reverse hydroxamates (*N*-hydroxyureas with a chiral centre e.g. BW70C) (Figure 14.11) were much less rapidly metabolised by glucuronidation and showed the opposite stereoselectivity with respect to metabolism by UGTs, i.e. the *S*-enantiomers were the preferred substrates.

A number of chiral substituted *N*-hydroxyureas which are 5-lipoxygenase (5-LO) inhibitors have been screened by Abbott as UGT substrates (Bouska *et al.*, 1997). For these compounds, glucuronidation was shown to be the major route of metabolism and this markedly limited the duration of action of the compounds *in vivo*. In addition, the first generation 5-LO inhibitor (zileuton) (Figure 14.11) was marketed as the racemic mixture. The *S*-enantiomer was metabolised at a greater rate (3.5x) by human liver UGT than the *R*-enantiomer. *In vivo*, the *S*-isomer was cleared more rapidly in humans indicating that metabolism by UGT was the major factor involved in clearance of zileuton (Sweeny and Nellans, 1995).

Salbutamol and many other β-2 agonists contain one or more asymmetric carbon atoms. Salbutamol is metabolised in man pre-dominantly by sulphation catalysed

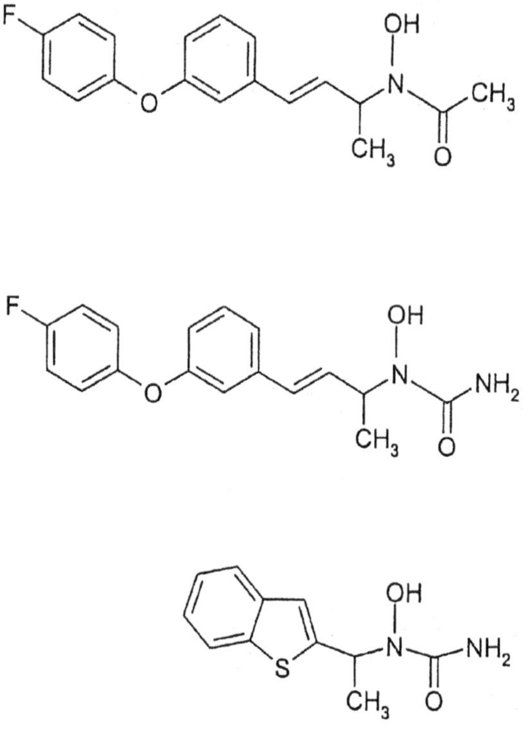

BW360C

BW70C

ZILEUTON

FIGURE 14.11 *The enantiomers of a series of reverse hydroxamic acids.*

by SULT isozymes. The formation of salbutamol sulphate has been shown to be stereoselective in human liver and intestine *in vitro* with a marked preference for the active (−) enantiomer (Walle *et al.*, 1993).

14.4.3 POLYMORPHISMS IN PHASE II ENZYMES

A number of Phase II enzymes have been shown to exist in multiple forms which elicit clinically relevant genetic polymorphisms. These include the UGT-glucuronosyltransferase (UGT1A1), *N*-acetyltransferase (NAT2), thiopurine methyltransferase (TPMT) and catechol *0*-methyltransferase (COMT) (reviewed in Parkinson, 1996; Evans and Relling, 1999).

UGT1A1, the enzyme responsible for the conjugation of bilirubin and certain xenobiotics, is subject to inter-individual variation. Thirty-one allelic variants have been identified by cDNA cloning which are implicated in the bilirubin conjugation disorders of Criggler-Najar and Gilberts syndrome. Patients with Criggler-Najar syndrome are deficient in UGT1A1 and hence lack the ability to conjugate bilirubin resulting in unconjugated hyperbilirubinaemia, which causes severe jaundice and often leads to death in infancy. In Gilberts syndrome, the milder form of the disease, patients have reduced levels of active UGT1A1 and hence reduced metabolic capacity so they experience a milder form of unconjugated hyperbilirubinaemia that often goes undetected for many years.

Slow acetylator phenotypes, poor metabolisers or PMs for the soluble enzyme NAT2, were originally suspected to be under genetic influence because of differences in the numbers of adverse effects in patients receiving the NAT2 substrate isoniazid in Japan and US. Orientals typically have $\leq$10 per cent of PMs whereas about 50 per cent of Caucasians have the PM genotype. In all cases, metabolism (N-acetylation) of amine-containing drugs by NAT2 results in deactivation of the compound and is thus a detoxifying pathway. Thus, PMs for NAT2 are at risk from a number of drug classes which are NAT2 substrates (e.g. dapsone, sulphonamides) which generate potentially toxic hydroxylamines via CYP-mediated metabolism.

TPMT-deficient patients are adversely affected by standard doses of anticancer drugs which contain a thiol group such as 6-mercaptopurine (6-MP) and 6-thioguanine (6-TG). These compounds are widely used in leukaemia therapy and a closely related compound azathioprine (which is metabolised to 6-MP) is an immunosuppressant. Patients with the wild-type TPMT enzyme are able to effectively methylate thiopurines such as 6-MP and 6-TG at the thiol group.

If the TPMT enzyme is missing or deficient, there is a major risk of thiopurine toxicity because of an accumulation of these toxic compounds. In addition the compounds are themselves carcinogenic which could lead to the development of further cancers if the thiopurines are not cleared because of this metabolic defect.

It should be noted that other major Phase II enzymes (SULTs, GSTs) also exhibit polymorphisms but an association with changes in the effects of drugs (as a result of changed metabolic capability of the mutant forms) has yet to be established. GST isoforms are known to be important in the detoxication of reactive species from environmental sources as well as reactive drug metabolites such as epoxides. However, GST polymorphism has yet to be unequivocally associated with changes in drug metabolism. There is evidence for an association of GST isoforms with several disease states (e.g. cancer susceptibility). SULT polymorphisms have been readily demonstrated in human platelets (Weinshilboum *et al.*, 1997). More importantly, large differences in the expression of SULT2A1 (DHEA ST) in human liver and intestine (major sites of sulphation activity *in vivo*) and of SULT1E1 (EST) in human small intestine suggest that polymorphic forms of human SULTs exist.

14.4.4 Drug–drug interactions

UGTs

A number of drugs are known to be cleared by UGT-mediated metabolism as a primary route of clearance (reviewed in Burchell *et al.*, 1995). Of these compounds one of the most extensively studied is the anti-HIV compound AZT (zidovudine).

Since AZT is routinely administered as part of a drug cocktail in AIDS therapy, the potential for drug interaction is large. A number of compounds have been shown to inhibit AZT glucuronidation *in vitro* in human liver microsomes but relatively few appear to have major clinical significance (Rajaonarison *et al.*, 1992). The UGT isoform involved in the metabolism of AZT is UGT2B7 (Barbier *et al.*, 2000).

Lamotrigine (LTG), the antiepileptic drug undergoes a number of drug–drug interactions with other anticonvulsant agents. LTG is metabolised primarily in man by N-glucuronidation, and is thought to be a substrate for UGT1A4. Both carbamazepine and phenytoin, both CYP inducing agents, have been shown to increase the clearance of LTG resulting in a corresponding reduced elimination half-life for LTG. This was considered to be due to induction of the UGT enzyme(s) catalysing the metabolism of LTG. In contrast, valproate, which is also metabolised in part by UGT, causes reduced clearance of LTG *in vivo*, by inhibiting the UGT responsible for LTG metabolism. In both cases, dosage adjustments for LTG are required to adjust the circulating levels of LTG in the presence of the inducing or inhibiting coadministered antiepileptic drugs (reviewed in Anderson, 1998).

A recent study to investigate the metabolism of an anticancer prodrug irinotecan was reported (Iyer *et al.*, 1998). The experimental approach was similar to that used extensively to implicate CYP isoforms in Phase I metabolism. Metabolism of the active (de-esterified) metabolite of irinotecan (SN-38) by a panel of human liver microsomes correlated with bilirubin (a UGT1A1 substrate) conjugation for those liver preparations and expressed human UGT1A1 (but not UGT1A4 or 2B7) catalysed the glucuronidation reaction. In addition, patients with Crigler-Najjar syndrome and Gunn rats (both of which are markedly deficient in UGT1A1) lacked glucuronidating activity towards SN-38. Thus various experimental approaches indicated that SN-38 was conjugated by UGT1A1, the major bilirubin UGT isoform. Patients with Gilbert's syndrome (which have partially impaired bilirubin UGT activity) would hence expect to have reduced levels of UGT1A1 and hence associated deficiency of SN-38 metabolism. Since SN-38 has been implicated with GI toxicity, it is apparent that impairment of its major route of metabolism would have undesirable side effects. Likewise, coadministration of other drugs which are substrates/inhibitors of UGT1A1 may lead to an unwanted drug–drug interaction.

SULTs

Sulphation plays an important role in the modulation of activity of many key endogenous compounds e.g. steroids and neurotransmitters such as dopamine. Thus interference with these functions could markedly affect homeostasis in the body. A number of commonly used drugs, such as clomiphene, ibuprofen chlorpromazine and tamoxifen have been shown to inhibit the sulphation of DHEA and oestrone by their respective SULT enzymes. Dietary chemicals such as vanillin and tartrazine are potent inhibitors of SULT isozymes. Various flavanoids such as quercetin are SULT inhibitors, and polyphenolic components of red wine are potent and selective inhibitors of human SULT1A1. Such compounds may act as chemical protectants against procarcinogens such as heterocyclic amines which require sulphation for activation (reviewed in Burchell and Coughtrie, 1997).

14.4.5 Induction

UGTs

A number of agents (particularly rifampicin and antiepileptic drugs) are known to induce UGT isozymes as well as CYP isozymes (especially CYP3A4) (Anderson, 1998; Tanaka, 1999). Oral contraceptive agents are also known to induce UGT isozymes. The ability of a compound to induce UGT has been used in a therapeutic situation. In Crigler-Najjar patients (which lack or are severely deficient in UGT1A1 which conjugates bilirubin), phenobarbital has been used to induce UGT1A1 *in vivo* and has been shown to induce this isozyme in human hepatocyte cultures. However, there is also a genetic influence in the degree of induction of UGT1A1 which can be achieved and recent work has shown that weak induction may in part be associated with variation in the UGT1A1 promoter sequence (Ritter *et al.*, 1999).

SULTs

SULT isozymes are generally considered to be refractory to induction by xenobiotics which induce CYPs and UGTs. However, Li *et al.* (1999) have recently reported induction of ethinyloestradiol sulphation in human hepatocyte cultures by rifampicin.

14.5 *Summary*

In summary, there is a rapidly growing knowledge base around the role of Phase II enzymes in the metabolism of xenobiotic and endogenous compounds. When new drugs are shown to undergo Phase II metabolism, we should be aware of the potential not only for drug–drug interactions via direct competition or effects on enzyme expression, but also the potential for interaction with endogenous compound metabolism which may affect physiological processes.

Differences in the gene expression of Phase II enzymes in the human population must also be taken into account when we assess human drug response where these enzymes are important for metabolic deactivation. New tools and technologies currently being developed, will allow us to probe further the understanding of the activity and function of these enzymes in the future.

14.6 References

Anderson, G.D. (1998) A mechanistic approach to antiepileptic drug interactions. *Ann. Pharmacother.* 32, 554–563.

Barbier, O. *et al.* (2000) 3′Azido-3′deoxythymidine (AZT) is glucuronidated by human UDP-glucuronosyltransferase 2B7 (UGT2B7). *Drug Metab. Dispos.* 28, 497–502.

Bouska, J.J. *et al.* (1997) Improving the duration of 5-lipoxygenase inhibitors – application of an in vitro glucuronosyltransferase assay. *Drug Metab. Dispos.* 25, 1032–1038.

Burchell and Coughtrie (1989) UDP-glucuronosyltransferases. *Pharmacol. Ther.* 43(2), 261–289.

Burchell, B. and Coughtrie, M.W.H. (1997) Genetic and environmental factors associated with variation of human xenobiotic glucuronidation and sulfation. *Environ. Health Perspect.* 105 (Suppl. 4), 739–747.

Burchell, B., Nebert, D.W., Nelson, D.R., Bock, K.W., Iyanagi, T., Jansen, P.L., Lancet, D., Mulder, G.J., Chowdhury, J.R., Siest, G. *et al.* (1991) The UDP-glucuronosyltransferase gene superfamily: suggested nomenclature based on evolutionary divergence. *DNA Cell Biol.* September; 10(7), 487–494.

Burchell, B. *et al.* (1995) Specificity of human UDP-glucuronosyltransferases and xenobiotic glucuronidation. *Life Sci.* 57, 1819–1831.

Dutton, G.J. (1966) Variations in glucuronide formation by perinatal liver. *Biochem. Pharmacol.* July; 15(7), 947–951.

Evans, W.E. and Relling, M.V. (1999) Pharmacogenomics – translating functional genomics into rational therapeutics. *Science* 286, 487–491.

Falany (1991) Molecular enzymology of human liver cytosolic sulfotransferases. *Trends Pharmacol. Sci.* July; 12(7), 255–259.

Falany, C.N., Vazquez, M.E., Heroux, J.A. and Roth, J.A. (1993) Purification and characterization of human liver phenol-sulfating phenol sulfotransferase. *Arch. Biochem. Biophys.* 1 May; 278(2), 312–318.

Glatt, H. (1997) Bioactivation of mutagens via sulfation. *FASEB J.* 11, 314–321.

Gordon G. Gibson and Paul Skett (1994) *Introduction to Drug Metabolism.* Blackie Academic & Professional.

Hayes and Pulford (1995) The glutathione *S*-transferase supergene family: regulation of GST and the contribution of the isoenzymes to cancer chemoprotection and drug resistance. *Crit. Rev. Biochem. Mol. Biol.* 30(6), 445–600.

Iyer, L. *et al.* (1998) Genetic predisposition to the metabolism of irinotecan (CPT-11) role of UDPGT isoform 1A1 in the glucuronidation of its active metabolite (SN-38) in human liver microsomes. *J. Clin. Invest.* 101, 847–854.

Li, A.P. *et al.* (1999) Effects of cytochrome P450 inducers on 17 alpha-ethinylestradiol (EE2) conjugation by primary human hepatocytes. *Br. J. Clin. Pharmacol.* 48, 733–742.

Meyer, B.F. (1993) Debrisoquine oxidation polymorphism: phenotypic consequences of a 3-base-pair deletion in exon 5 of the CYP2D6 gene. *Pharmacogenetics* June; 3(3), 123–130.

Miners and Mackenzie (1991) Drug glucuronidation in humans. *Pharmacol. Ther.* 51(3), 347–369.

Pacifici *et al.* (1988) Sulphation and glucuronidation of paracetamol in human liver: assay conditions. *Biochem. Pharmacol.* 15 November; 37(22), 4405–4407.

Parkinson, A. (1996) *Biotransformation of Xenobiotics in Casarett and Doull's Toxicology – The Basic Science of Poisons* (5th edn), Klaassen, C. (ed.) McGraw-Hill.

Rajaonarison, J.F. *et al.* (1992) 3′-Azido-3′-deoxythymidine drug interactions: screening for inhibitors in human liver microsomes. *Drug Metab. Dispos.* 20, 578–584.

Ritter, J.K. *et al.* (1999) Expression and inducibility of the human bilirubin UDP-glucuronosyltransferase UGT1A1 in liver and cultured primary hepatocytes: evidence for both genetic and environmental influences. *Hepatology* 30, 476–484.

Rushmore, T.H. and Pickett, C.B. (1993) Glutathione *S*-transferases, structure, regulation, and therapeutic implications. *J. Biol. Chem.* 5 June; 268(16), 11475–11478.

Spahn-Langguth, H. and Benet, L. (1992) Acyl glucuronides revisited: is the glucuronidation process a toxification as well as a detoxification mechanism? *Drug Metab. Rev.* 24, 5–48.

Sweeny, D.J. and Nellans, H.N. (1995) Stereoselective glucuronidation of zileuton isomers by human hepatic microsomes. *Drug Metab. Dispos.* 23, 149–153.

Tanaka, E. (1999) Clinically significant pharmacokinetic drug interactions between antiepileptic drugs. *J. Clin. Pharm. Ther.* 24, 87–92.

Tephly and Burchell (1990) UDP-glucuronosyltransferases: a family of detoxifying enzymes. *Trends Pharmacol. Sci.* July; 11(7), 276–279.

Vanstapel and Blanckaert (1988) Topology and regulation of bilirubin UDP-glucuronyltransferase in sealed native microsomes from rat liver. *Arch. Biochem. Biophys.* 15 May; 263(1), 216–225.

Vatsis, K.P., Weber, W.W., Bell, D.A., Dupret, J.M., Evans, D.A., Grant, D.M., Hein, D.W., Lin, H.J., Meyer, U.A., Relling, M.V. *et al.* (1995) Nomenclature for *N*-acetyltransferases. *Pharmacogenetics* February; 5(1), 1–17.

Walle, U.K. *et al.* (1993) Stereoselective sulphate conjugation of salbutamol in humans: comparison of hepatic, intestinal and platelet activity. *Br. J. Clin. Pharmacol.* 35, 413–418.

Weinshilboum, R.M. (1989) Methyltransferase pharmacogenetics. *Pharmacol. Ther.* 43(1), 77–90.

Weinshilboum, R.M. (1992) Methylation pharmacogenetics: thiopurine methyltransferase as a model system. *Xenobiotica*. September–October; 22(9–10), 1055–1071.

Weinshilboum and Otterness (1994) Human dehydroepiandrosterone sulfotransferase: molecular cloning of cDNA and genomic DNA. *Chem. Biol. Interact.* June; 92(1–3), 145–159.

Weinshilboum, R.M. *et al.* (1997) Sulfotransferase molecular biology: cDNAs and genes. *FASEB J.* 11, 3–14.

Wong, K.P. and Yeo, T. (1982) Importance of extrahepatic sulphate conjugation. *Biochem. Pharmacol.* 15 December; 31(24), 4001–4003.

CHAPTER 15

In vitro techniques for investigating drug metabolism

Graham Somers, Peter Mutch and Amanda Woodrooffe

15.1 *Introduction*

The use of *in vitro* techniques to study drug metabolism allows comparison of the metabolism of a compound across species prior to administration to humans. In addition, the use of human *in vitro* systems provides more relevant information on the metabolites likely to be formed in clinical studies. Therefore, interspecies comparisons of the metabolite profile of a drug candidate may assist rational selection of the most appropriate species for safety assessment studies. Finally, potential clinical interactions, i.e. the ability of a drug candidate to affect the pharmacokinetics of other coadministered therapies (induction or inhibition of drug-metabolising enzymes) can also be investigated using human *in vitro* systems.

The liver is a major site for the biotransformation of xenobiotics and so many models of drug metabolism have primarily focussed on the liver and the enzymes contained within it. Investigation of drug metabolism has involved the use of liver preparations which vary in their levels of cellular integrity. Systems range from the use of purified enzymes *in vitro* to whole liver perfusion *in situ*. For the purpose of this chapter, discussions will concentrate around the use of subcellular fractions (S9 and microsomes), isolated hepatocytes and liver slices.

The cytochromes P450 are a large family of enzymes involved in the metabolism of a wide range of structurally diverse xenobiotics. Cytochrome P450 enzymes are bound to the membranes of the endoplasmic reticulum, and concentrated sources used for the investigation of drug metabolism can be prepared from homogenised liver by differential centrifugation. The submitochondrial (S9) fraction of liver contains both cytosolic and membrane-bound enzymes but as a homogenate rather than an ordered cellular environment. The S9 fraction is prepared by sedimenting particulate matter, including cell nuclei and mitochondria, from homogenised liver at 9,000 $\times g$ and is a crude tissue preparation; the impure nature of this preparation may lead to analytical difficulties. However, a more refined enzyme may be prepared from crude liver S9 by further centrifugation. Fragments of the endoplasmic reticulum reform into vesicles known as microsomes. The microsomal pellet is produced by centrifugation of the S9 fraction at 100,000 $\times g$.

Microsomes are essentially an enriched source of the membrane-bound enzymes such as the cytochromes P450 and as such are probably the most commonly used system in the pharmaceutical industry to study *in vitro* cytochrome P450-mediated metabolism. Both S9 and microsomes retain enzyme activity following cold storage at $-80\,°C$. Therefore, S9 and microsome preparations may be made and stored ready for use, an advantage for cross comparisons of metabolism between species and in the case of humans between different liver donors.

The parenchymal cells of the liver (hepatocytes) are a rich source of cytochromes P450. Hepatocytes can be isolated from liver tissue by enzymatic dissociation using collagenase perfusion. Once isolated, hepatocytes can be used to study drug metabolism and induction or inhibition of drug-metabolising enzymes by xenobiotics.

The major advantage of hepatocytes over microsomes for the study of drug metabolism is that, as a cellular system, hepatocytes contain many enzymes and enzyme cofactors not present in the microsomal fraction of the cells. For example, several of the enzymes responsible for conjugation of xenobiotics, such as the sulphotransferases, are located in the cytoplasm of the cell (see Table 15.1). Although some Phase II metabolic pathways can be studied using microsomes supplemented with appropriate cofactors (e.g. glucuronidation), they may be more easily investigated using hepatocytes.

Hepatocytes may be used as short-term suspension cultures (four hours) or may be placed into culture for investigation of drug-related enzyme induction or enzyme inhibition that requires longer periods of exposure to the test compound. One issue with hepatocytes that are placed into culture is that they undergo de-differentiation, i.e. the loss of specific cell characteristics, and this results in a rapid decrease in their content and activity of drug-metabolising enzymes, notably the cytochromes P450. As such, primary cultures of hepatocytes are not routinely used for the study

TABLE 15.1 *Cellular location of the major drug-metabolising enzymes*

Reaction	Enzyme	Cellular location	Substrates
Phase I reactions			
Hydrolysis	Esterases	Cytosol Mitochondria Microsomes Blood	Esters
	Eposide hydrolase	Cytosol Microsomes	Epoxides
	Peptidase	Microsomes Blood Lysosomes	Peptides Glutathione conjugates
Reduction	Mixed function oxidases	Microsomes	Azo Nitro N-oxides Arene oxides Alkyl halogenides
	Alcohol dehydrogenases	Cytosol	Alcohols
Oxidation	Mixed function oxidases	Microsomes	Alkanes Alkenes Arenes Amines Thiones Thioesters
	Monoamine oxidases	Mitochondria	Amines
	Alcohol dehydrogenases	Cytosol	Alcohols
	Aldehyde dehydrogenases	Cytosol	Aldehydes
Phase II reactions			
Glutathione conjugation	Glutathione transferases	Microsomes	Electrophiles
Glucuronide conjugation	Glucuronyl transferases	Microsomes	Phenols Thiols Amines Carboxylic acid
Sulphate conjugation	Sulfotransferases	Cytosol	Phenols Thiols Amines
Methylation	Methyl transferases	Cytosol Microsomes	Phenols Amines
Acetylayion	Acetyl transferases	Cytosol	Amines
Amino acid conjugation	Transferases	Cytosol Mitochondria	Carboxylic acid Aromatic hydroxylamine

of species differences in drug metabolism but are much more valuable in the study of drug-related enzyme induction or enzyme inhibition.

Liver slices represent a greater level of structural integrity compared to sub-cellular fractions or hepatocytes and may be prepared using instruments such as the Krumdieck tissue slicer. Tissue slices have the advantage that, compared to hepatocytes, they retain an intact three-dimensional structure, allowing cellular architecture and hence intercellular communication to be maintained. This cell–cell contact between different hepatic cell types is important in maintaining cell differentiation. For studies using human liver, tissue slices offer a major advantage over the preparation of hepatocytes, in that samples encapsulated by the Glisson's capsule (required for hepatocyte isolation) are not necessary for the preparation of slices and therefore use can be made of any fresh human liver samples. Liver slices, like hepatocytes, are capable of performing both Phase I and Phase II biotransformations.

The preparation, uses, advantages and disadvantages associated with the use of S9, microsomes, hepatoctyes and tissue slices will be discussed in the next section. This chapter has primarily focussed on hepatic *in vitro* preparations; however, it should be noted that not only the liver but a range of other tissues such as kidney, lung and intestine contain drug-metabolising enzymes and carry out xenobiotic metabolism *in vivo*. Therefore, *in vitro* metabolic preparations, especially S9, and microsomes could be prepared from any tissue to study extrahepatic drug metabolism.

15.2 *Preparation of liver subcellular fractions and hepatocytes*

15.2.1 Preparation of subcellular fractions

The most commonly used subcellular fractions in industrial drug metabolism studies are the S9 fraction and microsomal preparations. Both preparations are produced using differential centrifugation of tissue homogenates. In addition, microsomes can be prepared from S9 by calcium aggregation.

In order to preserve enzyme activity, buffers, tools and centrifuge rotors should be maintained cold for the duration of the preparation procedure, either by storage on ice or within a refrigerator.

Excised livers (or portions of liver from larger animals and man) are weighed and washed in a suitable ice cold buffer at pH 7.4. The initial buffer is removed and the liver is added to the buffer to give a 25 per cent homogenate. The tissue is scissor minced and then homogenised using a suitable 'soft' homogenisation technique such as the 'pestle and mortar' Potter Elvhejam homogeniser. More aggressive tissue disruption methods tend to reduce the enzyme activity of the final preparation.

The crude tissue homogenate is then centrifuged at 9,000 × *g* for 20 minutes at 4 °C. This step pellets and therefore removes intact cells, cell debris, nuclei and mitochondria from the crude cell homogenate. The supernatant represents the sub mitochondrial fraction (S9), which may then be quickly frozen in liquid nitrogen and stored at $-80\,^{\circ}C$ prior to use.

The microsomal fraction may then be prepared from the S9 fraction by further centrifugation or by calcium precipitation. Centrifugation of the S9 at $100{,}000 \times g$ for one hour sediments the microsomal vesicles. After the supernatant is discarded, microsomes are resuspended in a volume of buffer (pH 7.4) equivalent to the original weight of tissue used. The centrifugation step may be repeated to further purify the preparation.

The preparation generally yields a protein concentration of a few milligrams of microsomal protein/millilitre tissue preparation. The purity and activity of the microsomal homogenate is dependent upon the preparation technique and will vary according to the aggressiveness of the homogenisation technique and subsequent temperature of the homogenate and degradation of the enzyme.

A number of additions to the preparation buffers have been suggested to increase the purity or enzyme activity of the final preparation. For example, the addition of EDTA in decreasing concentration to the preparation buffers (10 mM in homogenisation buffer, 1 mM in wash buffer and 0.1 mM in final buffer) is thought to stabilise flavin monooxygenase (FMO) activity (Sadeque *et al.*, 1992). The addition of potassium chloride (1.15 per cent w/v) to the homogenisation buffer further purifies the preparation by the removal of blood and cytoplasmic contaminants (Eriksson *et al.*, 1978). The addition of glycerol to the final storage buffer is thought to preserve enzyme activity on storage (Guengerich and Martin, 1998). Table 15.2 shows the composition of buffers used for the preparation of liver subcellular fractions.

An alternative method for the preparation of microsomes is to use calcium precipitation. This method is based on the calcium-dependent aggregation of the endoplasmic reticulum. Calcium chloride is added to the post-mitochondrial fraction to give a final concentration of 8 mM. The mixture is left to stand for five minutes with occasional mixing. Centrifugation at $27{,}000 \times g$ for 15 minutes will yield the microsomal pellet which may be resuspended as previously described.

The protein concentration of both S9 and microsomes should be determined prior to use in order to normalise incubation conditions between preparations (i.e. ensure the same amount of protein is added to each incubation). Protein measurement kits are commercially available and include the Lowry method (Lowry *et al.*, 1951) and the bicinchoninic acid method (Smith *et al.*, 1985).

TABLE 15.2 *Buffers used for the preparation of S9 and microsomes*

Homogenisation buffer	0.1 M phosphate buffer pH7.4 + 1.15% KCl (10 mM EDTA optional)
Wash buffer	0.1 M phosphate buffer pH 7.4 + 1.15% KCl (1 mM EDTA optional)
Storage buffer	0.1 M phosphate buffer pH 7.4 + 20% glycerol (0.1 mM EDTA optional)

The levels of active cytochrome P450 may be determined by the difference in spectrum (Omura and Sato, 1964). Determination of active cytochrome P450 gives an extra level of confidence in the activity of the preparation as well as greater consistency in incubation conditions if the incubations are normalised for cytochrome P450 concentration rather than microsomal protein concentration. In general, different spectra with S9 are not recommended as non-specific absorption and light scattering can occur due to the turbidity of this preparation.

Summary of the preparation of S9 and microsomal protein (by ultracentrifugation)

1 Carry out all steps at 4 °C.
2 Weigh the fresh or thawed liver sample.
3 Add four times the volume of homogenisation buffer to liver weight.
4 Scissor mince tissue then homogenise using a Potter Elvhejam or similar mechanical tissue homogeniser.
5 Centrifuge the homogenate at 9,000 × *g* for 20 minutes.
6 Combine the supernatants (S9 fraction) and snap freeze in liquid nitrogen. Store S9 fraction at −80 °C.
7 For the preparation of the microsomal fraction, centrifuge the S9 fraction at 100,000 × *g* for 1 hour.
8 Discard the supernatant and resuspend the pellet in buffer. Centrifuge the homogenate at 100,000 × *g* for 1 hour.
9 Discard the supernatant and resuspend the pellet in storage buffer (volume equivalent to the original tissue weight).
10 Snap freeze aliquots (1 or 2 ml) in liquid nitrogen and store at −80 °C

15.2.2 Preparation of hepatocytes

There are three methods routinely used for the preparation of hepatocytes. The methods involve removal of calcium from the tissue followed by treatment of the tissue with a solution containing collagenase. Calcium removal initiates the separation of cell–cell adhesion via calcium-dependent desmosomes. The collagenase treatment digests the architecture of the liver and allows the hepatocytes to be released. The first method is based on that of Berry and Friend (1969) and involves the perfusion of the liver *in situ*. The second technique was developed in 1976 by Fry and co-workers and involves digestion of liver slices, thus avoiding the need for perfusion. The benefit of this method is that an intact Glisson's capsule around the liver is not required, so use can be made of tissue that would otherwise be wasted. The third method is an adaptation of the *in situ* collagenase perfusion technique (Strom *et al.*, 1982; Oldham *et al.*, 1985). Small, end-of-lobe liver fragments surrounded by an intact Glisson's capsule are perfused by cannulating the exposed vessels on the cut surface of the sample. This third method is the method routinely used in our laboratories because it can be used to isolate hepatocytes from several different species, including human, with minimal changes to the basic technique. An *in situ* perfusion technique would not be suitable to use with larger species such as the dog.

The method described below is used for the isolation of hepatocytes from end-of-lobe liver samples (wedge biopsies). Table 15.3 details the composition of buffers and

TABLE 15.3 *Buffers and solutions for the isolation of hepatocytes*

Isolation buffer:	10 × EBSS	100 ml
Perfusion buffer	(without calcium and magnesuim)	30 ml
	7.5% sodium bicarbonate solution	870 ml
	purified water	pH adjusted to 7.4
Isolation buffer:	Perfusion buffer	490 ml
Chelating buffer	25 mM EGTA (in 0.1 M NaOH)	10 ml pH adjusted to 7.4
Isolation buffer:	Perfusion buffer	150 ml
Collagenase buffer	1 M $CaCl_2$	300 μl
	Trypsin inhibitor	~10 mg
	Collagenase H	12 units (rat) 24 units (dog, human, pig)
Dispersal buffer	Sodium chloride	4.15 g
	Potassium chloride	0.26 g
	HEPES	1.19 g
	Purified water	500 ml pH adjusted to 7.4
	BSA	5.0 g
Culture medium (for suspensions)	William's medium E	500 ml
	200 mM L-glutamine	10 ml
Culture medium (for monolayers)	William's medium E	500 ml
	200 mM L-glutamine	5 ml
	Penicillin (10,000 U/ml)/Streptomycin	5 ml
	(10,000 mg/ml)	0.5 ml
	Insulin (250 U/ml)	0.5 ml
	δ-aminolevulinic acid (1 mM)	0.5 ml
	Transferrin (5 mg/ml)	0.5 ml
	Hydrocortisone (3.6 mg/ml)	0.5 ml
	Zinc sulphate (5 μM)	
Culture medium (for monolayers)	Chee's essential medium	500 ml
	200 mM L-glutamine	5 ml
	Penicillin (10,000 U/ml)/ Streptomycin (10,000 mg/ml)	5 ml

solutions required for the isolation of hepatocytes. Figures 15.1 and 15.2 show the apparatus used for the isolation procedure and the perfusion of whole lobes of rat liver.

All buffers and solutions should be maintained at 37 °C with the exception of the dispersal buffer which should be kept at 4 °C. All buffers used during the perfusion should be maintained at pH 7.4 by continuous gassing with carbogen (95 per cent oxygen, 5 per cent carbon dioxide).

Exposed vessels on the cut surface of the liver tissue (or vessels entering the individual lobes for rat liver) are cannulated using 20 gauge (rat) or 16 gauge cannulae (human, dog, pig). The tissue is perfused with chelating buffer for approximately 5 minutes at a flow rate of approximately 6 ml/min/cannula (rat) or 12 ml/min/cannula (human, dog, pig). The chelating buffer is then washed out by perfusion buffer for approximately 5 minutes. The tissue is then perfused with collagenase buffer, which should be recirculated after 3–4 minutes. The collagenase perfusion should continue until the cells beneath the Glisson's capsule become spongy to the touch. This should take approximately 20–25 minutes for rat liver and anything up to 1 hour for the isolation of human hepatocytes. The time required for human hepatocyte isolation varies depending upon the age, status and fibrotic nature of the liver sample used.

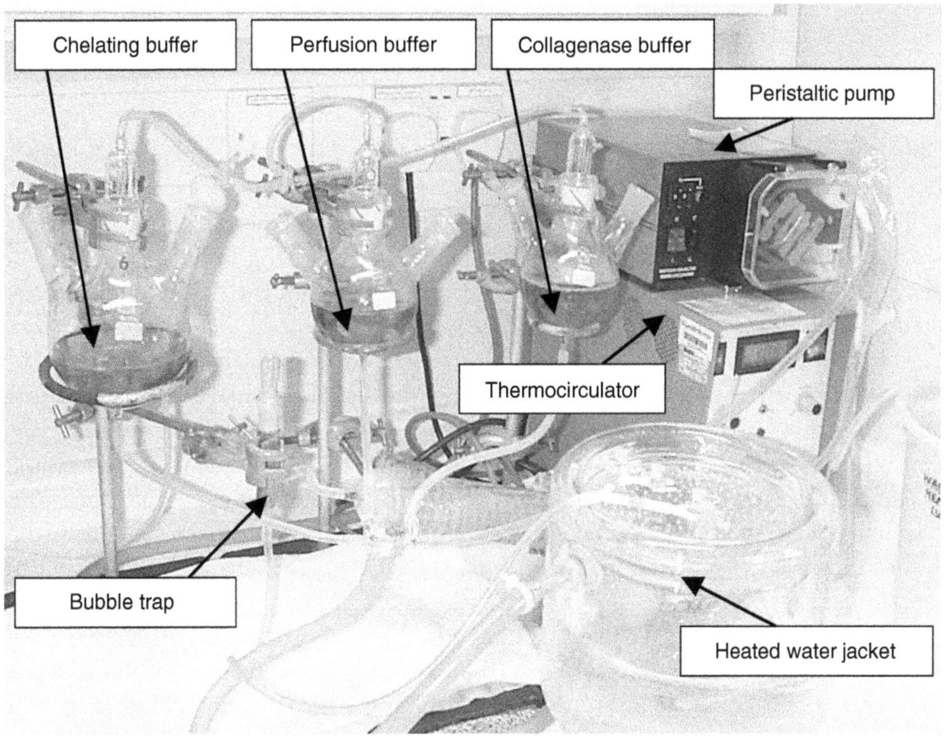

FIGURE 15.1 *Apparatus used for the isolation of hepatocytes.*

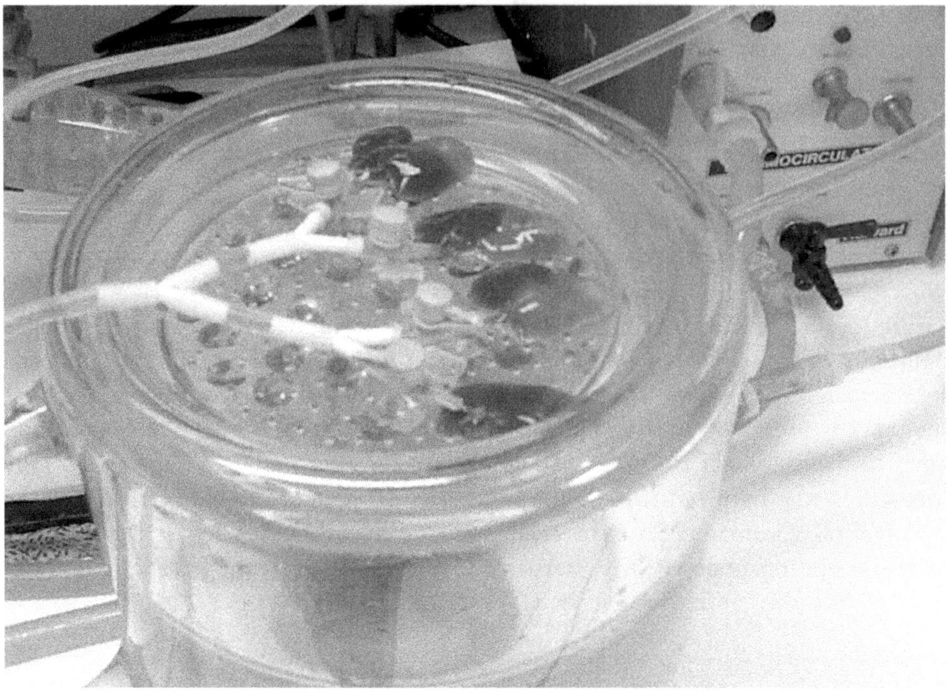

FIGURE 15.2 *Isolation of hepatocytes: perfusion of rat liver lobes.*

Once the extracellular matrix has dissociated sufficiently the perfusion is stopped, avoiding possible rupture of the Glisson's capsule.

The tissue is placed into a shallow dish containing dispersal buffer and using forceps, the Glisson's capsule is carefully peeled away releasing isolated cells into the dispersal buffer. The forceps can be used to gently 'comb' the cells to help release them from the tissue.

The cell suspension is filtered through nylon bolting cloth (64 μm pore size) pre-wetted with dispersal buffer containing DNAse I (5 mg/100 ml) to remove large clumps of tissue and cells. DNAse removes DNA that has been released from damaged cells which causes cells to clump together. All subsequent manipulations of the cell suspension are carried out at 4 °C. The low temperature minimises the activity of any cytotoxic enzymes that may have been released from damaged cells and to preserve drug-metabolising enzyme activity. Viable cells are sedimented by centrifugation ($50 \times g$ for 5 min) at 4 °C. The cells are washed twice more as previously described but without DNAse I in the final wash.

The final cell pellet is resuspended in a suitable incubation buffer such as William's medium E (plus appropriate supplements) and the viability of the preparation assessed using an appropriate cell viability test, of which the simplest is the trypan blue exclusion test. Trypan blue is a large molecular weight dye which is excluded from viable cells with an intact cell membrane. However, non-viable cells with a damaged membrane will take up the dye resulting in a blue-stained nucleus. After treatment with trypan blue, the total number of cells isolated in combination with the number of viable and non-viable cells can easily be determined using light microscopy and a haemocytometer. Generally, for small animal species, a viability of >90 per cent is required before use.

The remaining cell suspension is now ready to be diluted appropriately for use.

Summary of hepatocyte isolation (two-step collagenase digestion)

1 Perfuse tissue with chelating buffer.
2 Perfuse tissue with perfusion buffer.
3 Perfuse tissue with collagenase buffer until extracellular matrix has dissociated.
4 Place tissue into dispersal buffer.
5 Break open Glisson's capsule and tease out cells into the buffer.
6 Filter cells, with DNAse I and centrifuge (50 × *g*, 5 minutes).
7 Filter cells, with DNAse I and centrifuge (50 × *g*, 5 minutes).
8 Filter cells, without DNAse I and centrifuge (50 × *g*, 5 minutes).
9 Re-suspend cell pellet in medium.
10 Determine cell viability and total cell number using trypan blue exclusion.
11 Dilute remaining cells.
12 Use in suspension or plate cells out as monolayers.

15.2.3 Preparation of liver slices

There are a number of different techniques for producing liver slices, and a similar choice of incubation systems. A number of commercial tissue slicers are available, such as the Brendel-Vitron and Krumdieck machines, which allow thin slices of liver (thickness *ca.* 250 μm) to be reproducibly cut from cores of tissue. These cores may be prepared freehand or by using a mechanised borer. The cores are then placed in the machine, and slices cut using a microtome, which allows the thickness of the prepared slices to be controlled. The core, and the slices prepared from it, is kept submerged in ice-cold physiological buffer. Following this, prepared slices are harvested and used in the incubation system, the choice of which may depend on the aim of the experiment. If slices need to be prepared aseptically this may be possible as some mechanised slicers are autoclavable.

Summary of liver slice preparation

1 Obtain fresh liver.
2 Cut cylindrical cores from the tissue.

3 Place cores into the tissue slicer and prepare slices in ice-cold physiological buffer.
4 Transfer slices into incubation system of choice.

15.3 *Use of subcellular fractions, hepatocytes and liver slices to study drug metabolism*

15.3.1 Subcellular fractions

There are a number of uses for subcellular fractions within the pharmaceutical industry. However, the major uses within drug metabolism are to screen potential drug candidates for metabolic stability and as 'metabolite factories' to produce potential metabolites for identification with more ease than by extraction and analysis of drug-related material from biological fluids following *in vivo* drug administration.

Qualitative experiments investigating the metabolic profile of potential drug candidates (Adams *et al.*, 1981; Acheampong *et al.*, 1996) have been used to confirm the presence of metabolites in animals and man and therefore validate long-term and expensive toxicology testing.

Incubations are prepared by addition of the compound, enzyme preparation, buffer and appropriate enzyme cofactors. The addition of organic solvents to enzyme incubations should be kept to a minimum as organic solvents may affect enzyme activity (Chauret *et al.*, 1998). Choice of the appropriate enzyme cofactor is also an important consideration. For example, the preparation of microsomes produces an endoplasmic reticulum-rich fraction containing membrane-bound cytochromes P450. All soluble enzyme cofactors are lost during the process. Therefore, oxidations by cytochromes P450 will not proceed without the addition of the reduced form of the cofactor nicotinamide adenine dinucleotide phosphate (NADPH) or an NADP(H)-regenerating system to the microsomal incubations.

Following incubation, and simple 'cleanup' techniques such as the addition of organic solvents to precipitate proteins, the metabolites obtained may be analysed using high-performance liquid chromatography (HPLC), in conjunction with mass spectrometry (LC–MS) or nuclear magnetic resonance (LC–NMR). In this way, detailed information of the metabolic profile of a compound may be determined. Species-specific metabolism or the production of pharmacologically active or toxic metabolites may be quickly screened and investigated.

Quantitative metabolism may be used in the initial stages of research to screen and then rank potential drug candidates according to their metabolic stability. The advent of combinatorial chemistry has enabled chemists to rapidly produce large numbers of novel synthetic compounds. Metabolic stability (or instability) is a crucial factor in the development of any new medicine, so high-throughput methodologies employing subcellular fractions have now been developed to enable the metabolic stability of large numbers of compounds to be investigated in the minimum amount of time (Eddershaw and Dickins, 1999). Compounds with inappropriate metabolic stability can therefore be removed from research and development at an early stage.

15.3.2 Hepatocytes

Hepatocytes provide the pharmaceutical industry with a whole cell system to study the metabolism of drug candidates. Hepatocytes can be cultured in suspension in the presence of a test compound for up to 4 hours. The culture medium routinely used in our laboratories is William's medium E containing 4 mM L-glutamine. The medium does not contain phenol red as this indicator dye is metabolised by several Phase II drug-metabolising enzymes and therefore could compete for metabolism by these enzymes and prevent Phase II metabolism of the test compound (Driscoll *et al.*, 1982).

15.3.3 Liver slices

As a whole cell preparation, liver slices offer an alternative to hepatocytes and perfused liver in the study of metabolism.

Liver slices have a variety of uses in the study of drug metabolism. The ease and speed of their preparation facilitates the retention of metabolic activity and they are therefore useful as predictive tools when studying the biotransformations of drugs *in vitro*. They can be used as 'metabolite factories' to produce sufficient quantities of metabolite for characterisation and identification. Because the amount of liver tissue per slice will never be identical, however, there can be greater individual variability between slices compared with hepatocyte incubations when used in quantitative studies, for instance in drug interaction studies.

The choice of incubation system may depend on the aim of the experiment. A dynamic organ culture system may be used, where the slice is supported on a wire mesh in a vial-containing medium and placed on rollers in an oven maintained at 37 °C so that the slice moves in and out of the liquid phase (Smith *et al.*, 1986). Alternatively, slices may be placed in a conical flask, or in 12- or 24-well plates, and incubated with agitation in a temperature-controlled incubator. Whichever system is used, a pre-incubation of the slice in fresh culture medium (generally up to 2 hours duration) is carried out to allow sloughing of cells from the cut surfaces of the slice and ensure homeostasis. For short-term incubations, such as simple assessment of xenobiotic biotransformation in a manner similar to the use of hepatocyte suspensions, the slices may be incubated in a tissue culture medium such as

Williams' medium E (supplemented with glutamine) containing the test compound. Generally for a short-term culture, sufficient oxygen may be introduced to the system by pre-gassing the medium with carbogen. Alternatively, vials with a hole drilled in the lid to facilitate oxygen transfer may be placed in the incubator. For longer-term incubations, such as studying the biotransformation of slowly metabolised xenobiotics or the potential for induction of drug-metabolising enzymes (Lake *et al.*, 1997), the medium is usually supplemented with a number of additives such as foetal calf serum, hormones and antibiotics. In addition, for longer-term cultures, the medium may need to be changed regularly and adequate oxygenation maintained by placing the culture plates in a tissue culture incubator.

At the end of incubation both the medium and the slice are usually analysed, as metabolites may be retained within the slice.

15.4 *In vitro–in vivo correlations*

All the systems discussed so far can be used to measure the metabolic clearance of a compound *in vitro*. The data obtained from any of these systems can then be scaled using various models to provide an estimate of the clearance of that particular drug *in vivo*.

Subcellular fractions, especially microsomes (Houston, 1994; Houston and Carlile, 1997; Iwatsubo *et al.*, 1997) have been used to estimate rates of metabolic clearance of a particular drug *in vitro* in an attempt to estimate rates of metabolic clearance of a drug *in vivo*. This may be achieved either by quantifying rates of metabolite production, or by calculation of the rate of disappearance of substrate from the incubation by metabolism. Disappearance plots have the advantage that knowledge of the metabolic profile of a compound is not required before investigation commences, thus enabling the study of drug candidates whose metabolic profile is unknown. However, the disadvantage of this approach is that substrate may be removed from the incubation matrix by methods other than metabolism such as non-specific irreversible binding to cellular proteins.

The first step in quantitative prediction of the metabolic clearance of a drug candidate *in vivo* is achieved by determination of the intrinsic clearance of a drug. Intrinsic clearance is the ability of an enzyme system to metabolise a drug in the absence of any interfering constraints such as plasma protein binding or blood flow. Intrinsic clearance is quite simply the ratio of Michaelis Menton parameters K_m and V_{max}, as shown below.

$$\text{Rate of metabolism} = \text{intrinsic clearance} \times \text{substrate concentration } [S]$$

$$\text{Intrinsic clearance} = \frac{\text{rate of metabolism}}{\text{substrate concentration}}$$

Michaelis Menton states that

$$\frac{V_{max} \cdot [S]}{K_m + [S]}$$

When [S] is 10 per cent or less than K_m the equation reduces to

$$\frac{V_{max} \cdot [S]}{K_m}$$

Therefore intrinsic clearance = V_{max}/K_m

Once intrinsic clearance has been calculated as a rate (i.e. nmoles of parent turned over or metabolite produced/min/mg of microsomal protein), then the intrinsic clearance is scaled to predict clearance that would occur in the liver *in vivo*. For example, the literature average for the amount of microsomal protein is approximately 45 mg microsomal protein/g liver.

The effects of plasma protein binding and blood flow on the clearance process are then modelled using one of a number of liver models. The simplest model is the venous equilibration model shown below; however, more complex models including the parallel tube and dispersion models may also be used (Wilkinson, 1987; Saville *et al.*, 1992). Essentially the models vary in the estimation of the concentration drop of parent compound across the liver. This will be most important for highly metabolised compounds where the concentration drop across the liver will be greatest. Under these circumstances the venous equilibrium model will give the lowest prediction of clearance, the parallel tube model the highest prediction and the dispersion model prediction will be in between the two.

15.4.1 Venous equilibrium model

$$\text{Clearance } in\ vivo = \frac{Q \cdot Fu \cdot \text{intrinsic clearance}}{Q + Fu \cdot \text{intrinsic clearance}}$$

where Q = hepatic blood flow; Fu = unbound fraction of drug in the blood. The final result is an estimation of hepatic metabolic clearance which may then be used to predict the plasma pharmacokinetics of a drug in animals or man *in vivo*.

This technique, although at present used with caution, could in the future serve to estimate the metabolic clearance of compound in animals and man and reduce the need for widespread and intensive testing of the pharmacokinetics of compounds in animals. In theory, only compounds with appropriate kinetics would be investigated further leading to a reduction of research cost and effort.

15.4.2 Hepatocytes

Hepatocytes, like subcellular fractions, may also be used for both quantitative and qualitative studies and studies to examine drug interactions as previously outlined. The use of whole cells provides more metabolic pathways for metabolism of a test compound and as hepatocyte number in the whole liver is well established, the scaling from *in vitro* data generated in hepatocytes gives a better estimation of *in vivo* clearance.

15.4.3 Liver slices

Liver slices have also been used as a tool for the prediction of the intrinsic clearance of drugs, in a similar manner to hepatocytes (Worboys *et al.*, 1996). This application demonstrates one of the limitations of tissue slices, namely that the contribution of cells in the centre of the slice may be unrepresentative of the overall clearance due to the need for drug to diffuse to the centre. Also, although slices are cut very thinly (about 200–300 μm) and are maintained in conditions to maximise the supply of oxygen to the slice, the centre cells may become necrosed with time and thus not contribute to the turnover of drug. Finally, metabolites, or remaining parent drug, may be retained within the slice leading to over- or underestimation of clearance if only the medium, and not the contents of the slice itself, is studied at the end of the incubation period.

15.5 *Advantages and disadvantages of the* in vitro *systems used to study drug metabolism*

The cellular locations of the main enzymes responsible for xenobiotic metabolism have already been shown in Table 15.1. This table highlights the differences in the distribution of enzyme types between different *in vitro* liver preparations.

15.5.1 Subcellular fractions

The advantages and disadvantages of using subcellular fractions to study drug metabolism are summarised in Table 15.4. S9 is a crude cell preparation and contains a range of both cytosolic- and membrane-bound enzymes. Therefore, this fraction yields a wide range of biotransformation products. Whilst S9 is a crude preparation the microsomal preparation is a highly purified enzyme preparation that contains only those enzymes bound to the endoplasmic reticulum *in vivo*.

There is also a difference in the availability of cofactors for certain enzyme reactions between preparations. S9, as a crude preparation, should also contain the

TABLE 15.4 *The advantages and disadvantages of subcellular fractions for the study of drug metabolism*

	Advantages	**Disadvantages**
S9	Ease of preparation Contains soluble and membrane-bound enzymes Ease of storage Contains cofactors Prepared from frozen tissue	Crude preparation High protein concentration
Microsomes	Ease of storage Prepared from frozen tissue Membrane-bound enzymes	Requires ultracentrifuge No cofactors

necessary cofactors for enzyme activity. However, experience has shown that the addition of suitable cofactors (e.g. NADPH) may be important in retaining suitable cytochrome P450 activity.

Although microsomes contain cytochromes P450, the preparation will not carry out redox reactions *per se* due to the lack of cofactors available to aid in the reaction cycle. NADPH or an NADP(H)-regenerating system must be added to incubation mixtures for biotransformations to proceed. In addition, although microsomes contain membrane-bound glucuronyl transferases, the cofactor uridine diphosphate glucuronic acid (UDPGA) and also detergents need to be added for microsomes to carry out Phase II glucuronidation reactions. The detergents are required to release the enzyme from the centre of the microsomal vesicle where access to the substrate is impaired.

S9 and microsomes have the advantage that they may be prepared in large quantities from both fresh and frozen tissue. Once prepared, the tissue preparations may be stored at −80 °C without a significant drop in enzyme activity. This means that large numbers of experiments may be carried out using the same preparation facilitating comparison between experiments.

Disadvantages of using subcellular fractions include interactions due to large concentrations of non-specific protein within the matrix. Protein may bind and essentially remove the drug from the incubation medium leading to an overestimate of the stability of the drug. Concentrations of non-specific protein are much higher in the S9 fraction than in the microsomal fraction. Large amounts of protein may interfere with drug metabolism directly or hinder analysis of the experimental incubates.

Metabolism may also be impaired in subcellular fractions due to the build-up of Phase I metabolites which will effectively inhibit the turnover of parent material (product inhibition). This will lead to an underestimation of metabolic turnover.

In contrast, the intimate association of the drug with the enzyme under *in vitro* conditions with subcellular fractions may drive a reaction that may not occur *in vivo*. For example, a drug with a low volume of distribution may not become available within the cell for interaction with the enzyme *in vivo* and therefore the metabolic instability of a compound may be overestimated. In addition, the activity of drug transporters in the cell membrane may serve to regulate the intracellular levels of drug *in vivo*. This may lead to inaccurate estimations of metabolic clearance using subcellular preparations due to incorrect assumptions of the amount of drug interacting with the enzyme *in vivo*.

Finally, the activity of subcellular fractions is highly dependent upon assay conditions, for example, the activity of cytochromes P450 is dependant on buffer concentration and pH. Each cytochrome P450 has an optimum buffer and buffer concentration (Wrighton and Gillespie, 1998).

15.5.2 Hepatocytes

Advantages and disadvantages of using hepatocytes to study drug metabolism are shown in Table 15.5.

Hepatocytes may be used in short-term suspension incubations similar to those for subcellular fractions or may be kept in long-term culture. This section relates to short-term suspensions; hepatocyte culture will be discussed later.

Hepatocytes are structurally intact liver cells and therefore represent a step up in tissue integrity with respect to subcellular fractions. The presence of an intact cell membrane means that access of the drug to the drug-metabolising enzymes is controlled in a similar way to that *in vivo*. For example, access into or out of the cell may be controlled by the physical presence of the cell membrane and/or by drug transporters (both influx and efflux) present in the cell membrane.

Hepatocytes not only contain a full complement of enzyme activity but also the cofactors necessary for the completion of metabolic pathways. Hepatocytes therefore have advantages over the use of subcellular fractions with respect to Phase II and Phase III metabolism. In addition, because of the full complement of enzyme systems, metabolism can proceed normally from Phase I to Phase II metabolism and therefore build-up of Phase I metabolites (and therefore product inhibition) should not occur to the same extent as in microsomes.

Due to the presence of an intact cell membrane, enzyme activity in hepatocytes is much less dependent on the buffer or medium composition compared to subcellular fractions and, after centrifugation to lyse the cells, hepatocyte suspensions are much cleaner and therefore easier to analyse than subcellular fractions.

Table 15.5 *The advantages and disadvantages of using hepatocytes for the study of drug metabolism*

	Advantages	**Disadvantages**
Hepatocytes	Full enzyme compliment Culture methods available	Need fresh tissue Storage limited No cell–cell contact

Disadvantages of hepatocyte preparations include the need for fresh tissue for cell isolation, although a number of authors (Coundouris *et al.*, 1993; Zalenski *et al.*, 1993; Swales *et al.*, 1996) claim to have preserved the enzyme activity of isolated cells through cryopreservation, thus reducing the need for re-preparation of cells.

15.5.3 Liver slices

Table 15.6 highlights some advantages and disadvantages of liver slices in the study of drug metabolism. Their main advantage lies in the ease of preparation and the maintenance of cell–cell contact, and thus they offer a supplement or alternative to other whole cell systems for particular applications. The cryopreservation of liver slices has been investigated with a view to the long-term storage of human tissue which retains its drug-metabolising capacity, and results in this area, particularly using the vitrification technique, have been encouraging (de Kanter *et al.*, 1998). Further details on the use of tissue slices may be found in a number of articles (e.g. Parrish *et al.*, 1995; Bach *et al.*, 1996; Ekins, 1996; Thohan *et al.*, 2001).

15.6 *The study of drug interactions using* in vitro *systems*

Although this subject is dealt with in more detail in Chapter 16, it is also pertinent to mention in this chapter as *in vitro* drug interaction studies are generally carried out using either liver subcellular fractions or isolated hepatocytes.

15.6.1 Drug–drug interactions: subcellular fractions and hepatocytes

A number of clinically important drug interactions (reviewed by Landrum-Michalets, 1998) have highlighted the need to investigate the enzymology of drug metabolism reactions and determine whether potential drug interactions may occur in the clinic.

TABLE 15.6 *The advantages and disadvantages of using liver slices for the study of drug metabolism*

	Advantages	Disadvantages
Liver slices	Quick, easy to prepare Cell–cell contact No use of proteolytic enzymes All cell types present Cryopreservation potential	Need fresh tissue Necrosis of slice centre Long-term culture difficult Quantitative studies variable

Subcellular fractions and suspension cultures of isolated hepatocytes have been used for this purpose. Inhibition of the metabolism of drug A in the presence of drug B can be determined. Competitive inhibition of or by the drug candidate molecule can be established and any potentially dangerous interactions be further investigated. By investigating competitive inhibition using a competitor whose metabolism is attributable to a single cytochrome P450, such studies can also elucidate the cytochromes P450 involved in the metabolism of a potential drug candidate.

15.6.2 Drug interactions: monolayer culture of hepatocytes

One major disadvantage of primary culture of hepatocytes is the rapid loss of enzyme expression which occurs as the cultured cells undergo de-differentiation. In particular, there is a loss of cytochrome P450 expression in monolayer culture of hepatocytes.

Monolayer cultures of hepatocytes are therefore used most often to study enzyme induction and inhibition. Induction and inhibition of the levels of drug-metabolising enzymes present within a cell play a key role in some adverse drug reactions. Certain drug entities may induce or inhibit production of drug-metabolising enzymes, often via an effect on gene expression.

By placing hepatocytes into primary culture and providing them with substrata comprised of extracellular matrix proteins such as collagen, together with supplemented tissue culture media, hepatocytes can be maintained for several days or weeks. Because primary cultures can be maintained for these prolonged periods, changes in gene expression can be studied.

Freshly isolated hepatocytes can be plated out to form primary cultures. Hepatocytes placed into culture on collagen-coated plastic adopt a flattened morphology (see Figure 15.3). Hepatocytes do not proliferate in culture and so must be seeded at a density such that the cells form confluent monolayers once they have attached.

Monolayer cultures of hepatocytes are used to investigate the induction of cytochromes P450 by potential drug candidates. Despite the initial loss of cytochrome P450 activity in monolayer cultures of hepatocytes, the levels of individual cytochromes P450 can be increased again by treatment with certain chemical-inducing agents. Table 15.7 shows the most commonly used inducing agents together with the cytochrome(s) P450 that they induce.

To study the induction potential of a potential drug candidate, hepatocyte monolayers are prepared and left for 24 hours before treatment with known inducing agents or the potential drug candidates to be investigated. The cells are dosed daily for three days. Induction of the cytochromes P450 can be determined in several ways.

Increases in the catalytic activity of the cytochromes P450 in treated cells can be established by incubating the control and treated cells with a probe substrate

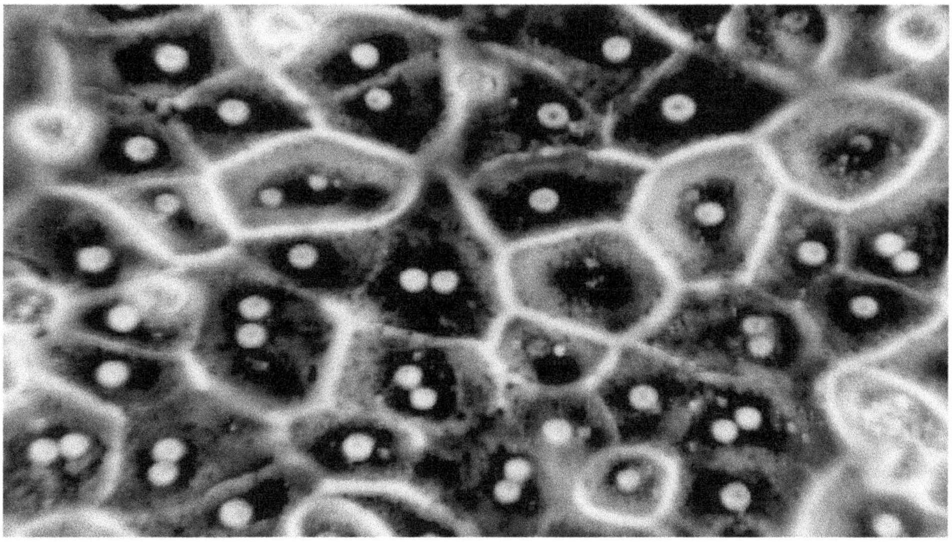

FIGURE 15.3 *Rat hepatocytes in monolayer culture. Cells were plated at* 1×10^5 *cells per* cm^2 *on collagen-coated dishes.*

specific for the cytochrome P450 of interest. Table 15.7 also shows probe substrates commonly used for assessing the activity of the different cytochromes P450.

Changes in the amount of cytochrome P450 protein can be determined by gel electrophoresis and Western blotting. Following treatment with the inducer or

TABLE 15.7 *Cytochromes P450: commonly used inducing agents and probe substrates*

Cytochrome P450	Inducing agent(s)	Probe substrate(s)
1A	*β*-naphthoflavone	7-ethoxyresorufin
	3-methylcholanthrene	Phenacetin
2A	Barbiturates (phenobarbitone)	Coumarin
2B	Phenobarbitone	7-pentoxyresorufin
		7-methoxyresorufin
2C	Rifampicin	Diclofenac (2C9)
		Tolbutamide (2C9)
		S-mephenytoin (2C19)
2D	None known	Bufuralol
		Debrisoquine
2E	Ethanol	Chlorzoxazone
	Isoniazid	*p*-nitrophenol
3A	Rifampicin	Testosterone (6*β*-hydroxylation)
	Dexamethasone	
	Phenobarbitone	Midazolam

potential drug candidate, the cells are harvested and the microsomal fraction prepared from the cells. Microsomal proteins are then separated using sodium dodecyl sulphate polyacrylamide gel electrophoresis (SDS-PAGE) and transferred electrophoretically to nitrocellulose. The nitrocellulose is then incubated with anti-cytochrome P450 antibodies, specific for each individual form. Once these antibodies have bound the cytochromes P450 on the membrane, the membrane is then incubated with secondary antibodies containing a linked enzyme such as alkaline phosphatase. Alkaline phosphatase is used to drive a colourimetric reaction which results in the formation of a coloured band where the cytochrome P450 band was transferred from the gel. The intensity of this coloured band is proportional to the amount of cytochrome P450 originally present in the sample. A similar method is used by cytochrome P450 ELISA kits although there is no need for gel separation as the antibody-binding steps are performed in 96-well plates. The basic principles of these techniques are depicted in Figure 15.4.

Basic protocol for induction studies using hepatocyte monolayers

1 Isolate hepatocytes and seed cells onto collagen-coated plasticware.
2 Seed cells in suitable tissue culture medium containing 10 per cent foetal calf serum (for example, William's medium E or Chee's medium).
3 Allow cells to adhere for 2 hours and replace medium with serum free medium.
4 After 24 hours, add inducing agents or test chemicals to culture medium.
5 Dose daily for three days.
6 Wash cell in PBS and incubate cells with a specific probe substrate. Analyse for metabolism of substrate and compare treated to untreated cells.
7 Harvest cells into PBS and prepare the microsomal fraction.
8 Separate the cytochrome P450 protein from other proteins using SDS-PAGE.
9 Analyse by Western blotting.

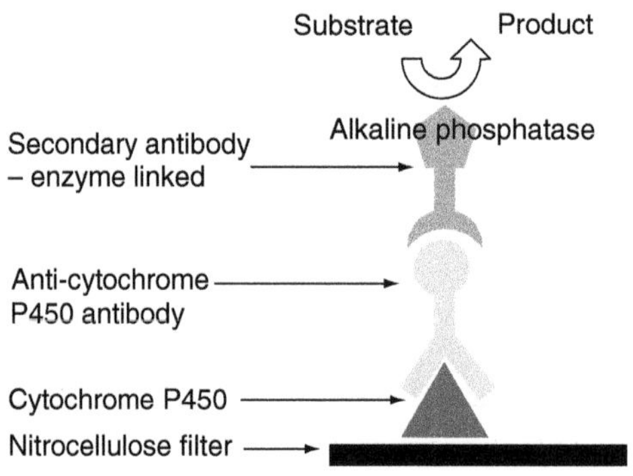

FIGURE 15.4 *Principles of blotting using enzyme-linked secondary antibodies.*

15.6.3 Drug interactions: liver slices

Liver slices can also be used to study the induction of cytochromes P450. They can be incubated in culture to examine the induction potential of xenobiotics on the cytochrome P450 enzymes of animal species (Lake *et al.*, 1993); however, this work has been extended to use liver slices to assess induction in human tissue (Lake *et al.*, 1996, 1997). Liver slices may also be used to assess the inhibitory potential of xenobiotics on drug-metabolising enzymes, particularly as slices retain both Phase I and Phase II metabolism *in vitro*.

15.6.4 Other *in vitro* models

So far this chapter has concentrated on the use of liver S9, microsomes, hepatocytes and liver slices and their use in studying drug metabolism. There are other *in vitro* models that can be used; however, these are not widely used by the pharmaceutical industry at present although may be more widely used in the future.

Due to the problems observed with hepatocytes when placed in culture, i.e. cell de-differentiation and subsequent reduction in the levels of cytochromes P450. A number of techniques have been developed to prolong the activity of hepatocytes in culture; these techniques include the use of liver spheroids, collagen sandwiches and hollow fibre bioreactors.

Hepatic cell lines have also been investigated for the study of drug metabolism. These techniques are briefly described below.

Liver spheroids

Liver spheroids are clusters of hepatocytes which are formed by culturing freshly isolated cells on dishes coated with poly-(2-hydroxyethylmethacrylate) (p-HEMA), a positively charged coating to which the hepatocytes are unable to attach. Gentle shaking on an orbital shaker encourages the hepatocytes to aggregate to form spheroids. Liver spheroids offer the advantage that, like liver slices, the cells are ultimately maintained in a three-dimensional structure allowing cell–cell communication to re-establish (Juillerat *et al.*, 1997). The spheroids are capable of metabolism for prolonged periods of time and the cytochromes P450 can be induced by chemical-inducing agents (Amman and Maier, 1997). Within the spheroids, functional bile canaliculi are formed (Hamilton, 1998).

Collagen sandwich cultures

Culturing hepatocytes in collagen sandwiches has been shown to extend the viability of cultured hepatocytes in terms of cell membrane integrity and P450 enzyme stability (Lecluyse *et al.*, 2000). Cells are cultured onto collagen-coated flasks in the normal way; however, after a period of time (*ca.* one day) the hepatocytes are immobilised in a further layer of collagen.

Hollow fibre bioreactors

Hollow fibre technology has been used clinically to provide extra-corporeal liver assist devices to maintain patients waiting for liver transplants or until spontaneous recovery due to hepatic regeneration occurs. Bioreactors have been seeded with human or pig hepatocytes and the cells perform the synthetic, metabolic, detoxification and excretion functions of the liver for patients with liver failure. Clinically, the devices are used for relatively short time periods (8 hours). However, as the system provides a dynamic culture environment for the culture of hepatocytes, it is under investigation for its suitability for use in the study of drug metabolism within the pharmaceutical industry. The bioreactor could be seeded with hepatocytes from a variety of species and if the system could be maintained for prolonged periods of time, in effect providing an artificial liver to work with, then it may be possible to study all aspects of liver function and in particular drug metabolism, induction of drug-metabolising enzymes and chronic hepatotoxicity.

Hepatic cell lines

There are several hepatic cell lines available for use in studying drug metabolism. Most have been derived from hepatomas or adenocarcinomas. Human hepatic cell lines, mainly HepG2 and Hep3B, are of particular interest to the pharmaceutical industry. One problem with using these cells, however, is that their complement of drug-metabolising enzymes does not reflect those present in freshly isolated human hepatocytes. HepG2, the more widely used human hepatic cell line, is suitable for investigating several of the Phase II pathways of metabolism and metabolism by cytochrome P4501A. However, there appears to be little catalytic activity of the other forms of cytochrome P450 in these cells. This may be due to a loss of expression of these forms as the cell line has been repeatedly passaged (undergone cell division) over the years.

15.7 *References*

Acheampong, A.A., Chien, D.S., Lam, S., Vekich, S., Breau, A., Usansky, J.M., Harcourt, D., Munk, S.A., Nguyen, H., Garst, M. and Tang-Liu, D. (1996) Characterisation of brimonidine metabolism with rat, rabbit, dog, monkey and human liver fractions and rabbit liver aldehyde oxidase. *Xenobiotica* 26, 1035–1055.

Adams, J.D., Baillie, T.A., Trevor, A.J. and Castagnoli, N. (1981) Studies on the biotransformation of ketamine: identification of metabolites produced in vitro from rat liver microsomal preparations. *Biomed. Mass Spectrom.* 8, 527–538.

Amman, P. and Maier, P. (1997) Preservation and inducibility of xenobiotic metabolism in long term cultures of adult liver cell aggregates. *Toxicol. In Vitro* 11, 43–56.

Bach, P.H., Vickers, A.E.M., Fisher, R., Baumann, A., Brittebo, E., Carlisle, D.J., Koster, H.J., Lake, B.G., Salmon, F., Sawyer, T. and Skibinski, G. (1996) The use of tissue slices for pharmacotoxicology studies: report and recommendations of ECVAM workshop 20. *Alternatives Lab. Anim.* 24, 893–923.

Berry, M.N. and Friend, D.S. (1969) High yield preparation of isolated rat liver parenchymal cells. *J. Cell Biol.* 43, 506–520.

Coundouris, J.A., Grant, M.H., Engeset, J., Petrie, J.C. and Hawksworth, G.M. (1993) Cryopreservation of human adult hepatocytes for use in drug metabolism and toxicity studies. *Xenobiotica* 23, 1399–1409.

Chauret, N., Gauthier, A. and Nicoll-Griffith, D.A. (1998) Effect of common organic solvents on in vitro cytochrome P450-mediated metabolic activities in human liver microsomes. *Drug Metab. Dispos.* 26(1), 1–4.

de Kanter, R., Olinga, P., Hof, I., de Jager, M., Verwillegen, W.A., Slooff, M.J.H., Koster, H.J., Meijer, D.K.F. and Groothuis, G.M.M. (1998) A rapid and simple method for cryopreservation of human liver slices. *Xenobiotica* 28, 225–234.

Driscoll, J.L., Hayner, N.T., Williams-Holland, R., Spies-Karotkin, G., Galletti, P.M. and Jauregui, H.O. (1982) Phenolsulfonphthalein (phenol red) metabolism in primary monolayer cultures of adult rat hepatocytes. *In Vitro* 18, 835–842.

Eddershaw, P.J. and Dickins, M. (1999) Advances in in vitro drug metabolism screening. *Pharm. Sci. Technol. Today* 2, 13–19.

Ekins, S. (1996) Past, present and future applications of precision cut liver slices for in vitro xenobiotic metabolism. *Drug Metab. Rev.* 28, 591–623.

Eriksson, L.C., DePierre, J.W. and Dallner, G. (1978) Preparation and properties of microsomal fractions. *Pharmacol. Ther.* 2, 281–317.

Fry, J.R., Jones, C.A., Wiebkin, P., Belleman, P. and Bridges, J.W. (1976) The enzymatic isolation of adult rat hepatocytes in a functional and viable state. *Anal. Biochem.* 71, 341–350.

Guengerich, F. and Martin, M. (1998) In: *Cytochrome P450 Protocols*, Philips, I.R. and Shephard, E.A. (eds), p. 35. Humana, New Jersey.

Hamilton, G. (1998) Characterisation and evaluation of liver spheroids as a model for long term culture of hepatocytes. PhD Thesis, University of Hertfordshire.

Houston, J.B. (1994) Utility of in vitro drug metabolism data in predicting in vivo metabolic clearance. *Biochem. Pharmacol.* 47, 1469–1479.

Houston, J.B. and Carlile, D.J. (1997) Prediction of hepatic clearance from microsomes, hepatocytes and liver slices. *Drug Metab. Rev.* 29, 891–922.

Iwatsubo, T., Hirota, N., Ooie, T., Suzuka, H., Shimada, N., Chiba, K., Ishizaki, T., Green, C., Tyson, C. and Sugiyama, Y. (1997) Prediction of in vivo drug metabolism in the human liver from in vitro metabolism data. *Pharmacol. Ther.* 73, 147–171.

Juillerat, M., Marceau, N., Coeytaux, S., Sierra, F., Kolodziejczyk, E. and Guigoz, Y. (1997) Expression of organ specific structures and functions in long term cultures of aggregates from rat liver cells. *Toxicol. In Vitro* 11, 57–69.

Lake, B.G., Beamand, J.A., Japenga, A.C., Renwick, A., Davies, S. and Price, R.J. (1993) Induction of cytochrome P-450-dependent enzyme activities in cultured rat liver slices. *Food Chem. Toxicol.* 31, 377–386.

Lake, B.G., Charzat, C., Tredger, J.M., Renwick, A.B., Beamand, J.A. and Price, R.J. (1996) Induction of cytochrome P450 isoenzymes in cultured precision cut rat and human liver slices. *Xenobiotica* 26, 297–306.

Lake, B.G., Ball, S.E., Renwick, A.B., Tredger, J.M., Kao, J., Beamand, J.A. and Price, R.J. (1997) Induction of CYP3A isoforms in cultured precision cut human liver slices. *Xenobiotica* 27, 1165–1173.

Landrum-Michalets, E. (1998) Update: clinically significant cytochrome P450 drug interactions. *Pharmacotherapy* 18, 84–112.

Lecluyse, E., Madan, A., Hamilton, G., Carroll, K., DeHaan, R. and Parkinson, A. (2000) Expression and regulation of cytochrome P450 enzymes in primary cultures of human hepatocytes. *J. Biochem. Mol. Toxicol.* 14(4), 177–188.

Lowry, O.H., Roseborough, N.J., Farr, A.L. and Randall, R.J. (1951) Protein measurement with the Folin phenol reagent. *J. Biol. Chem.* 193, 265–275.

Oldham, H.G., Norman, S.J. and Chenery, R.J. (1985) Primary cultures of adult rat hepatocytes – A model for the toxicity of histamine H2 receptor agonists. *Toxicol.* 36, 215–229.

Omura, T. and Sato, R. (1964) The carbon monoxide binding pigment of liver microsomes. I. Evidence for its hemoprotein nature. *J. Biol. Chem.* 239, 2370–2378.

Parrish, A.R., Gandolfi, A.J. and Brendel, K. (1995) Precision cut tissue slices: applications in pharmacology and toxicology. *Life Sci.* 57, 1887–1901.

Sadeque, A.J.M., Eddy, A.C., Meier, G.P. and Rettie, A.E. (1992) Stereoselective sulfoxidation by human flavin-containing monooxygenase. *Drug Metab. Dispos.* 20(6), 832–839.

Saville, B.A., Gray, M.R. and Tam, Y.K. (1992) Models of hepatic drug elimination. *Drug Metab. Rev.* 24, 48–88.

Smith, P.K., Krohn, R.I., Hermanson, G.T., Mallia, A.K., Gartner, F.H., Provenzano, M.D., Fujimoto, E.K., Goeke, N.M., Olson, B.J. and Klenk, D.C. (1985) Measurement of protein using bicinchoninic acid. *Anal. Biochem.* 150, 76–85 (published erratum appears in *Anal. Biochem.* 1987, 163, 279).

Smith, P.F., Krack, G., McKee, R.L., Johnson, D.G., Gandolfi, A.J., Hruby, V.J., Krumdieck, C.L. and Brendel, K. (1986) Maintenance of adult rat liver slices in dynamic organ culture. *In Vitro Cell. Dev. Biol.* 22, 706–712.

Strom, S.C., Jirtle, R.L., Jones, R.S., Novicki, D.L., Rosenberg, M.R., Novotny, A., Irons, G., McLain, J.R. and Michalopoulos, G. (1982) Isolation, culture and transplantation of human hepatocytes. *J. Nat. Cancer Inst.* 68, 771–778.

Swales, N.J., Johnson, T. and Caldwell, J. (1996) Cryopreservation of rat and mouse hepatocytes II. Assessment of metabolic capacity using testosterone metabolism. *Drug Metab. Dispos.* 24, 1224–1230.

Thohan, S., Zurich, M.C., Chung, H., Weiner, M., Kane, A.S. and Rosen, G.M. (2001) Tissue slices revisited: evaluation and development of a short-term incubation for integrated drug metabolism. *Drug Metab. Dispos.* 29, 1337–1342.

Wilkinson, G.R. (1987) Clearance approaches in pharmacology. *Pharmacol. Rev.* 39, 1–47.

Worboys, P.D., Bradbury, A. and Houston J.B. (1996) Kinetics of drug metabolism in rat liver slices II. Comparison of clearance by liver slices and freshly isolated hepatocytes. *Drug Metab. Dispos.* 24, 676–681.

Wrighton, S.A. and Gillespie, J.S. (1998) In vitro methods for predicting drug metabolism: the influence of assay conditions. *ISSX Proceedings* 13, 12.

Zalenski, J., Richburg, J. and Kauffman, F.C. (1993) Preservation of the rate and profile of xenobiotic metabolism in rat hepatocytes stored in liquid nitrogen. *Biochem. Pharmacol.* 46, 111–116.

CHAPTER 16

Drug–drug interactions: an in vitro *approach*

D.M. Cross and
M.K. Bayliss

16.1 *Introduction*

Drug–drug interactions are thought to be responsible for between 7 and 22 per cent of adverse drug reactions and underlie about 9 per cent of revisions to safety-related label warnings. The detection and characterisation of drug–drug interactions is a major concern to companies involved in the discovery and development of new medicines, and the regulatory authorities which police the healthcare business. Drug–drug interactions can occur when two or more drugs administered simultaneously mutually interact in a manner which results in alteration of the pharmacokinetic profile, pharmacological or toxicological response to one or both of the compounds. Drugs may interact via inhibition of absorption or elimination processes or induction of enzymes responsible for the metabolism of drugs. The consequences of such interactions may range from those of purely academic interest, such as minor changes in elimination or metabolite profiles, to overt toxicity or even fatal clinical outcomes. Drugs which interact with each other may cause loss or exaggeration of pharmacological effect, or confer an altered phenotype on the patient thus expanding the consequences of drug–drug interactions to apparently unrelated xenobiotic or endogenous metabolism. Interactions need not necessarily be confined to the effects of one drug on another: drugs may affect endogenous metabolic processes (e.g. 6β-hydroxyation of cortisol increases with cytochrome P4503A4 induction); drugs may interact with 'foodstuffs' (e.g. furafylline inhibits caffeine clearance) or 'foodstuffs' which contain potent pharmacological principles may interact with drugs (e.g. components of grapefruit juice can block terfenadine metabolism). The following discussion is essentially confined to drug–drug interactions.

16.2 *Clinical background*

The opportunity to investigate significant drug–drug interactions has in the past been almost entirely confined to clinical trials conducted during the latter stages of drug development. Drug–drug interaction trials rely on empirical observation of patients subjected to varying drug therapies in a clinical setting. During the pre-clinical development phase of a new chemical entity, knowledge about the potential for drug–drug interactions is limited to *in vitro* data. Furthermore, where the mechanism of action of the drug is novel, pre-clinical animal studies may have uncertain pharmacological or toxicological relevance to humans. For these reasons, clinical studies proceed gradually and with great caution.

Phase III clinical trials represent the culmination of the drug discovery/development process and are designed to establish the safety and efficacy of the putative treatment. These studies involve relatively large numbers of patients for the first time. To the pharmaceutical industry they represent the most expensive phase of development and consequently, failure at such a late stage can jeopardise substantial investments. Clearly, any early indicator of the risks likely to be encountered in clinical trials will be valuable in directing the design of studies, prevent inappropriate administration of the candidate drug and thus avoid unnecessary risk to patients participating in the trial. Pre-clinical and clinical interaction data are also contained on the label of new medicines and are therefore available to prescribers for the benefit of future patients in the healthcare market.

16.3 *The impetus behind an* in vitro *approach*

If conducted early enough in drug discovery, clinically predictive interaction studies may provide data able to assist in the design of new molecules with a reduced potential to cause adverse events. In recent years, the pharmaceutical industry has

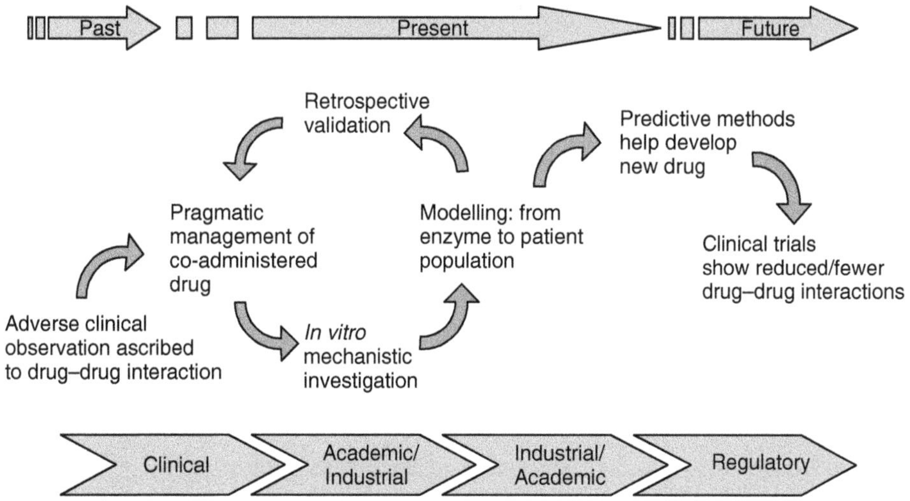

FIGURE 16.1 *A proposal for elimination of drug–drug interactions from new medicines.*

recognised the benefit from investigating the potential for drug–drug interactions early in the discovery–development continuum. Of the 194 new drug products approved by the US Food and Drug Administration between 1992 and 1997, about 30 per cent contained *in vitro* metabolism-based interaction studies, with the frequency of such studies generally increasing over time (Yuan *et al.*, 1999). Advances in experimental techniques and an improved understanding of the mechanisms underlying drug–drug interactions have enabled some relatively simple *in vitro* approaches to be rationalised against clinical outcomes in humans. Inevitably, much of the validation of such an approach has come from retrospective examination of the clinical interactions of existing drugs compared with *in vitro* data obtained subsequent to the drug being approved. The challenge for the pharmaceutical industry is to take this knowledge and make it predictive; the dilemma is that biological systems have evolved a capability to discern the smallest chemical and enantiomeric differences between molecules, such that data compiled for one drug are no certain guide to the properties of another (Figure 16.1).

16.4 *The mechanism behind drug–drug interactions*

Several mechanisms may underlie clinical drug–drug interactions. One or more of these mechanisms may operate at any one time since many drug molecules have the potential to be transported and metabolised by several different systems. Induction by xenobiotics can lead to increased metabolic activity of enzymes thus increasing the metabolism of the inducing compound (autoinduction) or other unrelated drugs and endogenous substrates. Reversible or irreversible inhibition of a single drug-metabolising enzyme will lead to a reduction in the capacity of that enzyme to clear drugs from the body. If the enzyme were a key determinant of drug clearance, then it would be reasonable to expect plasma drug concentration to become elevated or sustained, unless other enzyme systems can compensate for reduction in this key enzyme's intrinsic clearance. Thus enzymes that commonly metabolise drugs and therefore contribute to elimination of the pharmacologically or toxicologically active principle are a major source of drug–drug interactions and are discussed briefly below.

16.5 *Drug-metabolising enzymes*

The cytochromes P450 (CYP) are a diverse superfamily of enzymes which, taken together, are capable of metabolising a wide variety of endogenous and xenobiotic substances including drug molecules (Parkinson, 1996b). Some 11 different CYPs have been identified in the human liver and the majority of commonly prescribed drugs in the US are primarily cleared by CYP-mediated metabolism (Bertz and Granneman, 1997). The major CYP isoform in humans is CYP3A4 which is present in high concentrations in the liver and small intestine. The CYP3A4 present in both the intestinal mucosa and liver offers significant opportunities for drug–drug interactions (e.g. cyclosporin A and ketoconazole) and represents fundamental barriers to drug absorption and systemic exposure. CYP3A4 has a relatively broad substrate specificity capable of metabolising a wide variety of drugs and xenobiotics. Consequently, a large number of disparate therapeutic agents can be metabolised by this enzyme offering extensive opportunity for interactions. Another Phase I enzyme with a role to play is flavin-containing monooxygenase (FMO), a distinct class of flavoproteins capable of xenobiotic biotransformations. Current knowledge suggests there are relatively few forms of FMO which actively contribute to drug metabolism in humans, and that the apparent substrate specificity limits the number of therapeutic drugs which are metabolised by FMO. It has been proposed that one of the reasons ranitidine suffers relatively few drug–drug interactions in humans is that the drug is metabolised to a large extent by FMO, albeit with a low apparent affinity, for which relatively few co-administered drugs are substrates (Overby *et al.*, 1997). Phase II enzymes which typically conjugate drugs with highly water soluble sugar-derivatives, for example UDP-glucuronyltransferase (UGT) and sulphate, namely sulphotransferase (SUL) (Parkinson, 1996b), are also sources of potential drug–drug interactions. Clinical interactions based on Phase II enzyme interactions have been characterised for many drugs including lamotrigine (UGT), troglitazone (UDT and SUL) and salbutamol (SUL). Finally, acetylases, methylases, *N*-acetyltransferases, monoamine oxidases and esterases may be involved in metabolism of some drugs. For example, sumatriptan, a 5-hydroxytryptamine re-uptake inhibitor is metabolised by monoamine oxidase-A (MAO-A), an enzyme normally responsible for noradrenaline, adrenaline and serotonin catabolism. Other enzymes more commonly implicated in drug metabolism do not appear to be significantly involved. Therefore, the effective restriction of sumatriptan metabolism to MAO-A may be one theoretical factor acting to limit the potential for sumatriptan drug–drug interactions to a relatively small subset of drugs which are also metabolised by the same enzyme. Given such mechanistic knowledge, contra-indications for sumatriptan include MAO-inhibitors, ergotamines and other selective serotonin re-uptake inhibitors (Glaxo Wellcome, 1999). However, even where such interactions are thought to occur, such as with moclobemide, there appears to be scant evidence that they have any clinical significance (Stockley, 1999a).

16.6 *Drug transport systems*

Other systems, which do not themselves metabolise drugs, but which are critical to modulating systemic exposure can also be a source of drug–drug interactions (Sasabe *et al.*, 1997). The transport protein, *p*-glycoprotein (PGP), is present in especially high concentrations in the small intestine, and is often co-located with CYP3A4. Many substrates for CYP3A4 are also substrates or inhibitors of PGP, although this may be a fortuitous association (Thummel and Wilkinson, 1998) and inducers of CYP3A4 can also induce PGP (Ito *et al.*, 1998). Vinblastine is a substrate of CYP3A4 and PGP, whereas nifedipine is an inducer of CYP3A4 but an inhibitor of PGP. On the other hand, cyclosporin A (CsA) has been characterised as a substrate for CYP3A4 but a substrate and inducer of PGP. The net result of PGP activity is the transport of drugs out of cells, and therefore in the intestine PGP acts to prevent free access of some drug molecules, such as CsA, to the systemic circulation. Inhibition of PGP by co-administered agents, such as the antifungal ketoconazole can lead to elevated systemic exposure to CsA and potential toxicity. In the extreme cases, combination of PGP and CYP3A4 inhibition could lead to gross elevation of the systemic exposure (reduced first pass effect), or conversely, combined PGP and CYP3A4 induction could dramatically reduce exposure by increasing metabolism in the gut and liver (Ito *et al.*, 1998).

Facilitated uptake of drugs into the target tissue or eliminating organ also represents a potential source of drug–drug interactions. Carrier-mediated uptake of cimetidine into the liver can be inhibited by grepafloxacin (Sasabe *et al.*, 1997), similarly, non-steroidal anti-inflammatory compounds can inhibit the elimination of methotrexate via the kidney (reviewed in Ito *et al.*, 1998). Some drugs which reduce hepatic blood flow can affect the pharmacokinetics of co-administered high clearance drugs, for example cimetidine reduces propranolol clearance (Stockley, 1999b).

16.7 *Plasma protein binding*

The pharmacological or toxicological activity of drugs is often a function of the free drug concentration in the plasma and may relate to the unbound area under the plasma concentration–time curve (AUC) or steady-state unbound plasma concentration. Thus, protein-binding estimates can inform on the relationship between *in vitro* potency and *in vivo* efficacy. Drugs which bind extensively or avidly to plasma proteins such as albumin (e.g. warfarin) or α_1-acid glycoprotein (e.g. mibefradil) tend to have relatively high total concentrations of drug in blood compared with that unbound in plasma. Many drugs are highly plasma protein bound, with >99 per cent of the plasma drug concentration being associated with protein, and, moreover, drugs have the potential to compete with each other for plasma protein binding sites. *In vitro* experiments can be conducted which show significant changes in free drug concentrations when a second drug competing for protein binding is added. However, *in vitro* systems are an oversimplification of the living body, and many factors affect drug distribution and clearance *in vivo* which are absent *in vitro*. In the body, a complex equilibrium of drug distribution is established which is continuously modulated by absorption and elimination processes. For a highly bound drug, the volume of distribution (*Vd*) can become restricted in a way that reflects the distribution of albumin namely, drug and albumin are confined to the plasma and extravascular fluids ($Vd \sim 0.04$–0.3 L/kg). In the case of a drug with a low volume of distribution and where only the unbound fraction of the drug is pharmacologically active, then displacement of the bound-free equilibrium in favour of free drug by co-administration of another highly protein-bound therapeutic agent can increase the free fraction of the drug in plasma water. Where the therapeutic index is low, disturbance of the equilibrium can lead to toxicity, or where the concentration–response slope is steep, an exaggerated pharmacological response may ensue. *In vitro* data seem to support this hypothesis and such effects have often been reported when drugs are co-administered with the anticoagulant, warfarin (*Vd* 0.08–0.27 L/kg), which has a relatively narrow therapeutic index. However, an increase in the free fraction of drug through displacement from proteins also tends to result in increased clearance so that the bound-free equilibrium is rapidly re-established. The body therefore acts to buffer any changes in free drug so that any change in free fraction is transient. The converse situation can be envisaged where protein binding is high but *Vd* is large, then any free drug originating from displacement of bound drug will re-equilibrate into the tissues so that the fraction unbound in plasma remains essentially unaffected and interactions at the plasma protein binding level become irrelevant (Ito *et al.*, 1998). Whilst the theoretical consequences of this latter case may have limited clinical application, effects related strictly to displacement of protein-bound drug (the former case) appear to have been exaggerated in many cases through over-interpretation of *in vitro* data (McElnay, 1996; Stockley, 1999b). In general, for orally administered drugs, protein-binding interactions are typically transient in nature and probably originate from a mechanism other than the one related to displacement of protein-bound drug.

The nature of any clinical interaction is inevitably a balance of various relative interaction potentials for all the competing processes of disposition and elimination. Moreover, plasma proteins have a very high and largely non-selective capacity to bind drugs making the plasma proteins a sizeable reservoir for many circulating endogenous and exogenous substances.

16.8 *Drug concentration effects*

The exposure of the body to a drug is most often expressed in terms of plasma or serum concentration. However, interactions often occur in the eliminating organ, where drug concentrations may be significantly elevated over the plasma concentration (von Moltke *et al.*, 1998). This may affect the accuracy of *Km* and/or *Ki* determinations to which systemic or hepatic concentrations of drug may be related when predicting potential interactions (Ito *et al.*, 1998). Intact cell systems used *in vitro*, such as isolated hepatocytes or liver slices, may give a more accurate estimate of the physiologically relevant apparent kinetic parameters than human liver microsomes or expressed enzyme systems are capable of providing. For example, omeprazole appeared to be a more potent inhibitor of diazepam metabolism in liver slice compared with microsomal preparations, presumably through accumulation of omeprazole in the liver tissue (reviewed in Ito *et al.*, 1998). Liver slice parameters were closer to *in vivo* (rat) results. Similarly, cimetidine, which is widely known as an inhibitor of enzyme-mediated drug metabolism pathways is known to concentrate in liver cells thus increasing the concentration of inhibitor at its presumed site of action (Ito *et al.*, 1998).

Intracellular concentrations of drugs therefore vary, resulting in localised disturbance not only of elimination, but also of activity. Antiviral nucleoside analogues, such as zidovudine and lamivudine, undergo phosphorylation in the nucleus of target cells. The active triphosphate form of the drug becomes concentrated in the nucleus and is reported to have a longer half-life than the parent drug (Morse *et al.*, 1993). The presence of phosphorylated drug at relatively high concentrations and for extended periods offers the prospect of drug–drug interactions which may affect the efficacy of nucleoside analogues which are co-administered (Kewn *et al.*, 1997).

16.9 *Inhibition of drug-metabolising enzymes and its effect*

All the enzymes involved in the distribution and elimination of drugs have the potential to be inhibited by xenobiotics such as drug molecules, environmental

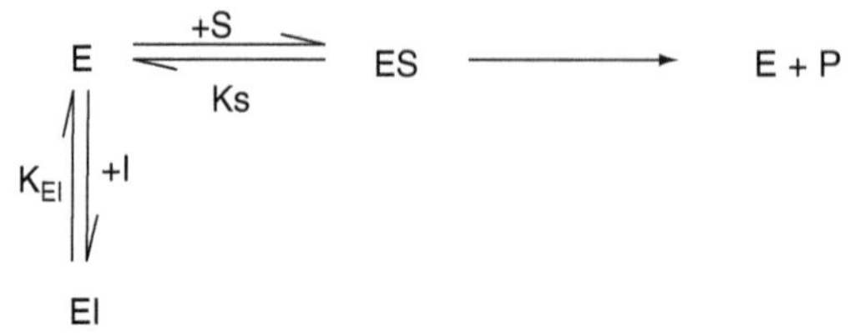

FIGURE 16.2 *Competitive inhibition; inhibitor (I) binds reversibly to enzyme (E) but does not influence enzyme–substrate complex (ES) formation such that* Km *for S is reduced but* V_{max} *is unaffected.*

chemicals and foodstuffs. In the following paragraphs we discuss some aspects of enzyme inhibition pertinent to drug–drug interactions.

Inhibitors which affect drug–drug interactions fall into the broad classification of reversible or irreversible. Reversible inhibitors may be competitive (HIV protease inhibitors) or non-competitive (ketoconazole and sulphaphenazole) in nature; a classification relating to the propensity for inhibitor (I) to compete directly with an alternative substrate (S) for the enzyme's active site (competitive, Figure 16.2) or with both enzyme and enzyme–substrate complex (non-competitive inhibition, Figure 16.3). Alternatively, inhibition may be irreversible ('mechanism-based', Figure 16.4), where the drug molecule binds to the enzyme in such a way that it

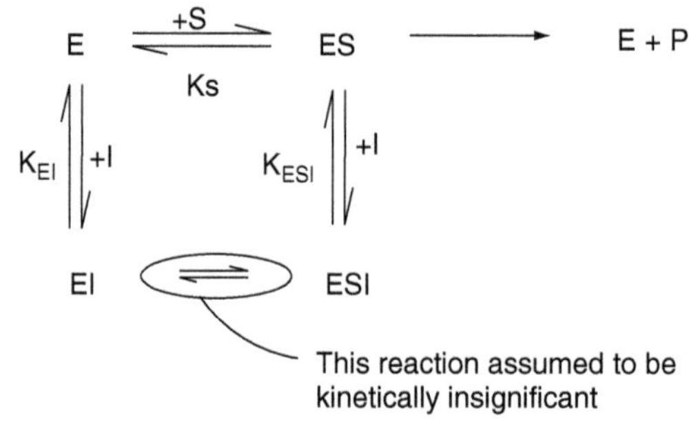

FIGURE 16.3 *Non-competitive inhibition; inhibitor (I) binds reversibly to enzyme (E) and enzyme–substrate complex (ES) with equal affinity such that* Km *for S is unaffected but* V_{max} *is reduced.*

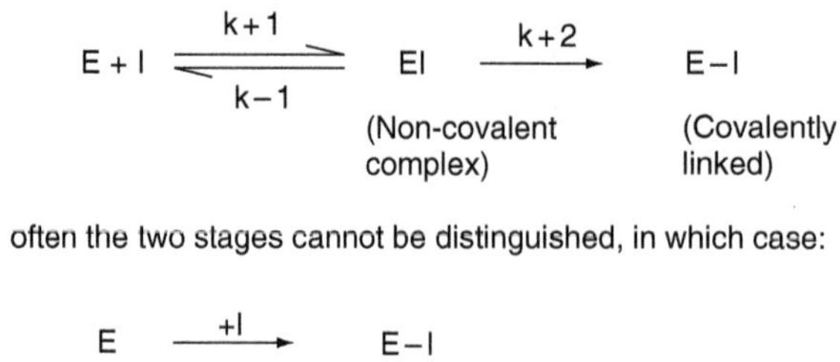

FIGURE 16.4 *Irreversible inhibition; inhibitor (I) binds covalently to enzyme (E) initially through a non-covalent complex.*

cannot be dialysed away, examples are mibefradil, furafylline and the active furanocoumarin of grapefruit juice (Ito *et al.*, 1998; Thummel and Wilkinson, 1998). Thus the rate of the enzyme-catalysed reaction can be dramatically reduced in the presence of inhibitor. The extent of inhibition depends on the relative affinity of inhibitor for enzyme and the concentration of inhibitor at the site of metabolism. For example, active constituents of grapefruit juice, such as 6′,7′-dihydroxybergamottin, appear to selectively inhibit CYP3A4 in the intestinal mucosa. However, it is possible that this apparent selectivity is a product of the relatively high concentrations of inhibitor presented to the enteric cells after oral ingestion, rather than a true discrimination between enteric and hepatic CYP3A4 (Dresser *et al.*, 2000).

Inhibition is most often determined as the percentage of a reaction inhibited by the addition of a fixed concentration of inhibitor. Within the pharmaceutical industry, this may well provide a suitable method for high-throughput screening when studying enzyme–inhibitor interactions; however, no predictions can be made concerning the way inhibition changes with compound exposure (systemic concentration or dose). A more informative measure of the potency of an inhibitor is the IC_{50}, characterised in terms of the concentration of inhibitor required to reduce the rate of metabolism of a fixed concentration of substrate to half its uninhibited value. However, only the inhibitor constant (Ki) is independent of substrate and inhibitor concentration, and therefore represents a measure of the intrinsic 'affinity' of the inhibitor for the enzyme. The relationship between IC_{50} and Ki depends on substrate concentration and inhibition type. If the substrate concentration (drug concentration) is very low ($\ll Km$) then the IC_{50} and Ki are approximately equivalent for the competitive and non-competitive cases. As substrate concentration ranges around the Km, the following relationships apply (Table 16.1).

Where non-competitive inhibition operates, the value of the IC_{50} is identical to the Ki at any substrate concentration. This is because the degree of non-competitive inhibition does not depend on the substrate concentration (Ito *et al.*, 1998). In the competitive case, IC_{50} values can grossly overestimate Ki if the substrate concentration is high relative to Km, but at substrate concentrations equal to or below Km, IC_{50} is no more than twice the Ki. In the uncompetitive case (Figure 16.5), the relationship between Km and Ki in terms of IC_{50} is the opposite of simple

TABLE 16.1 *The relationship between* IC_{50} *and* Ki *at varying substrate concentrations*

	IC_{50} in units of *Ki*		
Inhibition mechanism	**$[S] = \frac{Km}{10}$**	**$[S] = Km$**	**$[S] = 10\,Km$**
Competitive	1.1	2	11
Non-competitive	1	1	1
Uncompetitive	11	2	1.1
Irreversible	Inhibition is progressive, *Ki* value inappropriate		

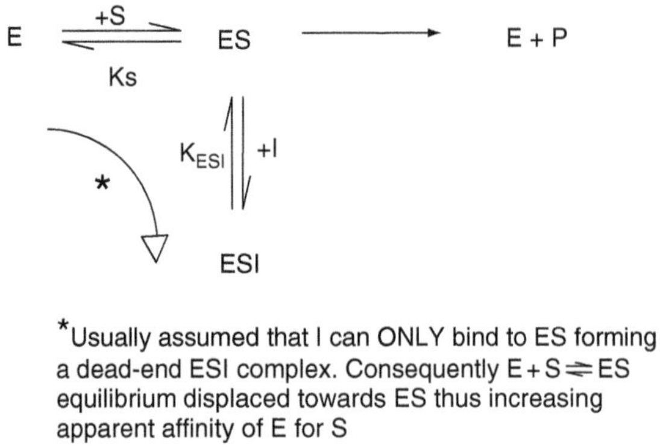
E
+S
Ks
ES
E + P
K_ESI
+I
*
ESI
*Usually assumed that I can ONLY bind to ES forming a dead-end ESI complex. Consequently E+S⇌ES equilibrium displaced towards ES thus increasing apparent affinity of E for S

FIGURE 16.5 *Uncompetitive inhibition; inhibitor (I) binds reversibly only to enzyme–substrate complex (ES).*

competitive inhibition (Rodrigues, 1999). Uncompetitive inhibition is a rare form and is described here only as a comparative case. Irreversible inhibition cannot be treated in the same way because often no detectable equilibrium is formed between the inhibitor and the enzyme so derivation of a *Ki* value is inappropriate for this mechanism. As seen in Table 16.1, for valuable estimates of *Ki* to be made from IC_{50} values, some knowledge of the inhibition mechanism is required and an estimate of the *Km* for the metabolism of the substrate. This kind of information is useful in gauging the extent or likelihood of drug–drug interaction from enzyme kinetic principles. For example, a knowledge of the kinetic constants underlying the interaction observed can be used to predict the percentage inhibition of a pathway likely to be observed *in vivo*. Taking the competitive case, the maximal inhibition possible in the absence of plasma protein binding is given by Equation 16.1 (Resetar *et al.*, 1991):

$$\%\text{Inhibition} = 100 \cdot \frac{[\text{I}]}{Ki\left(1 + \frac{[\text{S}]}{Km}\right) + [\text{I}]} \tag{16.1}$$

where *Ki* is the inhibitor constant, *Km* the substrate concentration at half $V_{\max}$ (the Michaelis-Menten constant), and [S] and [I] are the substrate and inhibitor concentrations, respectively.

If the substrate concentration at the site of interaction is very much lower than the *Km*, then Equation 16.1 simplifies to that shown in Equation 16.2:

$$\%\text{Inhibition} = 100 \cdot \frac{[\text{I}]}{Ki + [\text{I}]} \tag{16.2}$$

Similarly, the relationship between exposure, *Ki* and probability of interaction between co-administered drugs metabolised by the same enzyme can be summarised in Table 16.2.

TABLE 16.2 *Inhibition constant* (Ki) *and steady-state concentration of inhibitor as a fraction of its* Ki (C_{ss}/Ki) *considered as independent variables in the prediction of drug–drug interactions*

Ki (μM)	Interaction prediction	C_{ss}/*Ki*
<1	Likely	>1
1–50	Possible	1–0.1
>50	Unlikely	<0.1

C_{ss} as total systemic concentration of drug (bound and free) at the site of interaction.

Drugs which cause inhibition of a pathway are likely to have a significant interaction potential if they have a high affinity for the metabolising enzyme and a high concentration at the site of metabolism. Conversely, drugs which bind weakly to drug-metabolising enzymes and are present in the eliminating organ at low concentrations are unlikely to provoke drug–drug interactions by this mechanism. Estimates of IC_{50} for interaction of new chemical entities with purified CYPs offer an approach to quantifying risk of significant drug–CYP interaction, and thence potential drug–drug interaction, at an early stage of drug discovery/development. By this means, compounds with a propensity to inhibit metabolism of other drugs can be eliminated from development as early as possible.

Choice of substrate can be critical in designing *in vitro* assays to investigate drug–drug interactions. For example, *in vitro* testosterone 6β-hydroxylation as a measure of CYP3A4 activity is relatively easy to inhibit because the *Km* of CYP3A4 for testosterone is relatively high in humans (~50–100 μM) so even relatively poor inhibitors can produce significant percentage inhibition in this assay. Midazolam may be a more discriminating probe substrate because of its higher apparent affinity for CYP3A4; in human liver microsomes the *Km* value appears to be in the range 5–10 μM. *Ki* values are the most informative measures of inhibition potential because they are independent of substrate concentration. Although easier to measure, both IC_{50} and percentage inhibition determinations vary with substrate concentration and can be misleading when used to predict drug–drug interactions (Yuan *et al.*, 1999). For example, zidovudine, an antiviral nucleoside analogue also known as AZT, is predominantly eliminated in humans via glucuronidation, but with an apparently high *Km* (~4–5 mM). The glucuronidation pathway was studied *in vitro* using relatively high concentrations of zidovudine in the presence of various potential drug inhibitors, including antibiotics, antifungals, anticonvulsants, analgesics, calcium channel blockers and antidepressants (Rajaonarison *et al.*, 1992; Samplo *et al.*, 1995). Although some significant *in vitro* interactions were observed, including those with drug from several therapeutic classes including antifungals and anticonvulsants, it remains unclear whether these predicted *in vitro* interactions translate to clinically relevant effects after therapeutic dosing. In the case of ketoconazole and rifampicin, which were potent inhibitors *in vitro*, no evidence of adverse interaction was observed in clinical studies (Stockley, 1999c). Moreover, in clinical practice, the absorption of zidovudine is markedly reduced when taken with food, and exposure is increased with drugs which affect renal excretion, such as probenecid and trimethoprim (Somogyi, 1996). The latter effect may be mediated through modulation of zidovudine and zidovudine–glucuronide clearance in the kidney (Somogyi, 1996). However, mild to moderate inhibition of glucuronidation has been observed at high concentrations of zidovudine in human liver microsomes (Rajaonarison *et al.*, 1992). These data suggest the interaction may, at least in part, occur in the liver, rather than solely via renal secretion of zidovudine or its glucuronide. Clearly, reliance on *in vitro* models using only hepatic tissue may provide an incomplete view of the potential for zidovudine interactions.

16.10 *Induction of drug-metabolising enzymes and its effect*

The induction of drug-metabolising enzymes represents an important source of drug–drug interactions. Some CYPs, UGTs and, rarely, STs are susceptible to induction. Whilst not as common as interactions caused by inhibition, those resulting from induction may be just as clinically significant, particularly when oral contraceptives are involved. Drugs which are metabolised by inducible enzymes may be eliminated more rapidly if the enzyme activity is increased by induction, for example, oral contraceptives are eliminated more rapidly when coadministered with rifampicin. Thus, maintenance of pharmacologically active concentrations of drug may become increasingly difficult to achieve as induction proceeds. Furthermore, inter-individual variability in the rate of onset and extent of induction can render a nominal dosing regimen untenable for general administration to a patient population. Individual dose titration may be necessary requiring hospitalisation for the patient. Moreover, induction by a drug of its own metabolism is only part of the problem. Since many drug-metabolising enzymes have relatively broad substrate specificity, it is possible that co-administered drugs which are not themselves inducers can be cleared more rapidly thus reducing their effectiveness.

Another dimension to the problem of induction is that normally minor pathways can, in the induced state, become quantitatively important routes of elimination of parent compound. If the metabolites formed through such a pathway are toxic (e.g. nitrosamines) or lead indirectly to toxicity (e.g. paracetamol, procarcinogens), then the presence of elevated amounts of a once trivial metabolite may become highly significant (deBethizy and Hayes, 1994). By extension, the same is true of pharmacologically active metabolites which may have radically different pharmacokinetic properties or tissue distribution compared with the parent drug. For example, the half-life of the metabolite may be extended compared with the parent drug, as in the case of metyrapone and its metabolite metyrapol, or the metabolite concentrates in a particular tissue, for example, morphine-6-glucuronide may accumulate in the brain.

Rifampicin, a semi-synthetic antibiotic active in the treatment of tuberculosis, is a well characterised inducer of CYP3A4 in humans and is known to result in significant drug interactions with a diverse range of drugs, including anticoagulants, corticosteriods, oral contraceptives, oral hypoglycaemic agents, narcotics and analgesics. The intrinsic clearance of drugs by CYP3A4 appears to increase between 5- and 8-fold upon treatment with rifampicin, which is capable of causing a 20–40-fold reduction in plasma concentration of subsequently administered drugs which are substrates for CYP3A4, including oral contraceptives, cyclosporin, verapamil and nifedipine (Thummel and Wilkinson, 1998).

16.11 In vitro *approaches to investigating drug interaction*

In vitro techniques for the investigation of drug-metabolising enzyme induction and inhibition are becoming more widely accepted during the drug discovery–development process. The rationale for use of such techniques is based on an improved understanding of the mechanism underlying drug metabolism and disposition. The advantage to the pharmaceutical industry is that these methods can be applied earlier in the discovery–development process, allow refinement of the structure–function relationship before selection of the candidate drug for clinical investigation and are relatively inexpensive (Bertz and Granneman, 1997; Ito *et al.*, 1998).

16.11.1 The intact hepatocyte systems

The predominance of drug-metabolising enzymes in the liver has focused attention on this organ as the major target for drug–drug interaction studies. Isolated hepatocyte and liver slice preparations provide convenient *in vitro* systems which, for a short duration, retain the integrated Phase I and Phase II metabolic processes essential to replicating complex *in vivo* drug metabolism pathways. The preparation of hepatocytes and liver slices is applicable to a variety of species, including human, being limited only by tissue availability. However, technical shortcomings in the culture of isolated hepatocytes and liver slice preparations limit the duration of their effective use to, at most, a few days. Such a time frame may be sufficient to investigate enzyme induction, but the changing background status of enzyme expression during culture makes interpretation of the results hazardous. Nevertheless, intact cell preparations provide an experimental approach with exceptional relevance to the *in vivo* situation. Acute inhibition studies carried out in isolated cell or tissue slice preparations present the opportunity to study a complex interactive system in a controlled environment whilst retaining the feature of compound accumulation and disposition in the cell which may mimic the concentration of drug at the site of elimination *in vivo* (Cross and Bayliss, 2000).

16.11.2 Microsomes

A subcellular preparation widely used for the study of drug metabolism is the microsome. Again, the focus for drug metabolism studies is the liver; however, the intestinal mucosa is also a tissue requiring attention due to the increasing awareness of the potential for drug metabolism and interactions at this site. Microsomal preparations are disrupted endoplasmic reticulum which contain the major classes of Phase I activities and some Phase II enzymes. Not all the enzymes relevant to drug metabolism are present in these preparations, and some enzymes require special treatment to reveal their activity (e.g. glucuronyltransferases). Nevertheless, microsomal incubation conditions, including the drug and inhibitor concentration, can be manipulated with ease. Furthermore, microsomal preparations are amenable to extended storage at −80 °C or below. However, due to the absence of a cellular infrastructure, enzyme induction cannot be monitored in this system, although enzyme activation can be investigated. Hepatic microsome preparations reflect the enzyme activity profile of the donor, so in the case of human material, a broad spectrum of drug metabolism competency can be studied which mirrors the natural inter-individual variation in the population. The microsomal system also maintains the enzymology underlying some genetic polymorphisms in drug metabolism and the donor's response to previous pharmaceutical intervention resulting in induction and irreversible inhibition. In this way, a tissue bank of material can be built up that covers a range of typical drug metabolism activity and possibly some of the extreme cases likely to be encountered in the patient population.

One of the main values of examining drug metabolism in material from such a tissue bank is the identification of the enzymes involved in the metabolism of a prospective or existing drug. Inhibitors apparently specific to particular enzyme classes or isoforms have been used to assess the contribution of various drug-metabolising enzymes to drug elimination. Similarly, antibodies raised against specific enzymes such as individual CYPs have been used to illuminate the enzymology of drug metabolism, including the nature and extent of enzyme induction. One of the most powerful approaches using microsome preparations is to establish a correlation between the rate of test compound metabolism and the metabolism of a probe substrate specific to one CYP isoform. The strength of the correlation will be a function of the dynamic range of the activities present across the tissue samples, and thereby likely to be present in the patient population, and correspondence of metabolism by the same isoform (Parkinson, 1996a). A minimum of 20 preparations from individual donors should be sufficient for successful correlation analysis. The specificity of probe substrates and inhibitors is a continual source of uncertainty in these investigations. Drugs and chemical probes are often metabolised by more than one enzyme, so that only particular pathways appear to be catalysed by one isoform, for example, of the many possible pathways of testosterone metabolism, only testosterone 6β-hydroxylation is generally accepted to be CYP3A4-specific. The relative affinity of substrate for various drug metabolising enzymes may mean that a probe substrate is only specific at certain concentrations, e.g. ketoconazole is probably only specific for CYP3A4 at concentrations of $<1\ \mu M$. Antibodies may have limited specificity when used against orthologus enzymes from a second species. In the same way, chemical inhibitors validated in humans may not translate to other species in which pre-clinical testing is required. As knowledge is advanced, probe substrates and inhibitors once thought to be enzyme-specific have been found to have other non-specific activities or, on the other hand, metabolism of the probe substrate or inhibitor itself can lead to the formation of non-specific inhibitors. This latter point is well illustrated by the substrate methimazole previously used to characterise involvement of FMO in drug metabolism reactions. In addition to interactions with FMO, methimazole is now also recognised to strongly inhibit CYP3A4 and to be converted to metabolites which are non-selective P450 inhibitors (Guo *et al.*, 1997). The current consensus view of probe substrate and inhibitor specificity is defined by the level of our understanding and will inevitably change as more studies are conducted. Some recent opinions can be found in the recent scientific literature (for example, Parkinson, 1996b; Yuan *et al.*, 1999).

Knowledge of the enzymes involved in the metabolism of a drug is vital to understanding the mechanism of metabolism and hence the propensity for drug–drug interactions. Once the principal enzymes involved are established, consideration can be given to the implications for drug–drug interactions and future drug development. For example, extensive metabolism of a drug or candidate drug via CYP2D6 may represent a liability where the therapeutic index is low and the patient population contains extensive and poor metaboliser polymorphisms, e.g. mexiletine (Nakajima *et al.*, 1998). A consequence of this knowledge may be to ensure recruitment of *bona fide* extensive and poor metabolisers onto subsequent trials so that any liabilities of the candidate drug can be characterised in the most efficient way.

16.11.3 Sources of human tissue

One of the major impediments to conducting *in vitro* studies with human liver preparations is the supply of human hepatic material. Liver tissue can be obtained from unmatched transplant material or obtained in small amounts from surgical resection. Such material is often available only intermittently, making studies reliant on this supply vulnerable, and is subject to strict ethical and legal constraints. In the UK, distribution of tissue is channelled through non profit-making organisations under the control of government bodies. The availability of such precious material with such direct relevance to the human condition has had a complex impact on the pharmaceutical industry and academic world; at once fostering development of *in vitro* techniques predictive of human metabolism *in vivo*, and, through its limited supply, hampering the use of such techniques to forecast clinical interactions and toxicity which would help expedite the safer clinical evaluation of new medicines. Fortunately, academic advances in molecular biology have made human drug-metabolising enzymes available through cloning, thereby offering the prospect of a limitless supply of human enzymes for study. Unfortunately, these systems are at an early stage of development and are as yet not without significant liabilities, as discussed below.

16.11.4 Genetically engineered drug-metabolising enzymes

Human drug-metabolising enzymes have been cloned and expressed in mammalian, insect, yeast and bacterial cell culture systems. The resulting purified proteins or microsomal fractions are commercially available and represent an important source of material for the study of isoform-specific drug metabolism pathways and elucidation and/or characterisation of potential drug–drug interactions. The use of heterologous expression systems has made the supply of human CYPs effectively inexhaustible and relatively inexpensive. The potential to co-express various isoforms in the same cell, or mix single isoform-expressed CYPs to reflect known human hepatic microsomal activities, offers the opportunity to reconstitute some important aspects of liver function for use under controlled conditions. In this way, *in vitro* systems representative of individuals with any of the normal spectrum of CYP activities, an average of these activities, or a profile representative of a particular disease state or normal polymorphic state can be obtained. Thought must also be given to appropriate provision of required reductase, cytochrome b5 and cofactor generating systems in order to support optimal activities, and confirmation of the relevance of data generated by expression systems using primary human material *in vitro* or studies conducted *in vivo* (Rodrigues *et al.*, 1995).

However, the use of purified or expressed CYPs is not without its drawbacks. In the context of drug metabolism and interaction studies, these centre on the concentration of active protein present in the test system, and therefore impinge on the apparent V_{max} for a given enzyme-catalysed pathway. The use of enzyme concentrations *in vitro* which are higher than the normal physiologically expressed human levels may be advantageous in the generation and identification of metabolites, but can lead to overestimation of the importance of a particular pathway. Some correction factors are required to compensate for the activity of expressed CYPs *in vitro* versus their *in vivo* activity (e.g. Crespi, 1995). *In vitro*, at substrate concentrations very much less than the *Km* for the highest apparent affinity pathway, the contribution of any given enzyme to overall metabolism can be determined from Equation 16.3.

$$\text{Contribution} = \left(\frac{V_{max}}{Km}\right) \cdot \text{enzyme abundance} \tag{16.3}$$

Thus the principal enzyme, namely that which impacts most on the metabolism of a drug, is the enzyme with the highest contribution quotient. Modulation of the activity of the principal enzyme will have the greatest effect on the metabolic clearance of the drug and is likely to be the most sensitive target for drug–drug interactions. The above analysis assumes that expressed enzymes are present *in vitro* at their physiological concentrations and activities. If this is not the case, a further correction factor can be applied using an isoform-specific probe substrate to normalise activity *in vitro* to that obtained from a system with direct relevance to the *in vivo* CYP complement, such as human liver microsomes. The resultant term has been called the relative activity factor (*RAF*), as given in Equation 16.4:

$$RAF = \frac{\text{mean activity of isoform-specific probe substrate in human microsomes}}{\text{activity of isoform-specific probe substrate in expressed system}} \tag{16.4}$$

where 'activity' may be a rate at saturating substrate concentration or an intrinsic clearance value. (Only at saturating substrate concentrations does the enzyme-catalysed rate become directly proportional to the enzyme concentration, i.e. rate approached V_{max}.) *RAF* values, once derived for a standardised expression system against a panel of human liver preparations, can be applied to studies using non-saturating substrate concentration thereby gauging the relevance of studies with recombinant protein to the *in vivo* situation. The extrapolation may still be vulnerable, as demonstrated by the predicted contribution of CYP2C9 to terbinafine metabolism which may not be relevant *in vivo* (Vickers *et al.*, 1999) thus illustrating the problem of false positive results with recombinant systems.

Genetically engineered systems have also been constructed to express the orphan receptor hPXR, which appears to be involved in the early stages of CYP3A4 induction in humans. By linking the activation of hPXR by ligand (drug) binding to chloramphenicol acetyltransferase production, predictions of the potential for the drug to induce CYP3A4 can be made (Lehmann *et al.*, 1998). Other receptors involved in human CYP induction are under investigation, including the aryl hydrocarbon receptor (Frotschl *et al.*, 1998), in the hope of obtaining predictive models of human CYP1A2 induction *in vivo*. Presently, our understanding of the regulation of drug-metabolising enzyme activity by xenobiotics is expanding rapidly. So whilst current predictions of drug induction potential still often rely on assessment of structural similarity to known inducers, elucidation of the role of orphan receptors such as PXR, CAR and PPAR promises to revolutionise the quantitative prediction of induction potential (Waxman, 1999).

16.12 *A regulatory perspective*

Authorities that regulate the release of new drugs onto the healthcare market have recently started to appreciate *in vitro* drug interaction studies as valuable tools for the design of clinical studies, and moreover, promote the generation of such data for use in regulatory submissions. Quantitation of *Ki* values for the various enzymes involved in metabolism of a prospective drug, in combination with expected therapeutic steady-state plasma concentrations of the compound, has been used to identify appropriate substrates for interaction trials. Conversely, interactions which are unlikely to occur can also be identified *in vitro* and thus can be used to limit the extent of clinical trials undertaken.

The pharmaceutical industry is now provided with a means whereby well-executed *in vitro* studies are able to help clinical study design to impact directly on the labelling of medicines, rationalise the contra-indications offered and consolidate the patient group in which dosing is expected to be safe and efficacious (Davit *et al.*, 1999). Regulatory bodies are now encouraging the provision of *in vitro* data and have established tentative guidelines for their generation and predictive use (CDER guidelines for industry: www.fda.gov/cder).

16.13 *Some brief case histories*

In vitro predictions of *in vivo* drug–drug interactions are not always clear-cut. Some strong correlations have been observed which give confidence to our understanding of the metabolic processes involved, whilst other cases illustrate the highly complex nature of the interactions under investigation and the number of simultaneous but divergent processes to be considered. The following brief case histories exemplify some drug–drug interactions for which *in vitro* data has been correlated (Ito *et al.*, 1998; Thummel and Wilkinson, 1998; Davit *et al.*, 1999) and serve to illustrate the concepts discussed above.

16.13.1 Terfenadine

Terfenadine has been widely used for the treatment of seasonal allergic rhinitis. *In vivo*, the drug is rapidly converted to an active metabolite, fexofenadine, by CYP3A4-mediated metabolism. *In vitro*, ketoconazole, an azole antifungal, strongly inhibits CYP3A4 and so blocks terfenadine metabolism to the active fexofenadine thus dramatically reducing terfenadine elimination. In the clinic, co-administration of terfenadine and ketoconazole was found to result in excessively high exposure of patients to terfenadine which was capable of causing severe and sometimes fatal cardiac arrhymias. Such an interaction was found to be entirely predictable from *in vitro* studies conducted retrospectively. Subsequently, fexofenadine was developed and approved as a drug in its own right, and terfenadine was withdrawn from the US market. Fexofenadine in turn is not metabolised significantly by CYP3A4 *in vitro*, but ketoconazole still caused a significant increase in fexofenadine *AUC* in the clinic; a poor prediction from *in vitro* data. It was thought probable that fexofenadine absorption was enhanced by ketoconazole through inhibition of PGP (Davit *et al.*, 1999).

16.13.2 Ritonavir/saquinavir

Ritonavir and saquinavir are first generation HIV-protease inhibitors. *In vitro*, ritonavir (Rodrigues and Wong, 1997), is a potent, possibly irreversible inhibitor of CYP3A4, and saquinavir is >90 per cent metabolised by CYP3A4. Although saquinavir also interacts with CYP3A4, it is a 10–100-fold less potent inhibitor of this enzyme. In the clinic, ritonavir caused a 17-fold increase in saquinavir *AUC* with concomitant 14-fold increase in C_{max}, which was consistent with the inhibition of saquinavir metabolism by ritonavir; a good prediction from *in vitro* data.

16.13.3 Losartan

Losartan, an angiotensin II receptor antagonist, has been shown to be metabolised by CYP3A4 and 2C9 *in vitro*. *In vivo*, ketoconazole and itraconazole, antifungal agents capable of inhibiting CYP3A4 (Albengres *et al.*, 1998), had no effect on losartan pharmacokinetics because the *Km* for *in vitro* metabolism was relatively high compared with the therapeutic steady-state concentration of losartan (*Km* for metabolism ~20 μM and steady-state therapeutic plasma concentration *in vivo* <1 μM). Furthermore, alternative pathways for losartan metabolism were available *in vivo*. However, fluconazole, another antifungal agent, was found to block the conversion of losartan to its major active metabolite *in vivo*, so losartan *AUC* increased and the active metabolite *AUC* decreased in clinical interaction studies. Fluconazole is capable of inhibiting both CYP2C9 and 3A4, so in the case of this interaction, no alternative pathway was available for losartan metabolism and therefore elimination was significantly compromised. Rationalisation of the enzymology underlying both compounds led to a good prediction of *in vivo* effects from *in vitro* data.

16.13.4 Zafirlukast

Zafirlukast is a leukotriene LTD4 and LTE4 antagonist used in the treatment of asthma. *In vitro*, zafirlukast is metabolised by CYP3A4, 2C9 and 1A2. The *Ki* for each pathway was higher than steady-state plasma concentration for zafilukast by a factor of >2,000-fold for the unbound free fraction of parent drug or ≥2-fold for the bound plus free fraction. Parent drug was 99.9 per cent bound to plasma proteins. Additionally, a metabolite of zafirlukast showed significant inhibition of CYP2C9 *in vitro*, although the circulating concentration *in vivo* was not reported. Overall, no interaction was predicted based on this *in vitro* data because the free fraction of zafirlukast was so small. Clinical studies designed to investigate the possibility of interactions showed no clinical effect on terfenadine and theophylline, used as CYP3A4 and 1A2 probe substrates respectively; a good prediction from *in vitro* data. However, the same studies revealed a positive interaction with *S*-warfarin (CYP2C9) in spite of the *Ki* for *S*-warfarin being similar to that for terfenadine (poor prediction from *in vitro* data). A subsequent incident revealed an apparently idiosyncratic interaction of zafirlukast with theophylline demonstrating the diversity of individual responses possible in the patient population at large.

16.13.5 Grepafloxacin

Grepafloxcin, an antibacterial agent, displayed clinical C_{max} values substantially less than its *Ki* for inhibition of CYP1A2 or 3A4 as determined by monitoring theophylline N-demethylation and testosterone 6β-hydroxylation, respectively. Consequently, no interaction was expected with theophylline *in vivo*. However, grepafloxacin caused 50 per cent reduction in theophylline clearance after oral administration of the probe substrate in a clinical study (poor prediction from *in vitro* data), possibly because plasma concentrations of grepafloxacin were not indicative of those present at the site of interaction. Indeed, grepafloxacin has been shown to be actively taken up and concentrated by rat liver via a novel carrier-mediated active transport mechanism (Sasabe *et al.*, 1997).

16.13.6 Terbinafine

Terbinafine, an orally active fungicide, shows significant clinical drug interactions with co-administered drugs which are substrates for CYP2D6. This specific interaction was supported by *in vitro* (Vickers *et al.*, 1999) and *in vivo* (Abdel-Rahman *et al.*, 1999) studies in which terbinafine was shown to inhibit CYP2D6 (*Ki* 30 nM) in human liver microsome preparations and convert extensive metaboliser phenotypes to poor metaboliser phenotypes. In addition, some nitrogen-containing metabolites of terbinafine also inhibited CYP2D6. Such potent *in vitro* inhibition of CYP2D6 is a clear indication of potential interactions *in vivo* (Table 16.1). Volunteer studies revealed that a relatively acute treatment regimen with tebinafine essentially blocked conversion of dextromethorphan to dextrorphan which, under normal circumstances, is catalysed predominantly by CYP2D6. Inhibition was persistent after withdrawal of terbinafine, probably as a function of the extremely long elimination half-life of terbinafine in humans during therapeutic dosing (100 hours) (Abdel-Rahman *et al.*, 1999). Since the extensive metaboliser phenotype is pre-eminent in the normal population, comprising around 93 per cent of Caucasians, therapeutic administration of terbinafine presents a potential interaction hazard with other co-administered drugs which are CYP2D6 substrates, including antidepressants, antihypertensives and amphetamines (Nakajima *et al.*, 1998; Abdel-Rahman *et al.*, 1999).

Although a variety of other CYPs were also involved in the metabolism of terbinafine, interaction with individual pathways appeared not to result in clinically significant alterations in the pharmacokinetics of co-administered drugs (Vickers *et al.*, 1999). Conversely, co-administered cimetidine was found to affect terbinafine exposure, probably through simultaneous inhibition of more than one route of terbinafine clearance and possibly exacerbated by accumulation of cimetidine in liver cells. It is possible that the propensity for terbeinafine to be metabolised by a variety of CYPs may reduce the potential for clinically significant interactions, other than with CYP2D6. Inhibitors of specific CYPs used *in vitro* were liable to inhibit specific pathways of terbinafine metabolism, for example furafylline decreased dihydridiol formation, but the overall extent of metabolite formation was found to remain fairly constant, with alternative metabolic pathways compensating for the inhibited route. Poor inhibition of terbinafine metabolism in human liver microsomes by a CYP2C9-specific inhibitor, sulphaphenazole, indicated that this P450 isozyme did not play a major role in the metabolic clearance of the drug. However, studies with various human recombinant CYPs tended to suggest CYP2C9 was responsible for the majority of the predicted *in vivo* fractional intrinsic clearance when calculated via the appropriate relative activity factor. This discrepancy serves to highlight the pitfalls of over-reliance on quantitative metabolism studies using expressed enzymes, in spite of the application of correction factors relating *in vivo* to *in vitro* data.

16.14 *Overview*

Drugs may simultaneously act as both inhibitors (typically after acute administration for reversible inhibitors) and inducers (usually requiring chronic administration) both of drug-metabolising enzymes and transporters, such as PGP. Interaction studies carried out after a single dose of drug and inhibitor may provide evidence of the inhibition response (Dresser *et al.*, 2000), whereas prolonged repeat administration may become more difficult to interpret when the balance of induction and inhibition is unknown. In the latter cases, the clinical outcome of an interaction is extremely difficult to forecast from *in vitro* data. For example ritonavir, which is a potent inhibitor of CYP3A4 and an inducer of both Phase I and II drug-metabolising enzymes, including CYP3A4, had only a marginal effect on the clinical pharmacokinetics of alprazolam, which is itself mainly metabolised by CYP3A4 (Davit *et al.*, 1999).

In all cases, the interacting drugs should be administered in such a way that exposure is clinically relevant during the interaction study, and clinical results will inevitably take precedence over *in vitro* data. Clinical effects are often less extreme than expected from *in vitro* studies because interactions are buffered by the complexity of alternative and interacting pathways in the *in vivo* situation. The drug metabolism scientist must guard against over interpretation of *in vitro* data. Most correlations have been established for CYPs; more work needs to be done on other drug-metabolising systems, such as FMO and the enzymes-mediating Phase II pathways. Interaction studies *in vivo* carried out in volunteers using cocktails of simultaneously administered probe substrates, may become useful early indicators of potential clinical interactions. One advantage of using volunteer studies is that the doses can be minimised to prevent adverse toxicity, and the propensity for polypharmacy in the clinic is eliminated.

At the present time, *in vitro* data are most often produced to explain clinical observations as a retrospective investigation of the mechanisms underlying metabolism and interactions. The challenge of drug metabolism scientists today is to firmly establish the link between *in vitro* and *in vivo* data so enabling *in vitro* techniques to be used prospectively and with confidence. At best, *in vitro* studies currently provide a succession of narrow views onto the panoramic landscape of clinical medicine, of which the study of drug–drug interactions is only a small part. Nevertheless *in vitro* studies which exploit an understanding of the fundamental mechanisms of drug–drug interactions have engendered a progression away from the merely descriptive and have made truly predictive studies appear attainable.

16.15 *References*

Abdel-Rahman, S.M., Gotschall, R.R., Kauffman, R.E., Leeder, J.S. and Kearns, G.L. (1999) *Clin. Pharmacol. Ther.* 65, 465.

Albengres, E., Le Louet, H. and Tillerment, J.P. (1998) *Drug Saf.* 18, 83.

Bertz, R.J. and Granneman, G.R. (1997) *Clin. Pharmacokinet.* 32, 210.

Crespi, C.L. (1995) *Adv. Drug Res.* 26, 179.

Cross, D.M. and Bayliss, M.K. (2000) *Drug Metab. Rev.* 32, 219.

Davit, B., Reynolds, K., Yuan, R., Ajayi, F., Coner, D., Fadiran, E., Gillespie, B., Sahajwalla, C., Huang, S.M. and Lesko, L.J. (1999) *J. Clin. Pharmacol.* 39, 899.

deBethizy, J.D. and Hayes, J.R. (1994) In: *Principles and Methods of Toxicology* Hayes, W.A. (ed.), pp. 59–100. Raven Press Ltd, New York.

Dresser, G.K., Spence, D.J. and Bailey, D.G. (2000) *Clin. Pharmacokinet.* 38, 41.
Frotschl, R., Chichmanov, l., Kleeberg, U., Hilderbrandt, A.G., Roots, I. and Brockmoller, J. (1998) *Chem. Res. Toxicol.* 11, 1447.
Glaxo Wellcome (1999) In: *ABPI Compendium of Data Sheets and Summaries of Product Characteristics; 1999–2000*, pp. 493–494. Datapharm Publications Limited, London.
Guo, Z., Raeissi, S., White, R.B. and Stevens, J.C. (1997) *Drug Metab. Dispos.* 25, 390.
Ito, K., Iwatsubo, T., Kanamitsu, S., Ueda, K., Suzuki, H. and Sugiyama, Y. (1998) *Pharmacol. Rev.* 50, 387.
Kewn, S., Veal, G.J., Hoggard, P.G., Barry, M.G. and Back, D.J. (1997) *Biochem. Pharmacol.* 54, 589.
Lehmann, J.M., McKee, D.D., Watson, M.A., Willson, T.M., Moore, J.T. and Kliewer, S.A. (1998) *J. Clin. Invest.* 102, 1016.
McElnay, J.C. (1996) In: *Mechanisms of Drug Interactions*, D'Arcy, P.F., McElnay, J.C. and Welling, P.G. (eds), pp. 125–149. Springer-Verlag, Berlin.
Morse, G.D., Shelton, M.J. and O'Donnell, A.M. (1993) *Clin. Pharmacokinet.* 24, 101.
Nakajima, M., Kobayashi, K., Shimada, S., Tokudome, S., Yamamoto, T. and Kuroiwa, Y. (1998) *Br. J. Clin. Pharmacol.* 46, 55.
Overby, L.H., Carver, G.C. and Philpot, R.M. (1997) *Chem. Biol. Interact.* 106, 29.
Parkinson, A. (1996a) *Toxicol. Pathol.* 24, 45.
Parkinson, A. (1996b) In: *Casarett and Doull's Toxicology: The Basic Science of Poisons*, Klaassen, C.D. (ed.), pp. 113–186. McGraw-Hill, New York.
Rajaonarison, J.F., Lacarelle, B., Catalin, J., Placid, M. and Rahmani, R. (1992) *Drug Metab. Dispos.* 20, 578.
Resetar, A., Minick, D. and Spector, T. (1991) *Biochem. Pharmacol.* 42, 559.
Rodrigues, A.D. (1999) *Biochem. Pharmacol.* 57, 465.
Rodrigues, A.D. and Wong, S.L. (1997) *Adv. Pharmacol.* 43, 65.
Rodrigues, A.D., Mulford, D.J., Lee, R.D., Surber, B.W., Kukulka, M.J., Ferrero, J.L., Thomas, S.B., Shet, M.S. and Estabrook, R.W. (1995) *Drug Metab. Disposition* 23, 765.
Samplo, E., Lacarelle, B., Rajaonarison, J.F., Catalin, J. and Durand, A. (1995) *Br. J. Clin. Pharmacol.* 40, 83.
Sasabe, H., Terasaki, T., Tsuji, A. and Sugiyama, Y. (1997) *J. Pharmacol. Exp. Ther.* 282, 162.
Somogyi, A. (1996) In: *Mechanisms of Drug Interactions*, D'Arcy, P.F., McElnay, J.C. and Welling, P.G. (eds), pp. 173–212. Springer-Verlag, Berlin.
Stockley, I.H. (1999a) In: *Drug Interactions. A Source Book of Adverse Interactions, their Mechanisms, Clinical Importance and Management*, pp. 594–615, Pharmaceutical Press, London.
Stockley, I.H. (1999b) In: *Drug Interactions. A Source Book of Adverse Interactions, their Mechanisms, Clinical Importance and Management*, pp. 1–14, Pharmaceutical Press, London.
Stockley, I.H. (1999c) In: *Drug Interactions. A Source Book of Adverse Interactions, their Mechanisms, Clinical Importance and Management*, pp. 203–207. Pharmaceutical Press, London.
Thummel, K.E. and Wilkinson, G.R. (1998) *Annu. Rev. Pharmacol. Toxicol.* 38, 389.
Vickers, A.E.M., Sinclair, J.R., Zollinger, M., Heitz, F., Glanzel, U., Johanson, L. and Fischer, V. (1999) *Drug Metab. and Dispos.* 27, 1029.
von Moltke, L.L., Greeenblatt, D.J., Schmider, J., Wright, C.E., Harmatz, J.S. and Shader, R.I. (1998) *Biochem. Pharmacol.* 55, 113.
Waxman, D.J. (1999) *Arch. Biochem. Biophys.* 369, 11.
Yuan, R., Parmelle, T., Balian, J.D., Uppoor, S., Ajayi, F., Burnett, A., Lesko, L. and Marroum, P. (1999) *Clin. Pharmacol. Ther.* 66, 9.

CHAPTER **17**

Identification of drug metabolites in biological fluids using qualitative spectroscopic and chromatographic techniques

G.J. Dear and I.M. Ismail

17.1 *Introduction*

For the registration of any potential drug candidate it is essential to provide evidence that the compound's general metabolism in humans is similar to its metabolism in the animal species utilised for toxicological evaluation. To obtain this information, a number of studies are routinely performed using both radiolabelled and unlabelled compounds, thus enabling the analyst, as far as is reasonably practicable, to determine the metabolic fate of the new drug candidate.

Drugs are generally metabolised to generate more polar entities, which are more readily excreted. Drug metabolism can most simply be divided into two main phases: Phase I, functionalisation type reactions such as oxidation, reduction and hydrolysis; and Phase II, conjugative reactions such as formation of glucuronic acid (glucuronidation) and amino acid conjugates, sulphation, methylation and acetylation. In some instances, Phase III reactions also exist: these different types of biotransformation are described in more detail elsewhere in this book.

Conventionally, drug metabolite identification in the past has usually been based on the comparison of ultraviolet (UV) spectral data and high-performance liquid chromatography (HPLC) retention times of isolated 'unknown' metabolites with those of synthesised standards. Such a method of detecting and characterising drug metabolites is an uncertain, time-consuming and expensive process, as well as affording very limited structural information. Furthermore, Phase I metabolism of a drug candidate often results in only minor structural modification of the parent compound; these minor changes can make it particularly difficult to determine suitable chromatographic conditions to effect HPLC separation of metabolites. This chapter describes contemporary approach to the problem of characterising xenobiotic metabolites in complex biological fluids derived from drug metabolism studies.

17.2 *Mass spectrometry*

Mass spectrometry has contributed significantly to the structural determination and quantitation of drug metabolites. More recently, tandem mass spectrometry (MS–MS) has been increasingly used in both the characterisation and the quantitation of metabolites in complex biological matrices derived from both *in vitro* sources such as microsomal incubates and *in vivo* sources such as urine, blood, bile and faecal extracts. This section focuses on the role of mass spectrometry in the field of metabolite identification and cites two examples to illustrate the process.

Mass spectrometry is the analytical technique of choice for obtaining information on the atomic and molecular compositions of inorganic and organic materials. The mass spectrometer produces charged particles, which can consist of both the parent ion and ionic fragments of the original molecule and it separates these ions according to their mass/charge ratio (m/z). The resulting mass spectrum is a record of the relative intensity of these ions and is characteristic of every compound. In addition high-resolution mass spectrometry can even provide the elemental composition of the parent and fragment ions. The main advantage of a mass spectrometer as an analytical instrument is its inherent sensitivity. This is coupled with its specificity in being able to characterise unknowns and/or detect known compounds in complex mixtures. These features often enable the direct analysis of biological fluids such as urine and bile with little or no pre-treatment. The sensitivity results primarily from the action of the analyser as a mass/charge filter thereby reducing background noise and from the sensitive electron multipliers used for ion detection. The excellent specificity results from characteristic fragmentation patterns, which can give information about molecular weight and molecular structure. This specificity is enhanced by the use of on-line separation techniques such as HPLC. These fundamental features of a mass spectrometer make it an essential tool in any drug metabolism studies.

The parent drug and/or its metabolites are often present in the biological fluid at very low concentrations; hence reliable, sensitive and specific analytical techniques are required for their detection and characterisation. HPLC coupled to electrospray ionisation (ESI) mass spectrometry (LC–MS) has become increasingly popular for such tasks, since this soft ionisation technique is capable of generating ions that lead to data that can give both molecular weight and structural information. Typically the electrospray process generates ions through simple proton addition (MH+) or proton abstraction ($[M-H]^-$). The majority of quantitative and qualitative applications reported that ESI have been performed using a triple quadrupole mass spectrometer coupled to a conventional HPLC system operating in reverse-phase gradient mode, using columns of 4.6 or 2.1 mm internal diameter.

17.3 *Sample preparation*

Electrospray mass spectrometry requires the formation of analyte-related ions in solution which can be used to generate ions in the gaseous state for mass spectrometric analysis. For compounds that do not contain a charge or are not readily ionised, analyte-related ions are usually prepared by chemical means. For example, most basic drugs can be analysed in positive ion mode after being dissolved in a solution containing an acid (e.g. 0.1 per cent aqueous formic acid), to effect protonation (and hence the formation of a positive charge) of the basic group within the molecule. Similarly for an acidic drug, a basic solvent can be used (e.g. 0.05 per cent aqueous ammonia) to promote de-protonation of any acidic moieties (hence forming a negatively charged species), thereby allowing analysis in the negative ion mode. Acidic and basic modifiers can be added to HPLC solvents during LC–MS to promote the electrospray process. In this way electrospray-based techniques readily allow the coupling of reversed-phase HPLC and MS, the samples analysed usually being aqueous–organo mixtures. In drug metabolism, most samples are presented in liquid matrices derived from *in vivo* or *in vitro* experiments. Therefore urine and bile, for example, are often analysed directly by electrospray LC–MS, whilst analysis of plasma and serum samples usually requires that the proteins present be removed (e.g. protein precipitation, solid-phase extraction or ultrafiltration).

17.4 *Phase I*

There are many published examples of the use of MS in the identification of Phase I metabolites of drug molecules. As explained in more detail elsewhere in this book, Phase I metabolism predominantly includes oxidation, reduction, hydrolysis and hydration reactions. The most common metabolic pathways in xenobiotic metabolism are oxidative reactions followed by conjugation with various endogenous groups. The oxidative reaction usually results in the formation of a polar-oxygenated group on the substrate molecule. The metabolism of 1,2-amino-*N*-(4-(4-(1,2-benzisothiazol-3-yl)-1-piperazinyl)butyl benzamide, a potent serotonin 5-HT2 and dopamine D2 receptor antagonist (the structure is shown in Figure 17.1), being developed as a potential 'atypical' antipsychotic agent, is a representative example of a metabolic route dominated by oxidative reactions. In this instance metabolites of

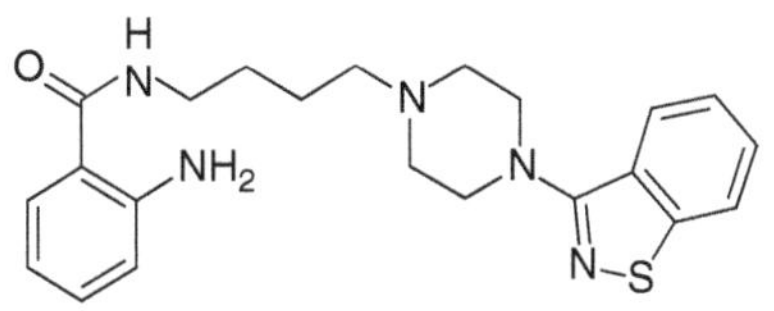

I (MW 409)

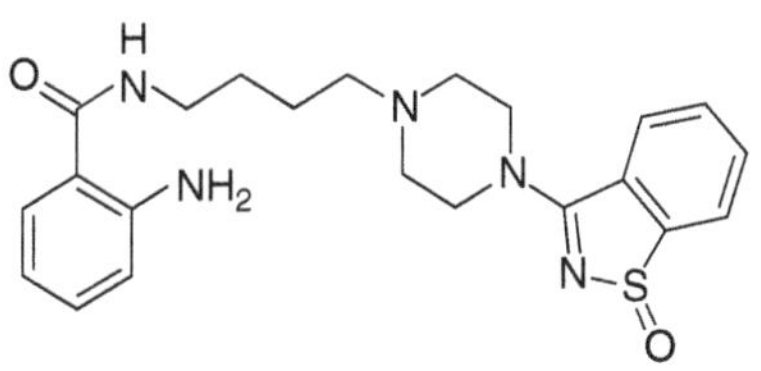

II (MW 425)

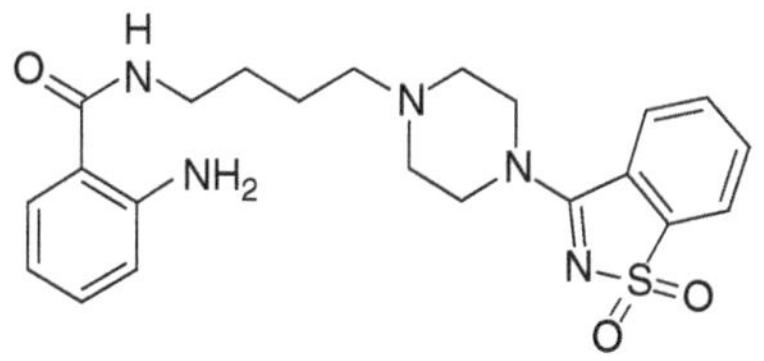

III (MW 441)

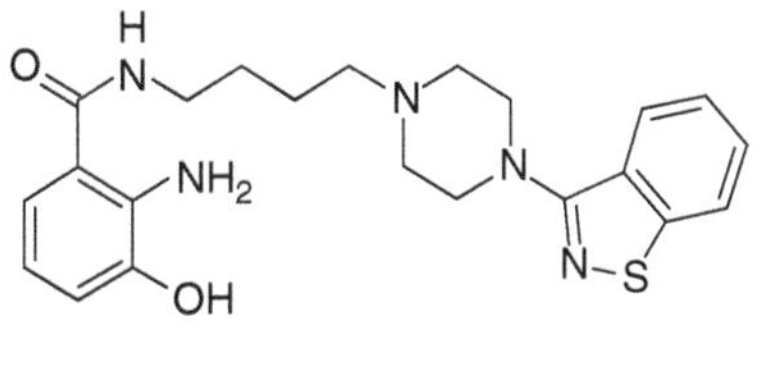

IV (MW 425)

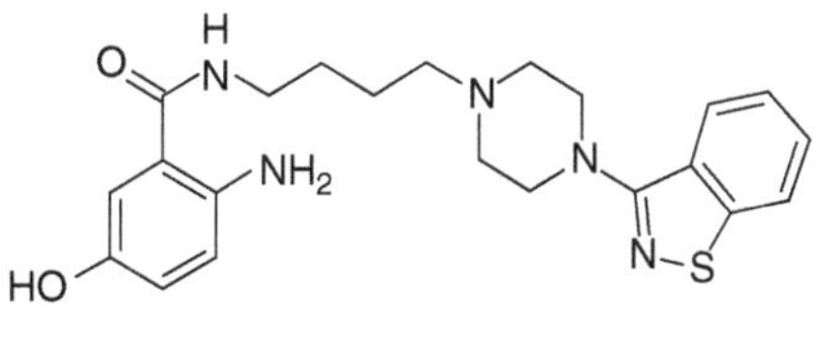

V (MW 425)

FIGURE 17.1 *The metabolism of 1,2-amino-N-(4-(4-(1,2-benzisothiazol-3-yl)-1-piperazinyl)butyl benzamide, a potent serotonin 5-HT2 and dopamine D2 receptor antagonist is a representative example of a metabolic route dominated by oxidative reactions.*

parent drug were identified in human urine and plasma by LC–MS using simple reverse-phase gradient chromatography coupled to an electrospray triple quadrupole instrument. Reverse-phase gradient elution is ideally suited for drug metabolite separation and/or isolation, since drugs and their metabolites can encompass a large range of polarities. As indicated above, urine samples were analysed directly, whilst plasma samples were analysed following simple protein precipitation with acetonitrile.

Initial *in vitro* work demonstrated that I is extensively metabolised in human liver microsomes, undergoing oxidation at the benzisothiazol sulphur atom to generate sulphoxide (II) and sulphone (III) metabolites. In addition, ring hydroxylations at either the 3- or 5-position of the benzamide ring gave rise to 3- and 5-hydroxyl metabolites, IV and V, respectively. The structures of I and its known Phase I metabolites are presented in Figure 17.1. As part of the clinical development of I, human urine and plasma samples, taken from a study of the safety and pharmacokinetics of an escalating single dose, were screened by LC–MS for potential *in vivo* metabolites.

Putative drug-related HPLC peaks were identified by a comparison of the post-dose sample with the corresponding pre-dose sample. In this approach each mass chromatogram over the chosen mass range is compared directly with an equivalent produced from a pre-dose sample. By default mass chromatographic peaks, which appear in the dosed sample but not in the control sample, are likely to be drug or dosage vehicle related. This process gives rise to molecular weight information (derived from the identified MH^+ or $[M-H]^-$ ions), which in some instances can be rationalised as a metabolic transformation (e.g. +16 amu metabolites, which characteristically indicate mono-oxygenation). Obtaining the molecular weight of a metabolite is usually the first and most critical step along the path, which leads to unequivocal structural elucidation. Table 17.1 presents some common metabolic steps and the subsequent effect on the molecular weight of the parent drug. The mass chromatographic comparison of dosed and control matrices can be performed manually, although computerised algorithmic pattern comparison software is available. In the case of known metabolites, such as II, these peaks can also be identified through a comparison of their retention and mass spectral characteristics with those of authentic materials, if available.

Extracted ion chromatograms from post-dose plasma and urine samples are given in Figures 17.2 and 17.3, respectively. In plasma, parent drug (I) and metabolite II were the only detectable drug-related peaks giving rise to MH^+ ions at *m/z* 410 and 426, respectively. Metabolite II also gave rise to discernible $[M+Na]^+$ and $[M+K]^+$ adduct ions. In Figure 17.2 these ions are summed together giving rise to a reconstructed mass chromatogram. Analysis of urine revealed the presence of I and metabolites II, III and V initially characterised *in vitro*. However, an additional drug-related peak was also detected in human urine (denoted VI), which did not co-chromatograph with any of the known metabolites, and which also gave rise to an MH^+ ion at *m/z* 426. Based on this mass difference (ΔMass = 16 amu cf. parent drug), VI was rationalised as a novel hydroxyl

TABLE 17.1 *Common metabolic reactions and their affect on molecular weight*

Metabolic reaction	**Formula**	**Affect on molecular weight of parent drug (M)**
Reduction	$+H_2$	M + 2
Methylation	$+CH_2$	M + 14
Hydroxylation	$+O$	M + 16
Hydrolysis of a ring	$+H_2O$	M + 18
Acetylation	$+C_2H_2O$	M + 42
Glycine conjugation	$+C_2H_3NO$	M + 57
Sulphate conjugation	$+SO_3$	M + 80
Taurine conjugation	$+C_2H_5NO_2S$	M + 107
S-Cysteine conjugation	$+C_3H_5NO_2S$	M + 119
Glucuronide conjugation	$+C_6H_8O_6$	M + 176
S-Glutathione conjugation	$+C_{10}H_{15}N_3O_6S$	M + 305
Alcohol to ketone	$-H_2$	M − 2
Demethylation	$-CH_2$	M − 14
Defluorination	$-F + H$	M − 17
Dechlorination	$-Cl + H$	M − 34

metabolite of I, i.e. not observed *in vitro*. No evidence was obtained for the formation of Phase II conjugates.

Confirmation of I, II and V in human urine was provided by LC–MS–MS, using their MH^+ ions as the precursor masses. The technique of MS–MS is well suited to mixture analysis, because of the fact that characteristic product ion spectra can be obtained for each component in a mixture without interference from other components, assuming that various parent ions are of different *m/z*. This is particularly important when dealing with samples from biological origin, in which many endogenous-interfering components may be co-eluting with the peak of interest. LC–MS–MS has proven to be a technique well suited to structural elucidation studies. The same fragmentation pattern that provides identification of a compound in a complex mixture also contains a wealth of information pertinent to the structure of the parent molecule. MS–MS product-ion spectra of I and its metabolites II and V in urine compared favourably to those of authentic material (see Figure 17.4). In all three cases, cleavage of the amide bond β to the terminal-substituted phenyl ring gives rise to a characteristic $ArC{\equiv}O^+$ fragment, resulting in product ions at *m/z* 120, for I and II, and *m/z* 136, in the case of V. Cleavage of the bond adjacent to the ring to form a fragment of the type $RC{\equiv}O^+$ is also apparent in the case of II, and gives rise to the product ion at *m/z* 333. Cleavage on either side of the secondary amine within the butyl linker chain, with concomitant charge retention on the benzisothiazol half of the molecule, generates the product ions at *m/z* 274 and 291, respectively, from both

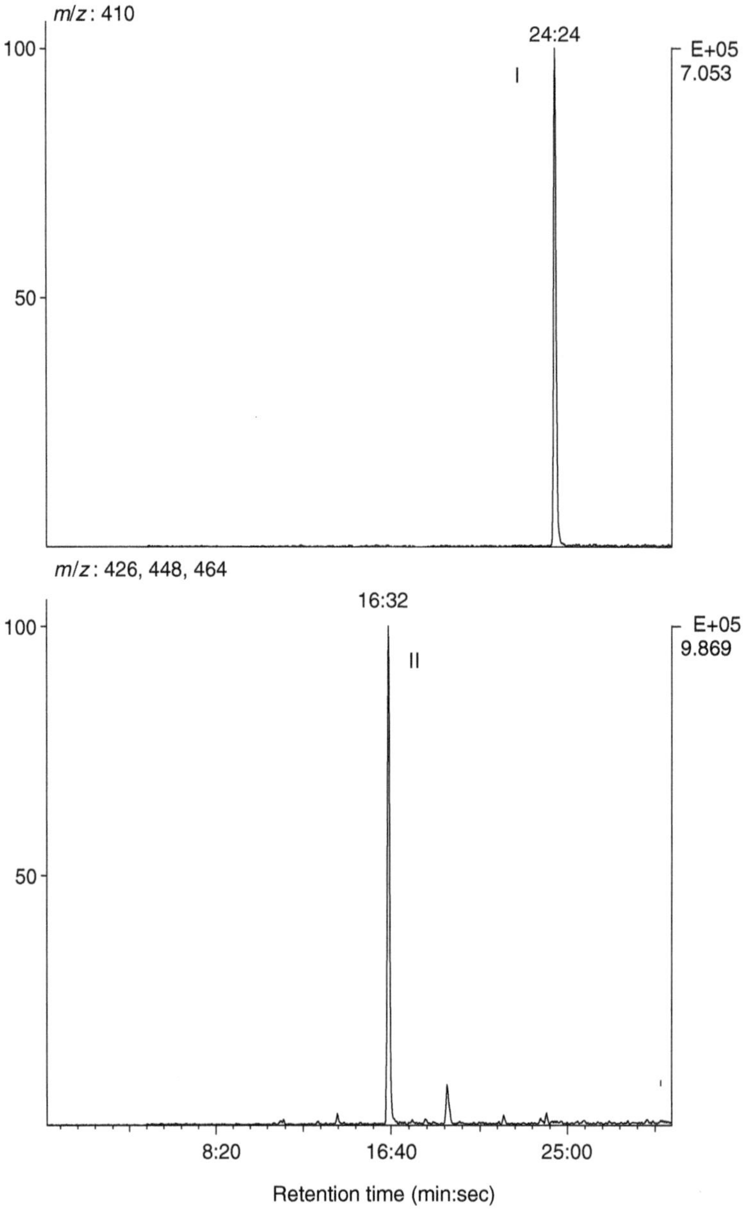

FIGURE 17.2 *Extracted ion chromatograms from post-dose plasma.*

I and V. Equivalent fragmentation gives rise to corresponding ions at *m/z* 290 and 307 in the case of II.

ESI MS–MS product-ion analysis was also used to obtain structural information on the novel metabolite, VI. Rationalisation of the resulting product-ion spectrum, shown in Figure 17.5, was assisted by comparison with those of authentic I and

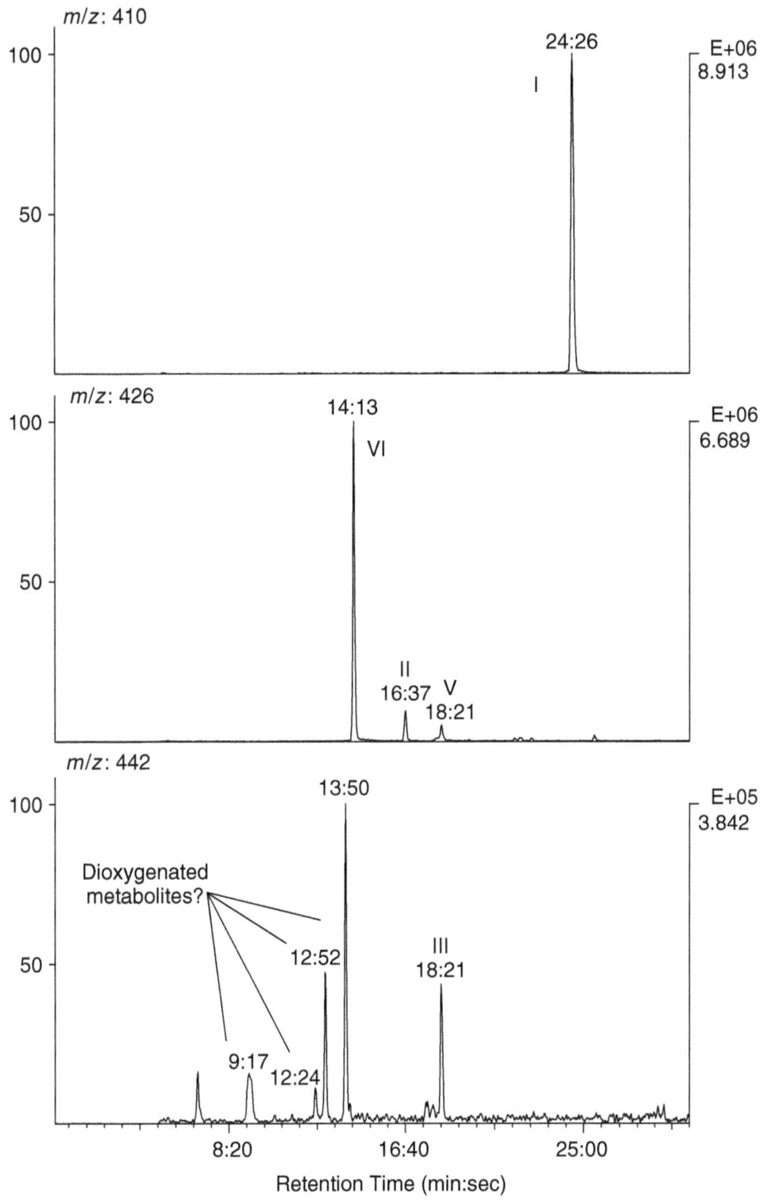

FIGURE 17.3 *Extracted ion chromatograms from post-dose urine samples.*

II–V. The major product ion at *m/z* 277 is not observed in the corresponding spectra of I or any of its known metabolites. However, the ion at *m/z* 120 is common with I, whilst the ions at *m/z* 219 and 234 are common with II. The product ions from VI can be rationalised in terms of a hydroxyl metabolite (as predicted) with the tentative site of oxidation being the benzisothiazol moiety (see Figure 17.6).

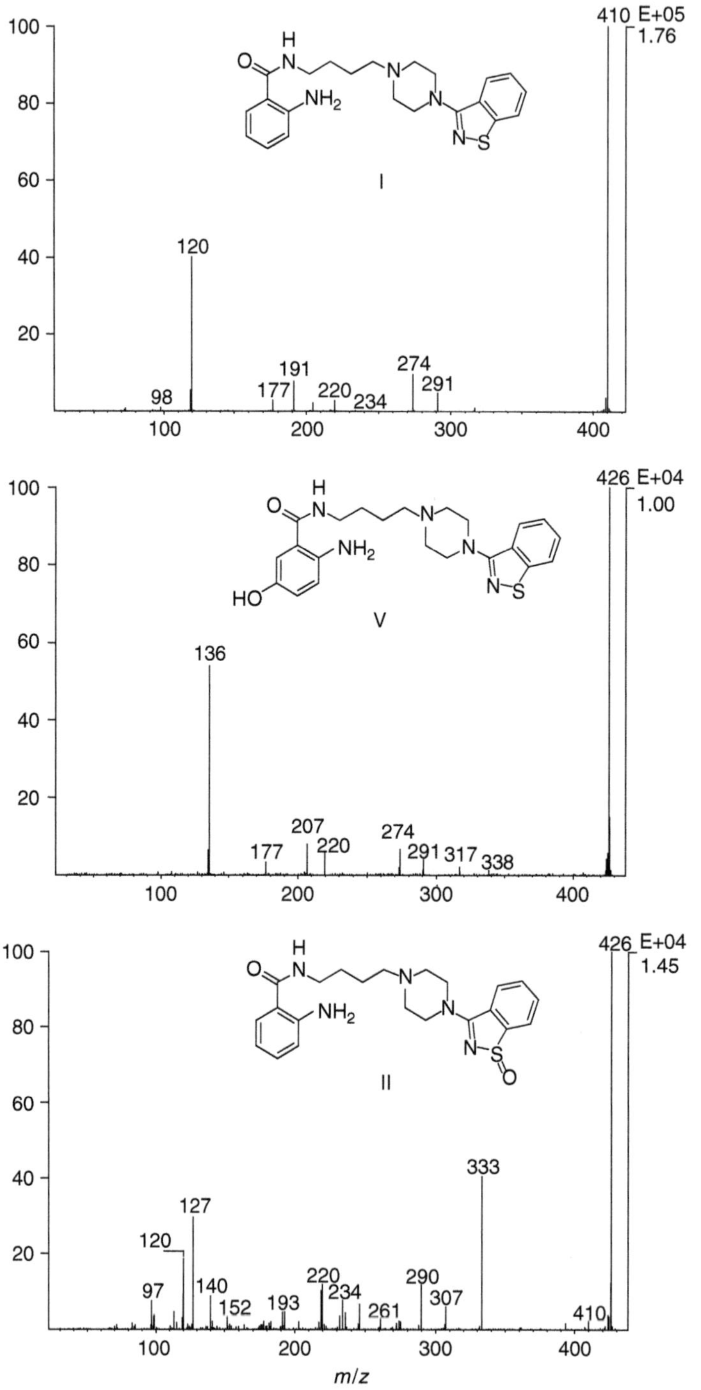

FIGURE 17.4 *MS–MS product-ion spectra of I and its metabolites II and V in urine, compared favourably to those of authentic material.*

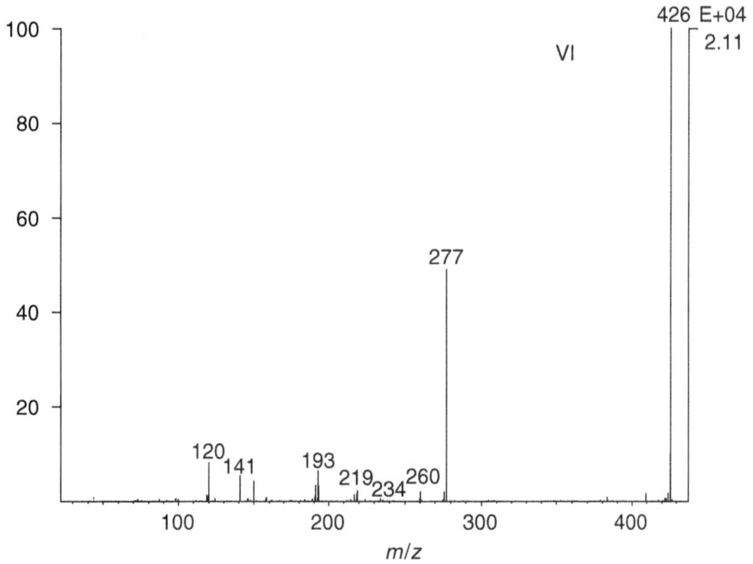

FIGURE 17.5 *ESI MS–MS product-ion spectrum used to obtain structural information on the novel metabolite, VI.*

Fragment ions can also be generated in the electrospray source by focusing ions through a potential gradient as they enter the mass spectrometer through the high-pressure region of the interface. Collisional activation in the high-pressure region of the API interface in combination with more conventional MS–MS enables second-generation product-ion spectra to be obtained. Using these techniques, further investigation of the *m/z* 120 product ion formed from both I and VI, and the *m/z* 277 product ion formed from VI alone, was possible. The resulting second-generation product-ion spectra of *m/z* 120 presented in Figure 17.7 are identical, being dominated by the ions at *m/z* 92 and 65, and therefore providing unequivocal confirmation that VI is drug-related. The second-generation product ion spectrum of *m/z* 277 (data not shown) exhibited ions at *m/z* 120 and 141, indicating that both these product ions are derived ultimately from *m/z* 277.

17.5 *Phase II*

Phase II metabolism is commonly classified as conjugative reactions in which parent drug or Phase I metabolites of parent drug are covalently attached to more polar endogenous functional groups such as glucuronic acid or sulphate. An additional but perhaps less common form of conjugation occurs through interaction with glutathione, an endogenous tripeptide (Gly-Cys-Glu). These conjugations make the drug molecule more polar in preparation for excretion. Most conjugation products are particularly labile molecules, which can be of an advantage in MS

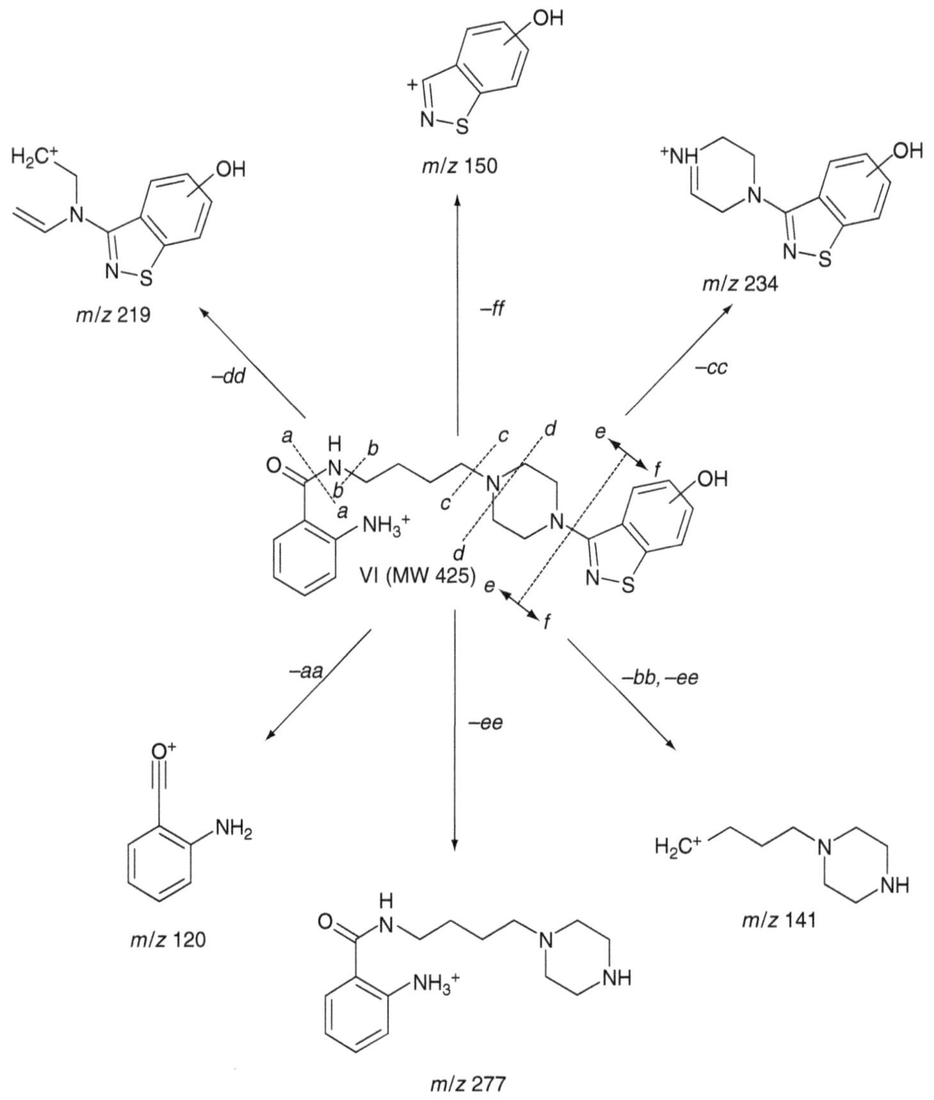

FIGURE 17.6 *The product-ions from VI, can be rationalised in terms of a hydroxyl metabolite (as predicted), with the tentative site of oxidation being the benzisothiazol moiety.*

studies. For example, in MS–MS experiments the conjugated entity will often dissociate leaving the original ionised parent drug or the Phase I metabolite to be detected. The analyst can take advantage of this, and use the constant neutral loss (CNL) mode of scanning for rapid screening of complex *in vivo* or *in vitro* matrices for conjugates. For example, the loss of a glucuronyl moiety during MS–MS experiments in almost all cases results in the loss of 176 amu from the parent ion under study, therefore CNL of 176 will enable the analyst to quickly pinpoint

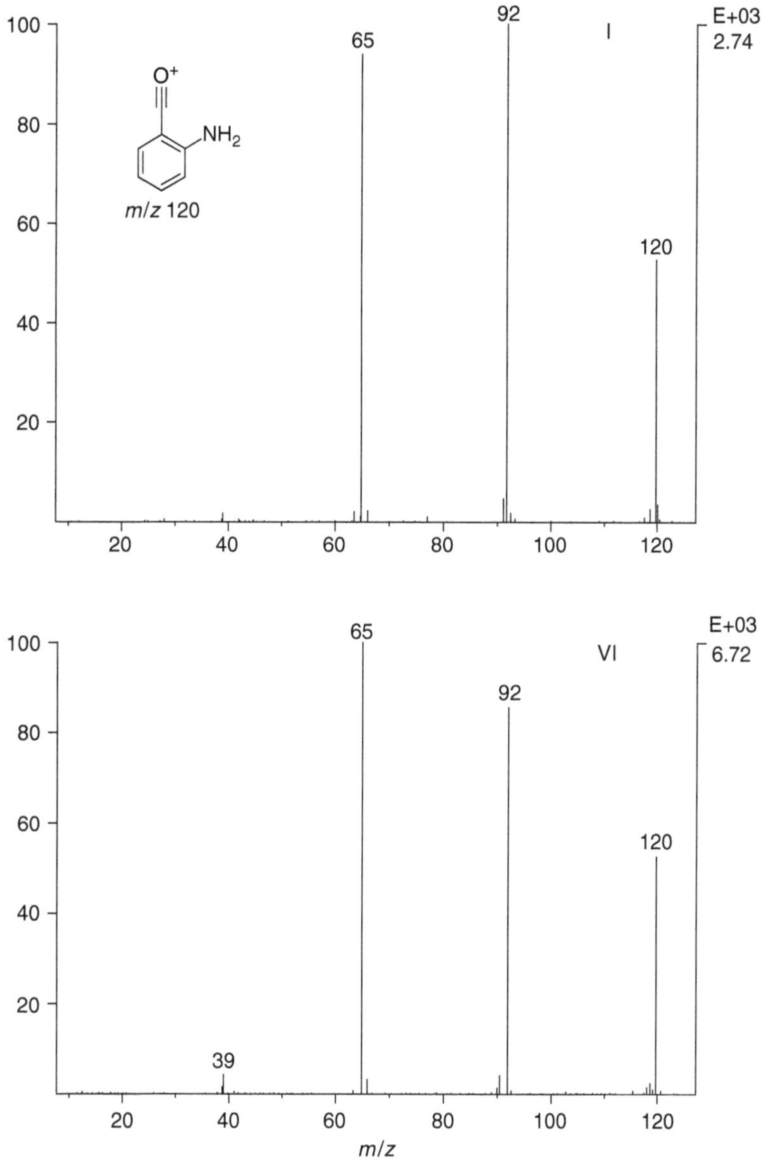

FIGURE 17.7 *Second-generation product-ion spectra of* m/z *120.*

possible glucuronide metabolites. These types of CNL screens are particularly effective when combined with HPLC using LC–MS–MS. In a similar manner, many conjugates give rise to common product ions; for example, aliphatic sulphates often exhibit an ion at *m/z* 97, corresponding to HSO_4^- in their associated MS–MS spectra. In these cases precursor ion scanning can enable the analyst to quickly screen samples for possible sulphate conjugates. Examples of CNL and precursor

TABLE 17.2 *Examples of CNL and precursor ions used in MS–MS drug metabolism studies*

Conjugate class	Ion polarity	Scan type
Glucuronides	+/−	CNL 176 amu ($-C_6H_8O_6$)
Phenolic sulphates	+	CNL 80 amu ($-SO_3$)
Aliphatic sulphates	−	Precursors of *m/z* 97 (HSO_4^-)
Sulphonates	−	Precursors of *m/z* 81 (HSO_3^-)
Sulphinates	−	CNL 64 amu ($-HSO_2$)
Acetamides	+	CNL 42 amu ($-C_2H_2O$)
Aryl-GSH	+	CNL 275 amu ($-C_{10}H_{17}N_3O_6$)
Aliphatic-GSH	+	CNL 129 amu ($-C_5H_7NO_3$)
N-acetyl cysteines	+/−	CNL 129 amu ($-C_5H_7NO_3$)
Taurine	+	Precursors of *m/z* 126 (Tau + H^+)
Phosphate	−	Precursors of *m/z* 63 (PO_2^-)
Phosphate	−	Precursors of *m/z* 79 (PO_3^-)

Adapted from T.A. Baille, *Proceedings of the 42nd ASMS Conference on Mass Spectrometry and Allied Topics* (1994), Chicago, Illinois, USA.

ion experiments used commonly within drug metabolism studies are detailed in Table 17.2.

In the following example, VII (1R, 1′R, 2R, 2′R)-2,2-[1,5-pentanediylbis-[oxy(3-oxo-3,1-propanediyl)]]bis[1-[(3,4-dimethoxyphenyl)-methyl]-1,2,3,4-tetrahydro-6,7-dimethoxy-2-methylisoquinolinium] dibenzenesulphonate, an intermediate-acting neuromuscular-blocking agent formed glucuronides in humans and dogs, but sulphate conjugates in cats. Initial *in vitro* work demonstrated that VII spontaneously degrades at physiological pH by Hofmann elimination to form products VIII (laudanosine) and IX (quaternary monoacrylate). Subsequent ester hydrolysis of IX generates X (quaternary alcohol). In plasma, VII is also metabolised by carboxyesterases to X and XI (quaternary acid), the former being rapidly hydrolysed further to the more stable XI. It has been reported that VIII can be further metabolised via N-demethylation to yield XII (tetrahydropapaverine). A schematic representation of the breakdown pathway is presented in Figure 17.8.

As part of the clinical development of VII, the disposition and metabolism of ^{14}C-VII following a single intravenous bolus dose was studied in various animal species and humans. Initial radiochemical HPLC profiling of human urine using an aqueous/acetonitrile reversed-phase gradient system revealed the presence of a major polar metabolite which did not co-chromatograph with any of the known metabolites or degradation products (assigned as XIII). These same samples were re-analysed using an identical HPLC system coupled to an electrospray triple quadrupole instrument, with on-line radiochemical detection. The radioactivity signal was connected to an analogue input channel on the MS data system, allowing simultaneous display of radiochemical and MS or MS–MS data (see Figure 17.9).

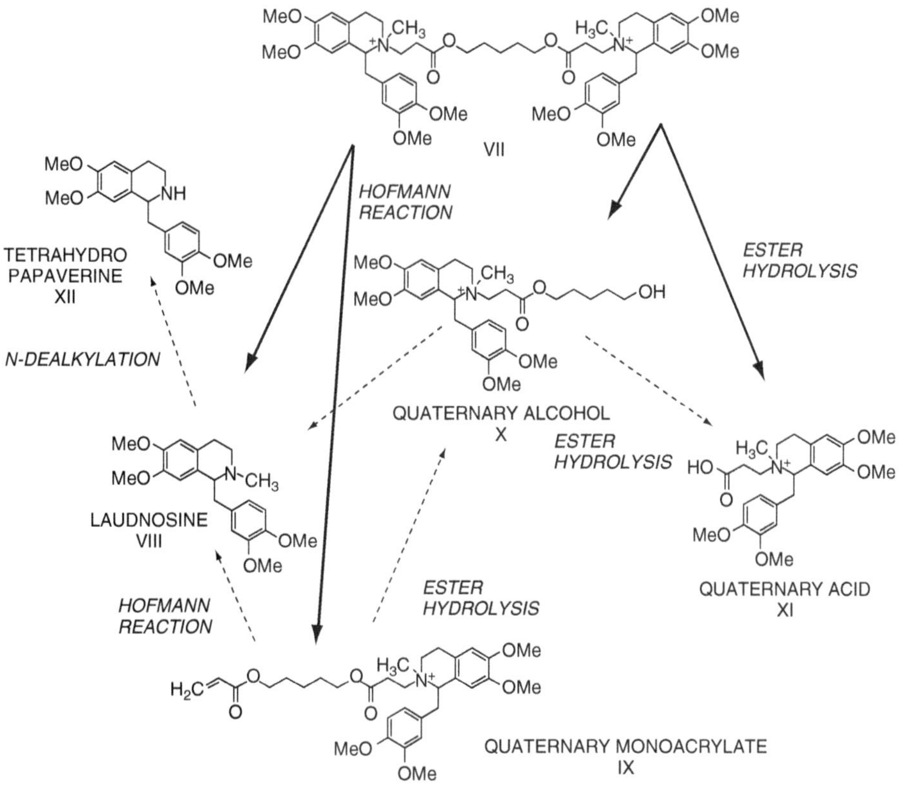

FIGURE 17.8 *A schematic representation of the breakdown pathway.*

Simultaneous detection of radiochemical and MS response provides an invaluable means to distinguish drug-related from endogenous, sample matrix-related, substances, and therefore vastly improves the efficiency of the metabolite identification process.

Under positive ion ESI parent VII is observed as its doubly charged molecular species, $M2^+$, at *m/z* 464, by virtue of its two quaternary nitrogen atoms. The metabolites IX, X and XI are observed as their singly charged molecular species, M^+, at *m/z* 570, 516 and 430, respectively. As neither VIII nor XII contain a quaternary nitrogen, these are observed as their protonated molecules, MH^+, at *m/z* 358 and 344, respectively. Representative spectra from human urine are given in Figure 17.10. All spectra are dominated by a single ion with no evidence of fragmentation. Two predominant ions, *m/z* 506 and 520, were found to contribute to the major unknown polar radioactive peak, XIII. These partially resolved ion peaks are clearly discernible in the extracted ion chromatograms in Figure 17.11. Based on molecular weight alone, these ions were tentatively assigned as the MH^+ species of co-eluting *O*-glucuronic acid conjugates of monodesmethyl XII and VIII, respectively (+176 amu, respectively). Several satellite peaks are visible in both the *m/z* 506 and 520 chromatograms, suggesting the presence of

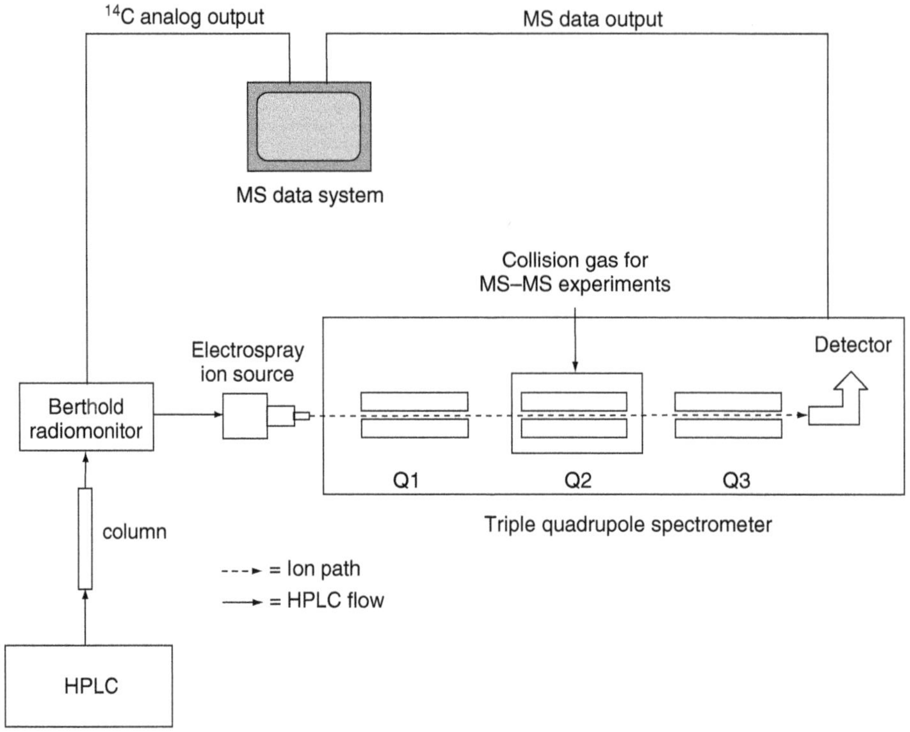

FIGURE 17.9 *Simultaneous detection of radiochemical and MS response.*

different positional isomers with respect to the site of conjugation. Indeed the four methoxy groups in both XII and VIII equate to four possible monodemethylated isomers, which can be subsequently conjugated (see Figure 17.12).

Product-ion MS–MS experiments were used to provide confirmatory evidence that the polar peaks identified were indeed glucuronic acid conjugates. Interpretation of product-ion spectra was assisted by comparison with those of authentic XII and VIII reference standards. MS–MS spectra of standard XII and VIII were dominated by product ions at *m/z* 206 and 192, respectively, which can be rationalised through cleavage of the benzylic bond linking the C-1 to the C-α position, resulting in a stabilised dihydroisoquinolium species.

Product-ion spectra of the major *m/z* 520 and 506 ions observed in human urine are shown in Figure 17.13. The product ions at *m/z* 344 and 300 observed in the MS–MS spectra of *m/z* 520 and 506 peaks, respectively, indicate that these were correctly assigned as glucuronyl-containing metabolites through the characteristic neutral loss of 176 amu from the parent ion. Fragmentation schemes for these conjugates are given in Figure 17.14. The product ion at *m/z* 206 indicates that glucuronidation has occurred on the dimethoxy phenyl group of VIII following O-dealkylation, while the *m/z* 192 ion supports glucuronidation on the 6,7-dimethoxy isoquinoline group of VIII following O-dealkylation. An equivalent

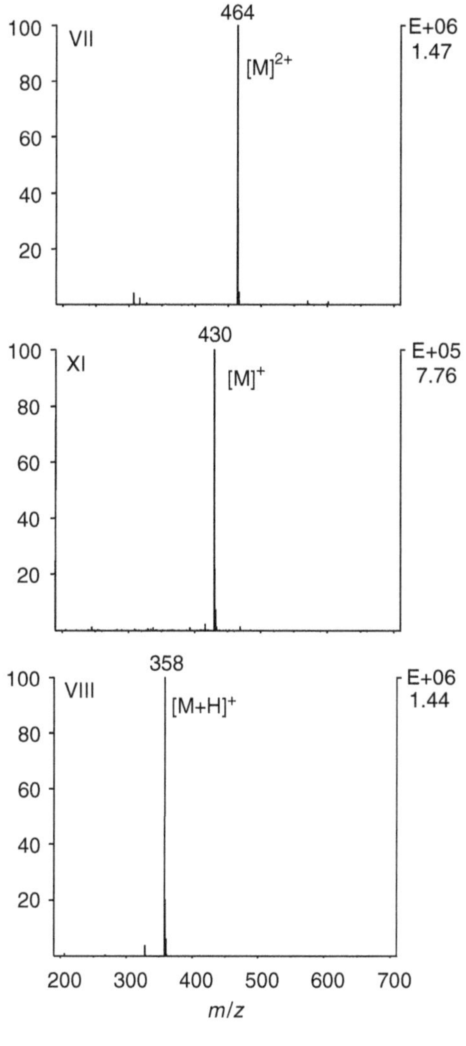

FIGURE 17.10 *Representative spectra from human urine.*

ion at *m/z* 178 is formed from the *O*-glucuronic acid conjugate of monodesmethyl-XII. The presence of these conjugates was also confirmed by enzyme digestion studies with β-glucuronidase.

Similar metabolite profiles were observed in dog urine and dog bile although sulphate conjugation of monodesmethyl-VIII was confirmed as the major route of excretion in cat bile. The MS–MS spectrum of this metabolite exhibited the loss of 80 amu, which as highlighted in Table 17.2 is diagnostic of phenolic sulphate conjugates. The identified sulphate conjugate was detectable in both positive ion and negative ion electrospray LC–MS–MS, giving rise to MH^+ and $[M-H]^-$ ions.

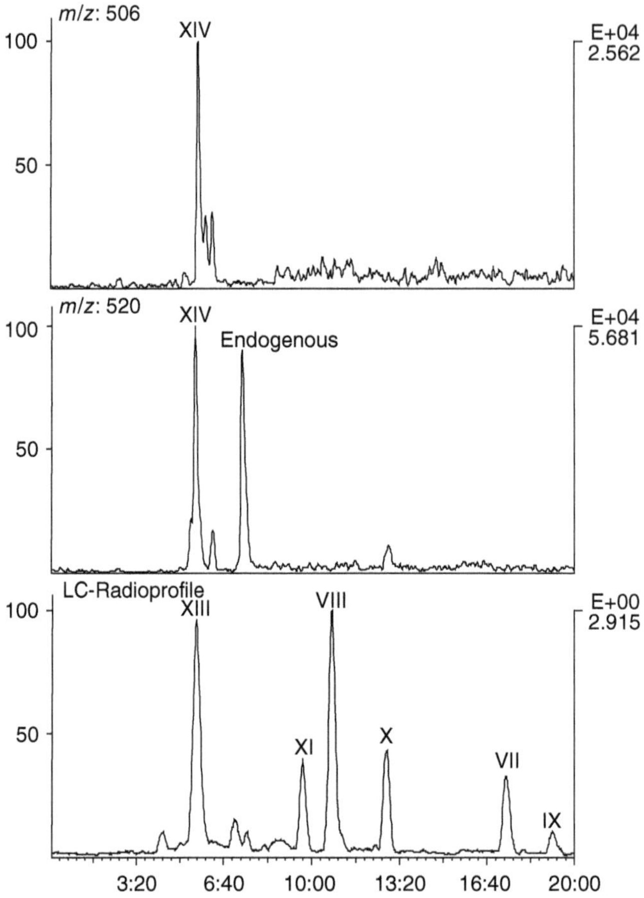

FIGURE 17.11 *Partially resolved ion peaks are clearly discernible in the extracted ion chromatograms.*

The examples above have highlighted the now common use of LC–MS and LC–MS–MS for metabolite identification in complex biofluids, using conventional chromatography coupled to a tandem quadrupole mass spectrometer via an API interface (usually electrospray, or some variant of this source). Although this general approach has found a secure place in many of the drug metabolism laboratories across the pharmaceutical industry, the technique is constantly under review and advancement. These include the increased use of LC–MS with ion trap and time-of-flight mass spectrometers, the former providing a means to further investigate fragmentation fingerprints of metabolites using MSn scanning and the latter providing on-line accurate mass measurements for the elucidation of empirical formulae.

However, mass spectrometry does not always allow unequivocal structural confirmation, and in these instances NMR spectroscopy is often needed to provide conclusive structural information, particularly with regard to stereochemistry.

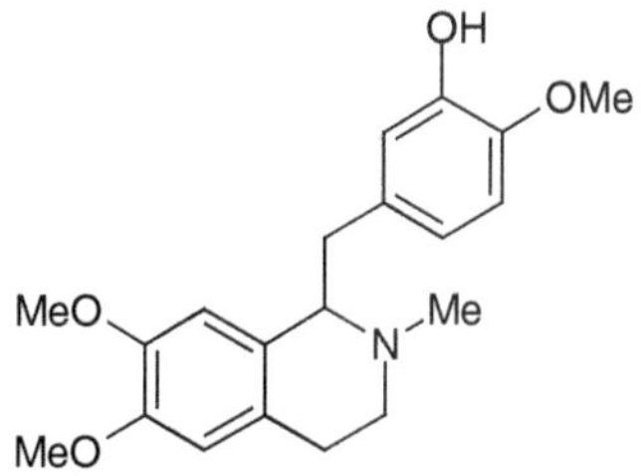

Laudanine

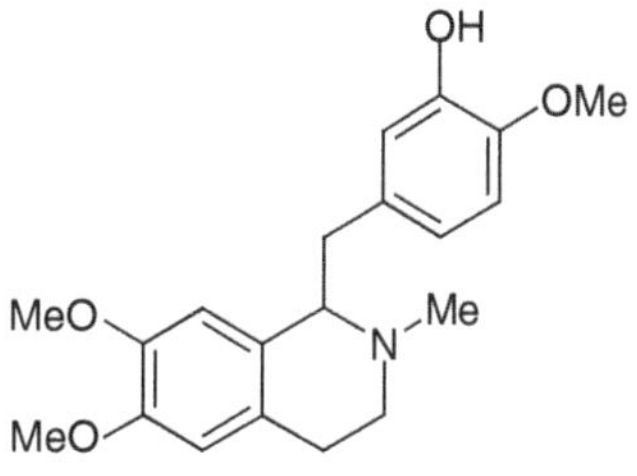

Pseudolaudanine

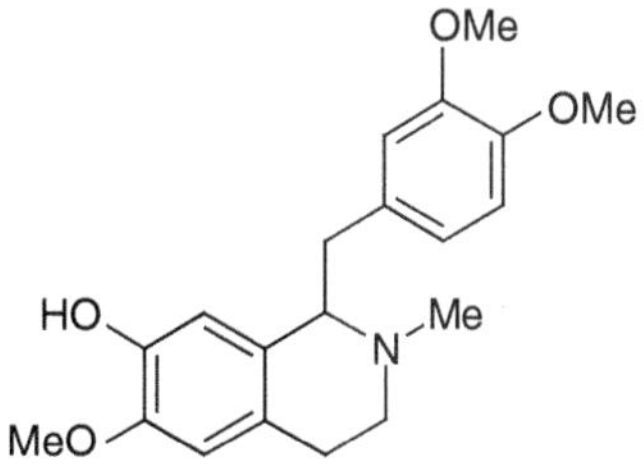

Codamine

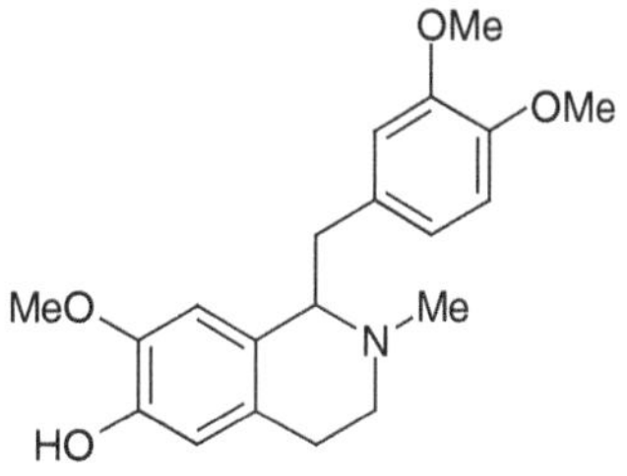

Pseudocodamine

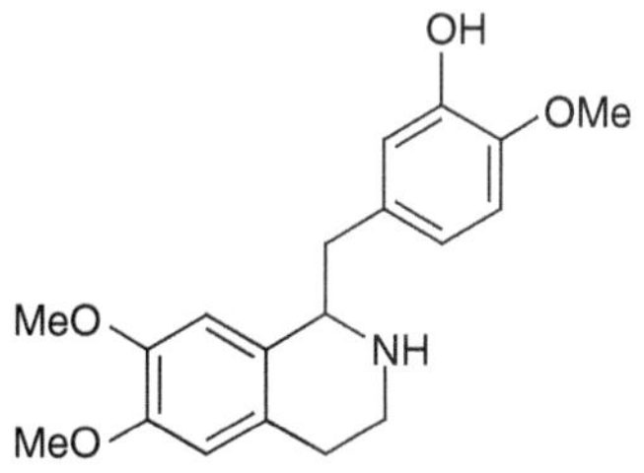

N-norlaudanine

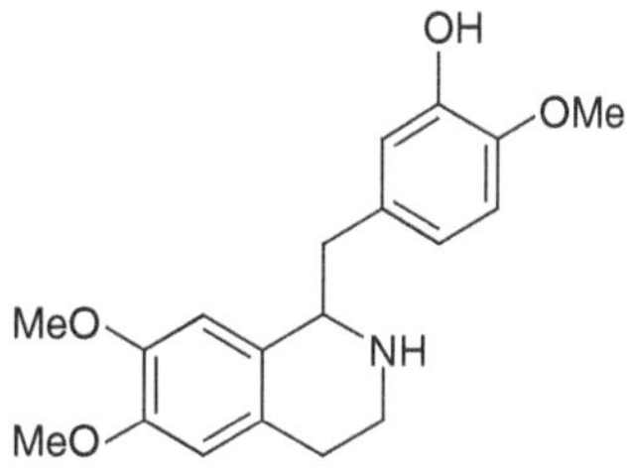

N-norpseudolaudanine

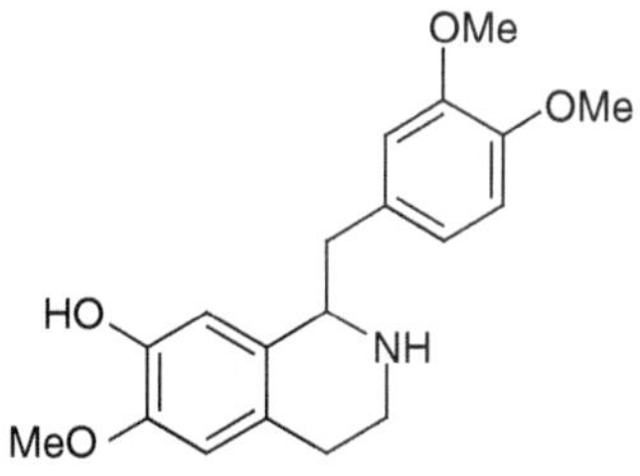

N-norcodamine

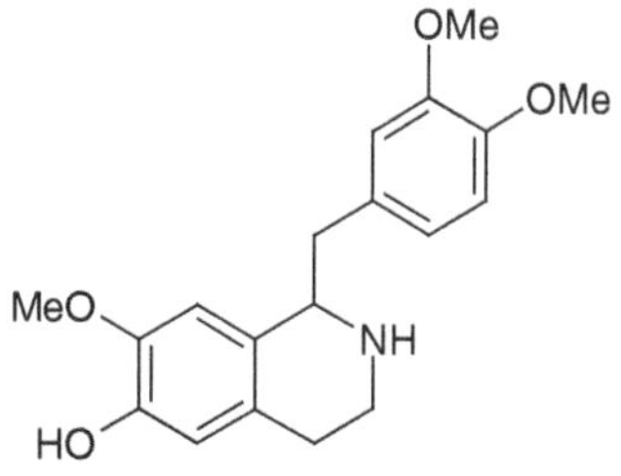

N-norpseudocodamine

FIGURE 17.12 *Four methoxy groups in both XII and VIII equate to four possible monodemethylated isomers, which can be subsequently conjugated.*

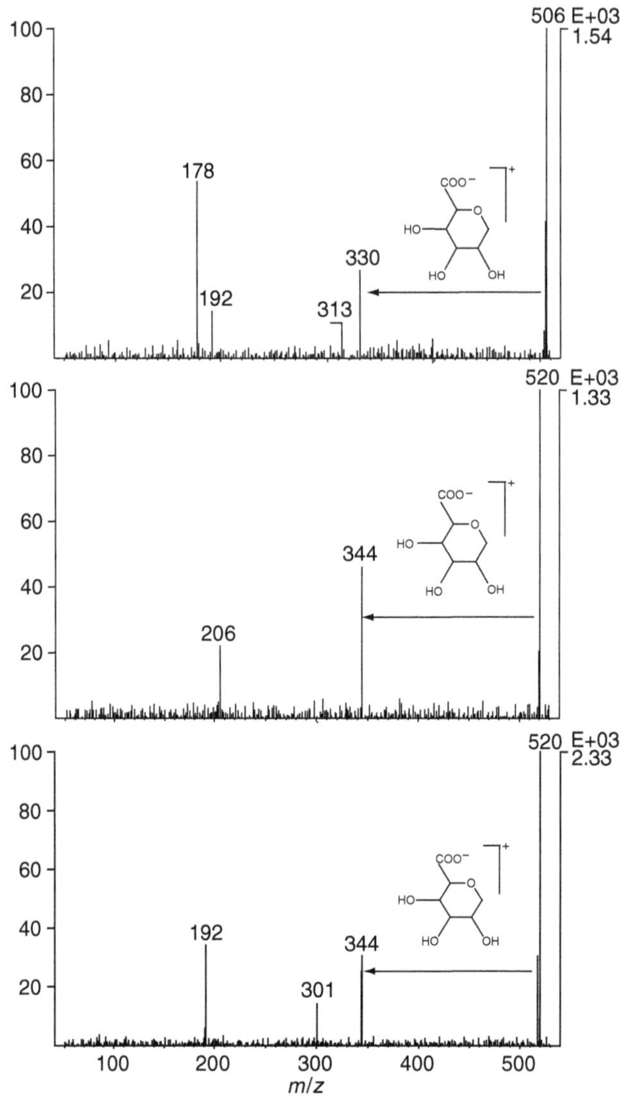

FIGURE 17.13 *Product-ion spectra of the major* m/z *520 and 506 ions observed in human urine.*

17.6 *NMR spectroscopy*

Nuclear magnetic resonance or NMR spectroscopy is a spectroscopic technique that arises from the magnetic properties of spinning atomic nuclei when placed in an external magnetic field. The most useful nuclei in NMR spectroscopy terms are those nuclear isotopes possessing a spin quantum number (I) value of 1/2 such as ^{1}H, ^{13}C, ^{19}F and ^{31}P and of these ^{1}H is by far the most important and widely used. However, as will be seen later in this article, NMR is a versatile technique and

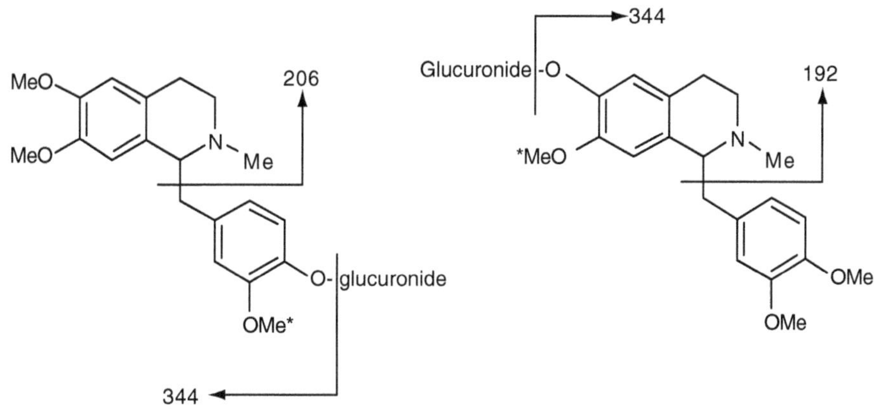

Isomeric *O*-glucuronide conjugate of
monodesmethyl laudanosine (*m/z* 520)

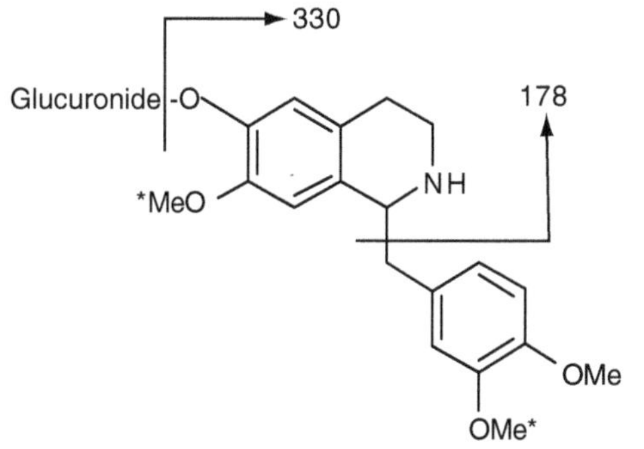

O-glucuronide conjugates of
monodesmethyl tetrahydropapaverine (*m/z* 506)
*– denotes alternative sites of putative conjugation

FIGURE 17.14 *Fragmentaion schemes for the glucuronyl-containing conjugates.*

where appropriate other nuclei such as ^{19}F can be usefully applied in drug metabolism studies where appropriate.

^{1}H NMR has long been a standard tool for organic structure determination. This is mainly because several valuable unique pieces of structural information are readily obtained from the parameters measured in NMR spectra. These include the chemical shift (δ in ppm), the spin–spin coupling pattern (multiplicity), the coupling constant (J in Hz), nuclear Overhauser enhancement (NOE) and signal integration.

Encoded within the chemical shift δ values of each and every proton in a molecule is information that gives an indication of the nature of the magnetic and hence the chemical environment that is experienced by that individual proton. The through bond spin–spin coupling constants and the multiplicity of the signals (i.e. whether the signals are singlets, doublets, triplets or more complicated so-called second-order patterns) enable the determination of not only the number of other protons that are in the immediate vicinity but also their relative stereochemistry, since the magnitude of the coupling constants is dependent on the angle between the protons.

As the measurement of signal intensities in the NMR spectrum enables the determination of the number of protons contributing to that signal it is possible to determine the number of protons in a molecule by comparison of the relative signal intensities.

Performing NOE experiments enables the determination of the relative through-space proximity of protons to each other, information that is only otherwise available by means of laborious and complicated crystal structure studies.

The information from these parameters makes NMR spectroscopy one of the most information-rich qualitative analytical techniques available for the characterisation of novel drug metabolites. There are many excellent NMR references that discuss these parameters as well as the theoretical and quantum mechanical basis of NMR spectroscopy, and the authors would refer the student to one of these publications for further and more involved discussion.

As NMR is a technique that is dependent on the properties of individual nuclei in molecules the range of compounds that can be analysed is not limited by factors such as volatility, presence of chromophores or polarity which can limit the application of other analytical techniques. In fact ^{1}HNMR spectroscopy can justly lay claim to be being almost a 'universal detector' as most drug substances are likely to be proton-containing organic compounds and as such will give rise to ^{1}H NMR signals. This ability of NMR to be a 'non-selective detector' and to obtain signals from all proton-containing material in the sample can in fact be a double-edged sword. On the positive side it allows a specific and simultaneous determination of a number of metabolites without any preconceptions or prior assumptions about their nature and thus maximising the chance of identifying important but unexpected or previously unknown metabolites. As such it is particularly valuable for acquiring metabolite profiles on samples where prior knowledge is limited, and the advantages afforded by NMR methods should facilitate new progress in metabolic and biochemical research. However, definitive metabolite structural characterisation can rarely be acquired directly from crude biological fluid samples without some form of sample preparation to reduce the intense signals that arise from the matrix.

In addition, NMR spectroscopy is non-destructive which allows samples to be further purified if necessary and subsequently analysed by other techniques. In fact MS and NMR data have long been used in conjunction with each other and with separation techniques, usually HPLC in the characterisation of novel drug molecules but not until recently have they been used as combined hyphenated techniques such as LC–NMR. Indeed reports exist where all three techniques have been linked to generate LC–NMR–MS systems.

17.6.1 Sample preparation and isolation

The isolation procedures used in the isolation of drug metabolites from biological matrices need to deliver samples for analysis that are relatively pure for the purposes of analysis and structural elucidation by ^{1}H NMR. And in this respect ^{1}H NMR spectroscopy, unlike mass spectrometry is relatively unforgiving and the background signals arising from the endogenous components of the matrix or other impurities associated with the isolation procedures can totally obscure the drug-related peaks of interest. Therefore great care must be taken to produce samples that are as pure as possible to ensure a successful outcome to the analysis.

Only in cases where there is a fluorine atom in the molecule, and as there are no naturally occurring endogenous fluorine containing molecules, is it possible to analyse samples directly in biological matrices by the use of ^{19}F NMR. The usefulness of this approach is illustrated later in this chapter.

The isolation and purification of drug metabolites from biological matrices for ^{1}H NMR analysis has traditionally been carried out using techniques such as solid phase extraction and HPLC. This process has been a relatively time-consuming and therefore expensive affair and has often been a constraining factor in the use of ^{1}H NMR in drug metabolite characterisation.

The identification of the metabolites of a novel non-nucleoside reverse transcriptase inhibitor, XIV, (S)-2-ethyl-7-fluoro-3-oxo-3,4-dihydro-2H-quinoxaline-carboxylic acid isopropylester (see Figure 17.15) will be used to describe an alternative

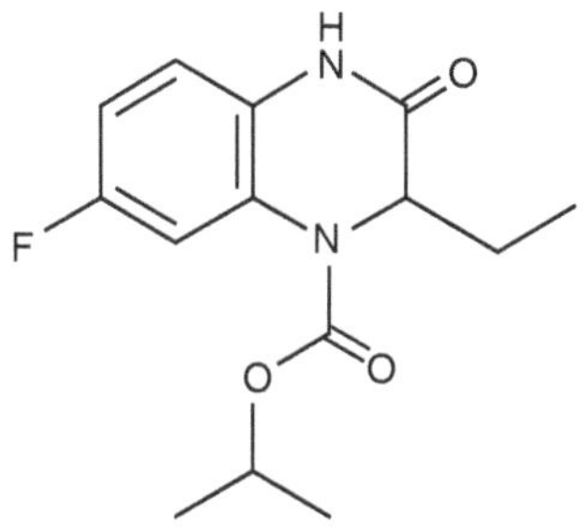

XIV

FIGURE 17.15 *A novel non-nucleoside reverse transcriptase inhibitor, XIV (S)-2-ethyl-7-fluoro-3-oxo-3,4-dihydro-2H-quinoxaline-carboxylic acid isopropylester.*

and rapid approach to drug metabolite identification, using preparative scale HPLC followed by NMR and LC–NMR combined with MS data.

Pooled urine samples collected following oral administration of XIV to animal test species and man were separately freeze-dried then reconstituted in distilled water to give a final volume equal to one-tenth of the initial volume. Injections of the concentrated urine samples were made onto a preparative HPLC column and analytes separated with reversed-phase gradient elution. The column eluent was collected into 96-well micro-titre plates using 15-second time slice fractions. Collected fractions were evaporated to dryness and then re-dissolved in 50:50 acetonitrile:deuterium oxide. The resulting dissolved fractions were transferred individually to 5 mm NMR tubes for analysis.

Isolated fractions were analysed by ^{1}H and ^{19}F NMR spectroscopy for the presence of drug-related material. The resulting NMR spectra were used to ascertain the distribution of drug-related material in the processed fractions. This was achieved initially through the presence of a signal in the ^{19}F NMR spectrum and subsequently by a comparison of the ^{1}H NMR spectra with that acquired for the authentic parent compound. The ability to process large volumes of biological fluids, using preparative scale HPLC, makes the interpretation of the resulting NMR spectra easier, since bulk levels of metabolite(s) can be isolated. Since NMR spectroscopy is an inherently insensitive technique, the provision of relatively large amounts of isolated metabolite material (micrograms) enables high-quality spectra to be acquired in a relatively short time.

17.7 *Characterisation of metabolites by ^{1}H NMR*

Examples of the use of ^{1}H NMR spectroscopy in the characterisation of Phase I and Phase II metabolites are outlined below using the most common metabolic pathways as illustrative examples.

17.7.1 Phase I

Aromatic hydroxylation

The hydroxylation of aromatic moieties within drug molecules is one of the most common metabolic transformations. The confirmation of the position of substitution on an aromatic ring is an excellent example of the use of the information-rich content of ^{1}H NMR spectroscopy. The site-specific information that can often only be obtained from an NMR spectrum is probably the most common use of ^{1}H NMR spectroscopy in drug metabolite structural elucidation.

The confirmation of the individual positional isomers formed following the aromatic hydroxylation of *XIV* gives an excellent illustration of the use of ^{1}H NMR spectroscopy in resolving the identity of the individual isomers. ^{1}H NMR spectra of isolated metabolites (see Section 17.6.1) were compared to the ^{1}H NMR spectrum of authentic parent drug, *XIV* (see Figure 17.16). The ^{1}H NMR spectrum of parent drug can be characterised by amongst others the aromatic protons in the region δ 6.9–7.0, corresponding to 5-H and 6-H as defined in Figure 17.16 and the methine proton 12-H at δ 4.95. The 8-H aromatic proton was detected as a broad singlet at δ 7.4, as a result of restricted rotation about the carboxylic acid isopropylester side chain.

Changes to the aromatic resonances (e.g. coupling, chemical shift and integrals) corresponding to 5-H, 6-H and 8-H in the ^{1}H NMR spectra of aromatic-hydroxylated metabolites, can thus be used to identify the position of substitution. In this instance the number of aromatic-hydroxylated metabolites formed was further increased by the occurrence of an NIH shift (named after the National Institute of Health where this migration was first observed) whereby the fluorine atom migrates in the ring to generate further metabolites (see Figure 17.17).

Aliphatic hydroxylation

As above, aliphatic hydroxylation can be assigned by changes and/or disappearance of proton resonances within the ^{1}H NMR spectrum. A simple example of this type of metabolite occurs in the hydroxylation of the isopropyl methyl groups of *XIV*. In this example, comparison of the integrals in the aliphatic region of the spectrum of the isolated metabolite at δ 1.26 (data not shown) with those of authentic parent drug (see Figure 17.16) indicated the loss of one of the isopropyl methyl groups. Hydroxylation at the isopropyl group would generate a CH_2OH group whose protons should be evident in the NMR spectrum at approximately δ 3.5 but these could not be clearly observed as the signals from the H2–H4 protons of an attached glucuronyl moiety were in this region. The integral value of the protons in this region showed the presence of five protons, which supported this hypothesis. Based on this assignment and subsequent MS data (not shown) a definitive structure could be assigned (Figure 17.18).

De-alkylation, ester hydrolysis and other losses from the NMR spectrum

The loss of *N*-alkyl, *O*-alkyl or *S*-alkyl substituents is readily discerned in the ^{1}H NMR spectrum. The loss of an alkyl group from any of the above functional groups will be primarily evident in the NMR spectrum through the loss of the signals attributable to methyl or ethyl protons. In the case of *N*-dimethyl groups where only one of the methyl groups is lost through metabolism and replaced with a proton there may be additional information in the spectrum through the presence of additional coupling if the NH is not lost through exchange with the deuterated solvent.

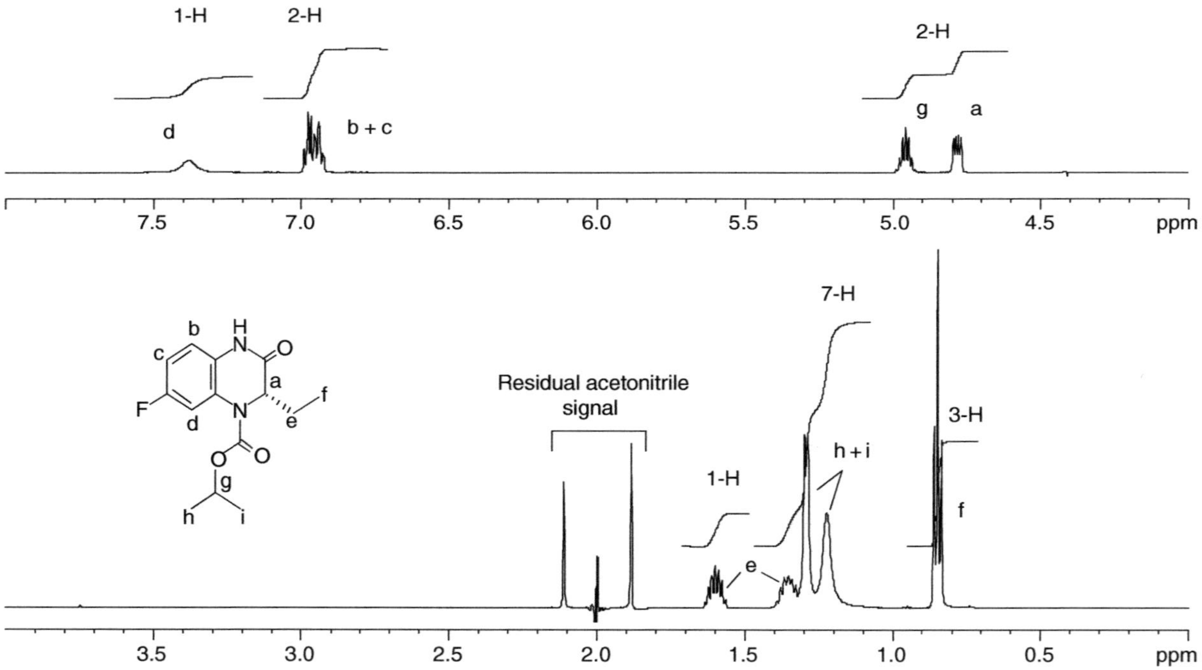

FIGURE 17.16 *^1H NMR spectra of isolated metabolites were compared to the ^1H NMR spectrum of authentic parent drug, XIV.*

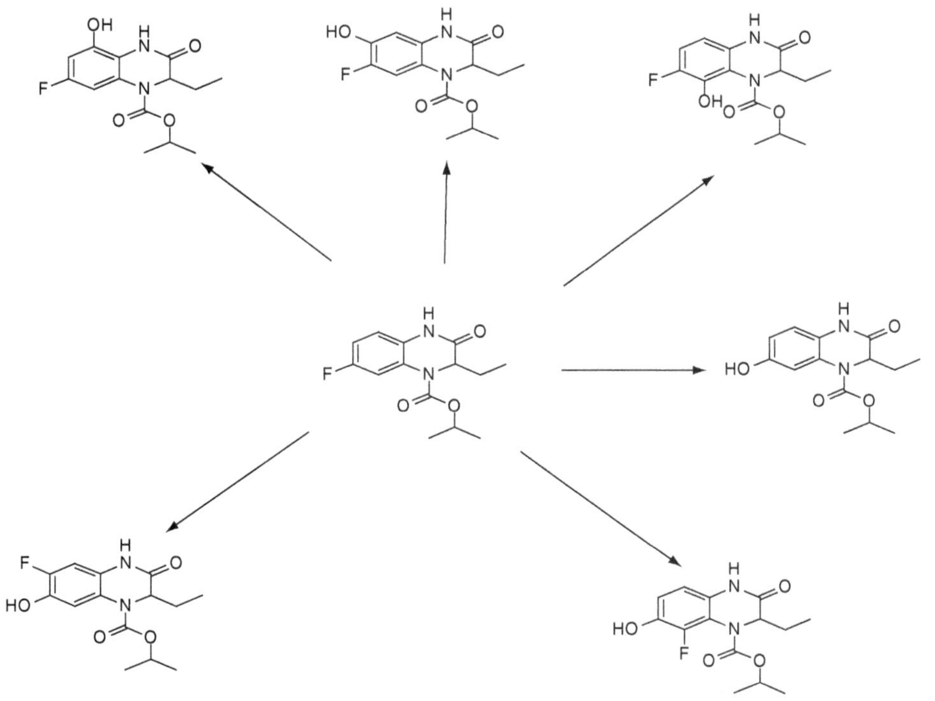

FIGURE 17.17 *Proposed position of substitution aromatic hydroxylated metabolites.*

Additionally the loss of a methyl group from a molecule may cause changes in the chemical shifts of nearby protons. Similarly the loss of any ester group might be indicated by the absence of any characteristic signals in the NMR spectrum attributable to the ester group.

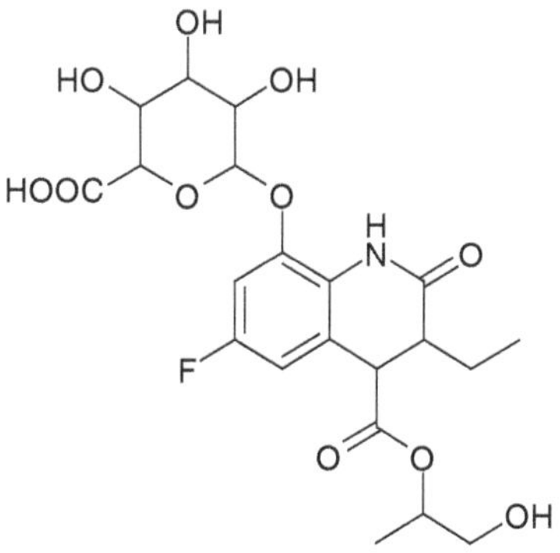

FIGURE 17.18 *Assigned structure.*

N- and *S*-oxidation

N- and *S*-oxides formed as a result of the oxidation of primary, secondary and tertiary nitrogen or sulphur atoms are common metabolic products. However, as no protons are directly involved in these bio-transformations, characterisation based on the ^{1}H NMR spectra of these metabolites is obtained indirectly from protons adjacent to the sites of metabolism which are affected by the formation of the *N*- and *S*-oxides.

17.7.2 Phase II

As outlined above, Phase II metabolism or conjugation generally involves the covalent addition of endogenous compounds, which lead to the formation of highly water-soluble products.

Glucuronic acid conjugates

Glucuronide formation is the most common form of conjugation of xenobiotic drug substances. Glucuronides can be *O*-linked when formed through conjugation to alcohols and phenols to form 'ether' glucuronides, and carboxylic acids to form 'ester' glucuronides. Similarly, *N*-linked glucuronides can be formed through conjugation to primary, secondary and quaternary amines. *S*-linked glucuronides occur through conjugation with sulfonamides and thiols.

The presence of a glucuronide metabolite can usually be rapidly determined by the occurrence of specific and diagnostic proton resonances within the ^{1}H NMR spectrum. For example, the H1 anomeric signal is typically evident as a doublet in the region δ 4.0–5.5. Similarly the remaining glucuronyl protons are usually evident clustered around δ 3.0–4.0. In addition the chemical shifts of the evident glucuronyl protons can often provide information regarding the nature of the glucuronide (e.g. ester or ether).

The diagnostic chemical shifts of the anomeric H1 proton for a number of common glucuronic acid conjugates are given in Table 17.3 to illustrate the utility of the anomeric proton's chemical shift.

The ^{1}H NMR spectrum of an isolated glucuronide metabolite of *XIV* clearly indicated a glucuronide conjugate that is substituted in the aromatic region (see Figure 17.19a). The ^{19}F NMR data (not shown) which produced a signal at about δ 135 for this metabolite is consistent with an aromatic ^{19}F ortho to oxygen. In the ^{1}H NMR spectrum shown in Figure 17.19, the size of the coupling constant on the observed aromatic proton at δ 6.88 is 11.0 Hz, which is consistent with an ortho ^{19}F$-^{1}$H coupling. On warming the sample, the aromatic proton signal for 8-H at δ 7.44 which is normally broad, through restricted rotation of the isopropyl group

TABLE 17.3 *Characteristic ^{1}H chemical shifts of the H1 anomeric proton of some common glucuronide conjugates*

Functional group – glucuronide conjugates	Characteristic chemical shift ^{1}H (ppm)	Functional group – glucuronide conjugates	Characteristic chemical shift ^{1}H (ppm)
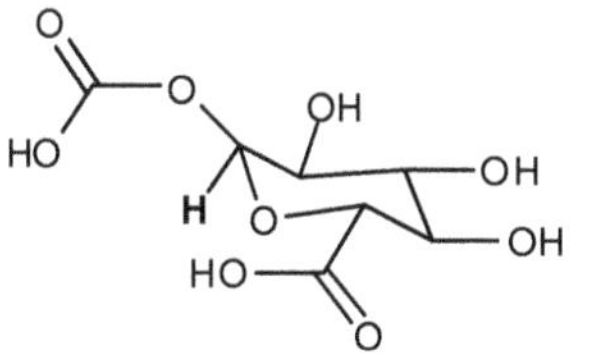	5.4–5.5	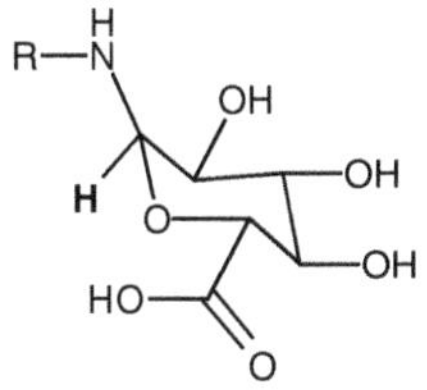	5.0–5.1
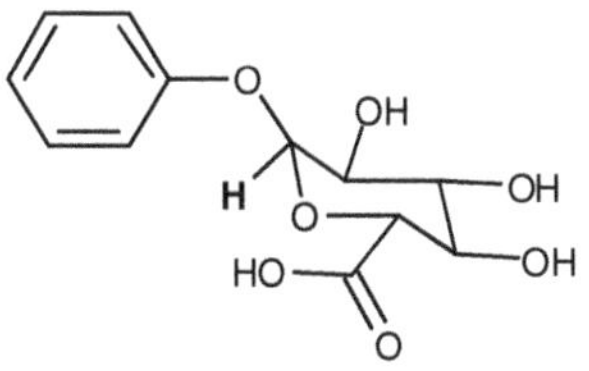	4.7–5.35	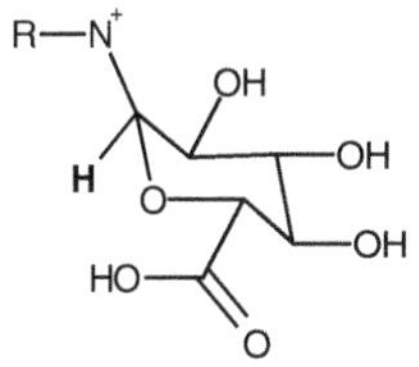	5.25–5.7
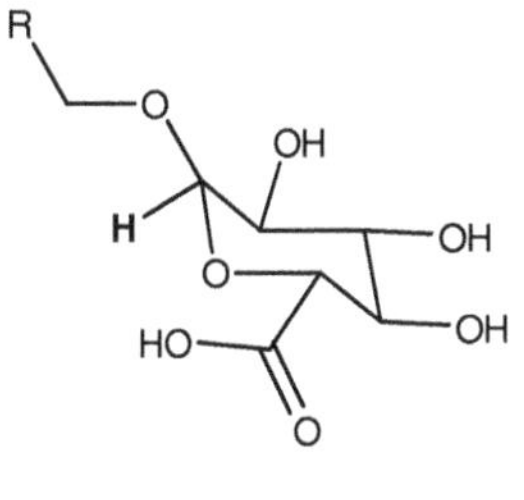	4.0–4.6	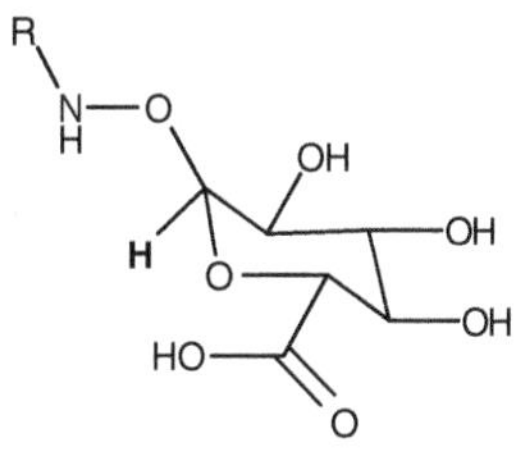	4.6–5.7

is sharpened sufficiently to observe coupling (see Figure 17.19b). A coupling constant of 6.14 Hz was recorded which is consistent with a meta $^{19}F-^{1}H$ coupling. Further confirmation of the structure was provided by a positive NOE from the anomeric H1 glucuronide proton at δ 4.95 to the 8-H aromatic proton at δ 7.44 (see Figure 17.19c), confirming the close proximity of the 8-H proton and the anomeric proton. This result strongly suggests that the fluorine and the hydroxyl groups (and thus the glucuronide) are at the 6- and 7-positions, respectively, and thereby confirm the metabolite as a 6-fluoro-7-hydroxyglucuronide.

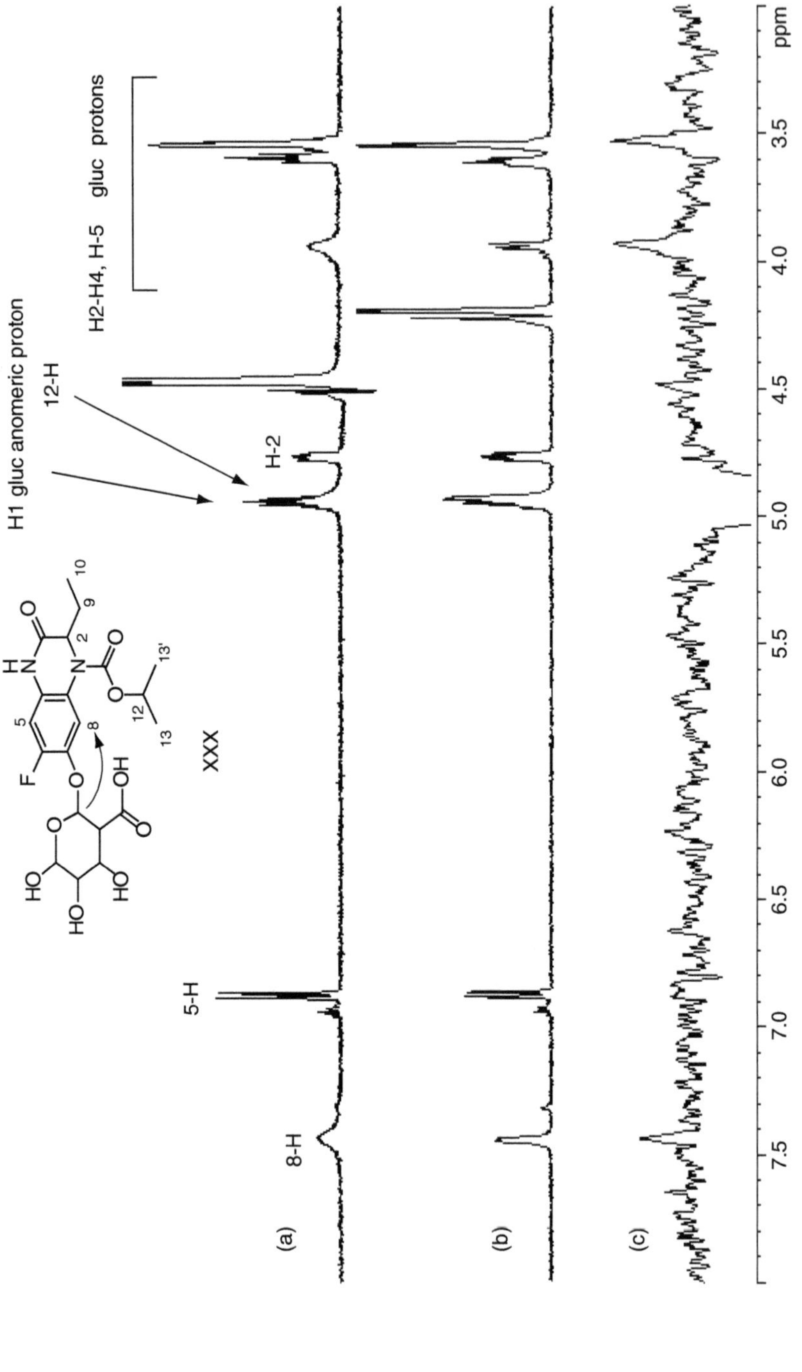

FIGURE 17.19 *The ^1H NMR spectrum of an isolated glucuronide metabolite.*

Other conjugates

Additional types of conjugation are also common, and examples include glycosylation, acetylation, amino acid conjugation (e.g. taurine) and glutathione conjugation. Covalent attachment of such groups to the parent drug molecule, as

TABLE 17.4 *Common ^{1}H NMR diagnostic signals indicative of metabolism*

Functional group	Characteristic chemical shift ^{1}H (ppm)	Functional group	Characteristic chemical shift ^{1}H (ppm)
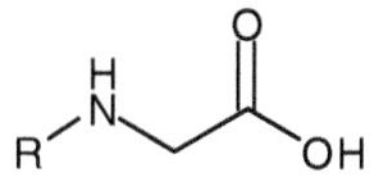 Glycine conjugation	3.45–4.1	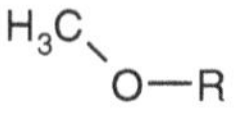 O-methylation	3.7–4.1
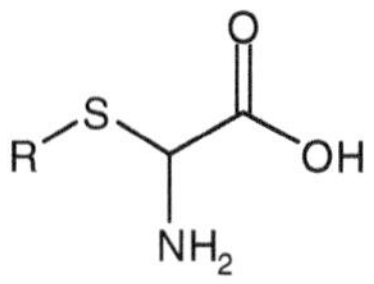 Cysteine conjugation	CH 3.7–4.45 CH_2 3.0–4.0	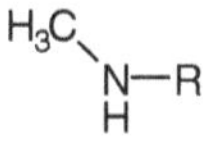 N-methylation	2.9–3.3
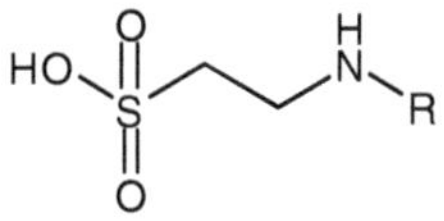 Taurine conjugation	2.95–3.7	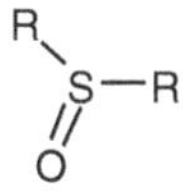 Sulphoxide formation	Formation of sulphoxide induces 0.2–1.3 downfield shift in adjacent protons
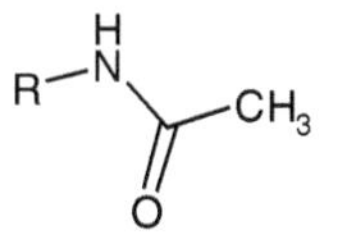 Acetate conjugation	1.9–2.7	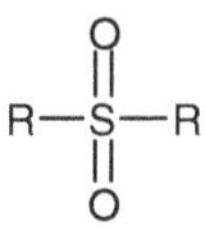 Sulphone formation	Formation of sulphoxide induces 0.5–0.7 downfield shift in adjacent protons
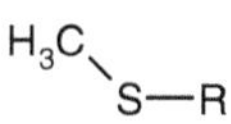 S-methylation	1.8–1.87		

described for glucuronidation, typically gives rise to diagnostic signals within the ^{1}H NMR spectra of such metabolites (see Table 17.4). For example, acetylation usually results in a distinctive singlet around δ 2.00, corresponding to the acetyl methyl group.

Sulphate conjugation, which is a very common means of metabolism, is transparent in the ^{1}H NMR spectrum due to a lack of observable protons of the sulphate group. The protons of the sulphate group are too labile to be observed in the spectrum as they undergo exchange with the deuterium of the NMR solvent. Therefore sulphate conjugation cannot be directly observed from the sulphate group. As in the case of *N*-oxide and *S*-oxide metabolites, characterisation can be obtained indirectly from protons adjacent to the sites of metabolism. This combined with complimentary MS data is usually sufficient to characterise such conjugates.

17.8 *^{19}F NMR metabolite profiling*

The absence of an endogenous fluorine background in biological matrices enables ^{19}F NMR spectroscopy to be used in the same fashion as a radiochemical label if a fluorine atom is present in the candidate drug molecule. Therefore the presence of drug-related material in any biological fluid may be determined simply by running a ^{19}F NMR spectrum of the biological fluid without any pre-treatment or isolation. Additionally as ^{19}F NMR spectroscopy has quite a large chemical shift range it is therefore sensitive to changes distant from the fluorine atom. The fluorine atom may therefore be used to determine the number of metabolites that are generated, and by comparison of the integral values of the metabolites against a suitable standard it is even possible to perform mass balance studies by ^{19}F NMR spectroscopy.

An example of the use of ^{19}F NMR in drug metabolism studies is shown in Figure 17.20 where the number and relative proportion of fluorine-containing species may be determined directly by ^{19}F NMR measurement of untreated human urine following the administration of a drug substance containing a fluorine atom.

17.9 *Conclusions*

Mass spectrometry and NMR spectroscopy both provide an effective and efficient means of characterising drug metabolites in complex biofluids. It is clear that both techniques benefit from some form of sample separation (e.g. analytical or

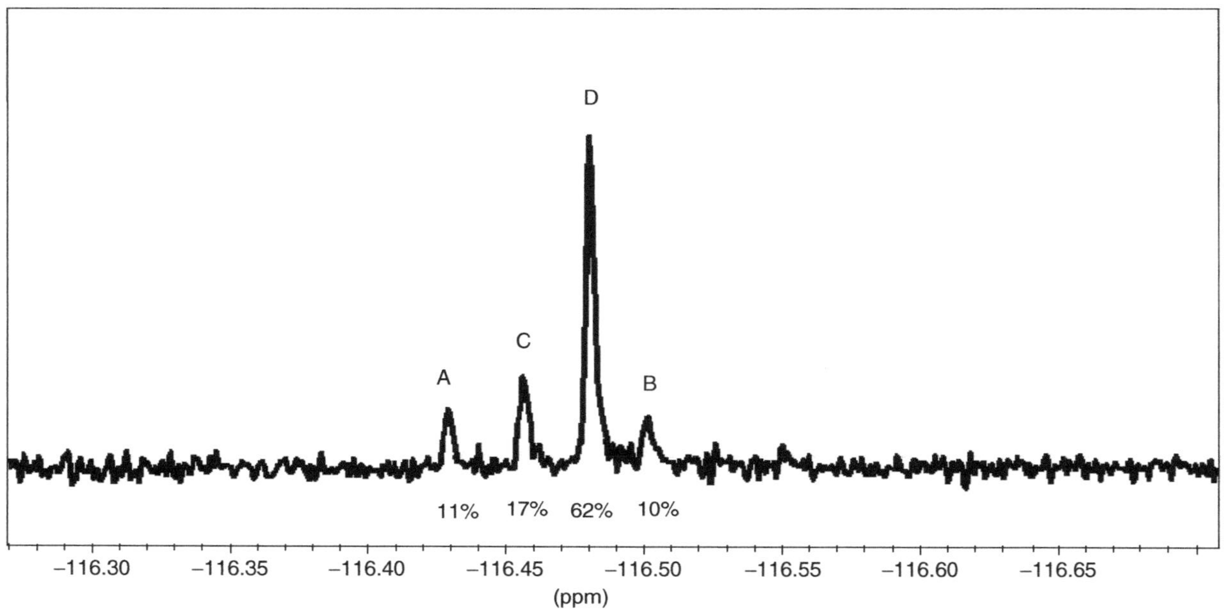

FIGURE 17.20 *An example of the use of* ^{19}*F NMR in drug metabolism studies is shown where the number and relative proportion of fluorine-containing species may be determined directly by* ^{19}*F NMR measurement of untreated human urine following the administration of a drug substance containing a fluorine atom.*

preparative scale HPLC) prior to analysis. Although there are many examples where the techniques have been used in isolation with great success, it has become apparent to the authors that the accuracy and efficiency of the structural elucidation process is enhanced by the concurrent use of both mass spectrometry and NMR spectroscopy.

CHAPTER 18

Molecular biology

Steve Hood

18.1 *Introduction*

Molecular biology is now a recognised facet of modern pharmaceutical research, from the discovery of novel compounds to the pre-clinical evaluation of new drugs. The basic principles and common protocols are now incorporated in many undergraduate teaching programmes and the introduction of pure molecular biology degree courses has established a skill base within industry and academia.

To fully cover 'what you should know' could run into several books. This chapter aims to give an overview of the underlying science of molecular biology and then highlights its uses within the field of drug metabolism.

This chapter has been divided into three sections. The first section covers the underlying theory that is the basis of the molecular biology used in a modern drug metabolism lab. The remaining sections address the two major questions that molecular biology can help to answer: which enzyme metabolises my drug and does my drug induce or suppress the metabolism of another coadministered drug.

18.2 *Basic molecular biology*

In 1944, Oswald Avery provided evidence that DNA may play a role in the genetic information of the cell, but it was not until 1953 that Watson and Crick (with Franklin and Williams) proposed their model for the structure of DNA, and the science of molecular biology was born. It was realised that this simple, self-replicating molecule comprising four bases and a sugar–phosphate backbone could encode for all the diverse proteins found within a living organism. Because the structure consisted of two antiparallel strands of nucleotides, such molecules could be unwound and duplicated, thus explaining the principles of heredity and cell division.

The backbone of the nucleic acid is made up of a chain of ribose sugar units linked by phosphate residues in the 3- and 5-positions of the ring. In RNA the sugar exists as a ribose residue while in DNA the sugar is reduced further to the deoxyribose form. Attached to the 1-position of the ribose is one of the four bases, adenine, guanine, cytosine and thymine (or uracil in RNA). A cytosine residue can pair with guanine residue on the other strand by means of three non-covalent hydrogen bonds while adenine and thymine pair with two such bonds. It therefore requires more energy (as heat) to break a GC bond as is required for an AT bond, and this is an important factor in techniques which require strands to hybridise to each other. This is shown in Figure 18.1.

The genetic information is arranged into genes, each gene coding for a single protein. Eukaryotic genes have some common features in their structure. At the front (5′-end) of the gene there is a region of DNA called the promoter. This is the on/off switch for the gene and can be regulated by a series of proteins inside the nucleus of the

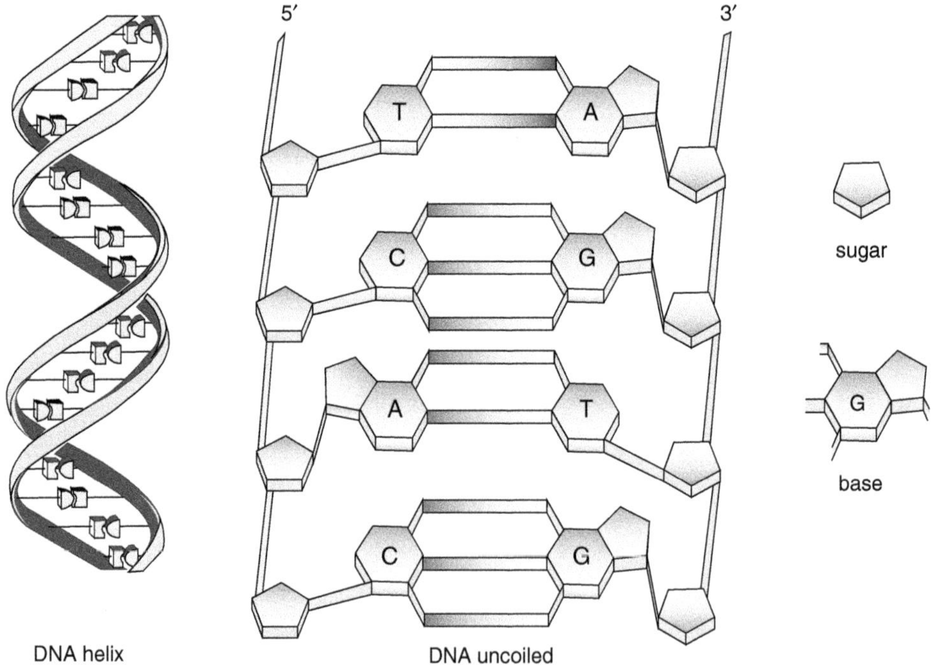

FIGURE 18.1 *The base pairing of the DNA double helix.*

cell. The genetic information of the gene is grouped in regions called exons. These exons are separated by regions of non-coding 'junk' DNA (introns) which are not involved in the production of the final protein. In prokaryotic genomes, where space is limited, there are no introns (see Figure 18.2). When the gene is activated, RNA polymerase binds to the promoter and proceeds to make a single-stranded RNA copy of the coding strand of the DNA. This process is known as *transcription*. The introns are then cut out of this new RNA strand in a process called splicing. The resulting strand contains information derived from the exons only and is called messenger RNA (mRNA). The mRNA is then exported from the nucleus where it is used as a blueprint to make the protein. This process is known as *translation* and is performed by the ribosomes. The bases on the mRNA are read in groups of three, known as codons, each group coding for an amino acid or a ribosomal command (e.g. 'start' or 'stop' translation). The ribosomes run along the mRNA molecule with the growing protein chain until the stop signal is reached, when the ribosome drops off the chain and the protein is finished. The single-stranded RNA molecule is prone to rapid degradation and therefore the amount of protein produced is closely regulated at the transcriptional level. The processes of transcription and translation are collectively known as gene expression.

The workhorse of the molecular biologist is the bacterium and as this is a prokaryotic organism, it cannot perform intron splicing. Therefore genomic DNA cannot be used for expression in these cells as the introns would also be translated leading to the production of a 'nonsense' protein. The instability of RNA limits its use as a template for expression in bacteria and so another form was required. Virologists, working on a group of viruses that carried their genetic information as RNA (the Retrovirus), discovered that the life cycle includes a conversion of the single-stranded RNA into a double-stranded analogue. The enzyme responsible for this

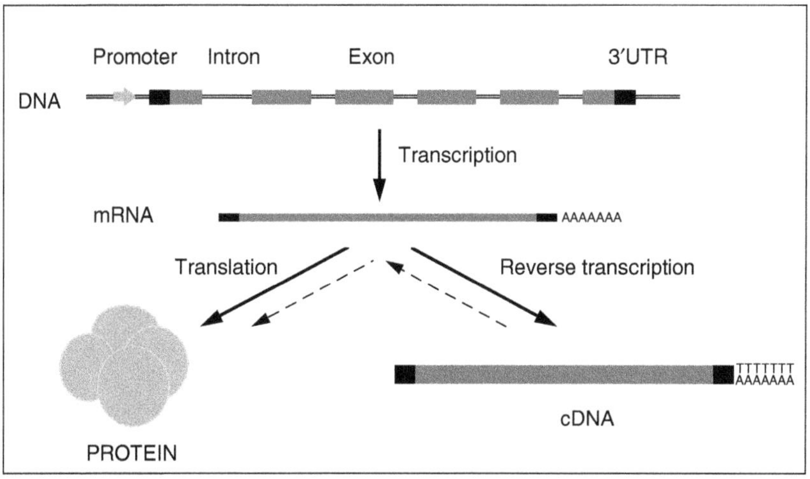

FIGURE 18.2 *The flow of genetic information from DNA (and cDNA) to protein.*

step was isolated and named *reverse transcriptase*. By using this enzyme, it is possible to convert eukaryotic mRNA into a more stable double-stranded molecule with the properties of DNA. This molecule is known as *complementary DNA (cDNA)* and is equivalent to the corresponding genomic DNA but without the introns or promoter. This can then be used for expression in a prokaryotic (or eukaryotic system). The relationship between DNA, RNA, cDNA and protein is shown in Figure 18.2. The underlying principle in genetic manipulation is that if you insert a fragment of DNA into a host cell, it will be duplicated as the cell divides and therefore you will increase the number of copies of your fragment. In order to perform this amplification, the DNA must be inserted into a suitable part of the host cell's genetic material so that it will be duplicated along with the endogenous DNA during cell division. DNA suitable for the insertion of foreign material is known as a vector; the most commonly used vectors are plasmids.

Plasmids are small (2–3 kb) loops of DNA found in bacteria and yeast. They were first discovered when it was noticed that bacteria could pass antibiotic resistance from one colony to another. This was shown to be mediated by plasmids containing genes for enzymes that de-activated the antibiotics. While plasmids were being investigated, other groups had isolated enzymes that cut DNA at specific sequences (restriction endonucleases) and other enzymes that could rejoin these cuts again (DNA ligases).

The principles of cloning are shown in Figure 18.3. Both vector and insert are cut with the same restriction enzyme, purified and then incubated together with a ligase that reforms the backbone of the plasmid. The resulting recombinant DNA is inserted into bacterial cells which then multiply. Each cell can contain 50–100

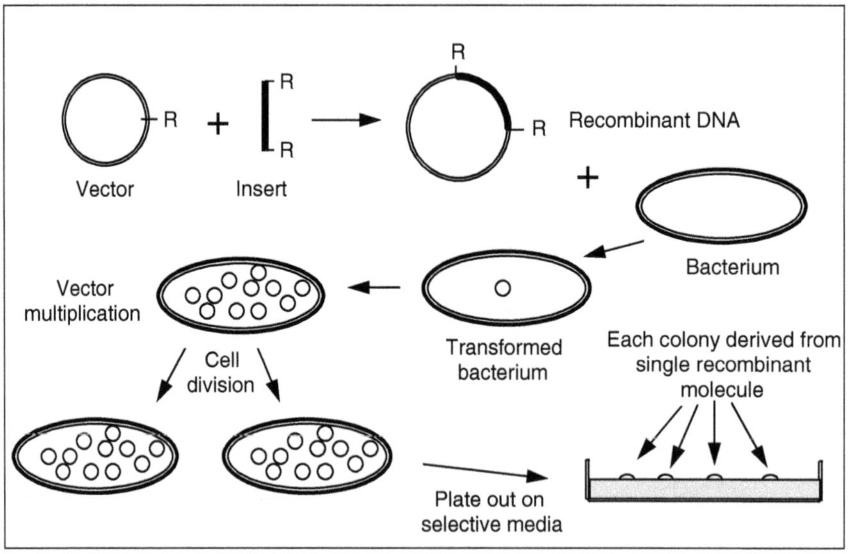

FIGURE 18.3 *Cloning and selection of recombinant DNA.*

copies of the recombinant plasmid and can duplicate every 20–30 minutes. Most plasmids have been engineered to contain one or more antibiotic resistance gene which protects the cells when they are grown on selective agar plates. Once selected, the cells can be grown up in liquid culture and the plasmids re-isolated, purified and studied further.

18.3 *Which enzyme?*

The identification of the route of metabolism is a key part of the regulatory package of a new drug compound and this work can be approached from two directions.

The first, and simplest option, is to use heterologous systems containing a single-expressed enzyme and examine if the drug is turned over in such a system. This approach allows the kinetics of the drug to be examined in isolation from any competing reactions.

The alternative approach is to look at the complete metabolism system, e.g. human liver microsomes, and to knockout single enzymes. By determining the metabolism that does not occur in the inhibited state, it is possible to extrapolate the role of that isoform in the metabolism of the compound. This approach can be achieved by the use of specific chemical inhibitors (e.g. ketoconazole for 3A4) or inhibitory antibodies raised to specific epitopes on the target enzyme and is discussed in other chapters in this volume. However, molecular biology will allow us to generate transgenically altered animals where the enzyme of interest has been removed (currently only available in mice).

18.4 *Expressed enzymes*

18.4.1 Introduction

Heterologously expressed enzymes have become important tools for the study of Phase I and Phase II drug metabolism. While the majority of the work has been focused on the cytochrome P450 family, the approach has successfully been utilised for the expression of sulphotransferases (STs), flavin mono-oxygenases (FMOs) and UDP glucuronosyltransferases (UGTs). The role of these enzymes in the activation and detoxification and clearance of xenobiotics make them important targets for understanding and predicting drug metabolism. In order to characterise the activity of these enzymes, it is necessary to produce quantities of pure protein, both for catalytic activity studies, the production of metabolites (bioreactors) and for the production of antibodies which can be used to characterise the levels of expression of the protein in other tissues.

Traditionally this has been achieved by isolating and purifying the enzymes from hepatic microsomes prepared from animals that had been pre-treated with inducing agents. The purification procedure involves a series of fractionation steps involving a range of gel-filtration and affinity columns. However, even after extensive purification, it is still not possible to separate closely related but distinct isoforms. This approach is not suitable for the isolation of human isoforms as the availability of human tissue for the preparation of microsomes is limited, and the induction of donors to enrich the levels of poorly expressed isoforms is both unethical and impractical. This problem has been addressed by several groups, and human drug-metabolising enzymes have been expressed in bacteria, yeast and cultured cell lines. This is known as heterologous expression as the gene from one species (e.g. man) is expressed in another (e.g. *Escherichia coli*).

Heterologous expression is extensively described in *Methods in Enzymology* (1996) vol. 27.

18.4.2 Why use expressed enzymes?

Expressed enzymes are becoming increasingly popular as tools for metabolism studies and are used to replace human liver microsomes (HLMs). Their utility can be identified by the following properties:

User-friendly – The enzymes are supplied as membrane preparations or purified protein and can therefore be used directly in existing metabolism incubation protocols.

High activity – Because each enzyme is overexpressed in the heterologous system there is a high specific activity. This is significant for isoforms expressed at a low level in human tissue. Expressed enzymes do not display inter-individual variation seen with HLMs.

Single enzyme in each batch – The lack of any competition between different isoforms within the heterologous system allows a more accurate assessment of the contribution of that isoform to the metabolism of the test compound.

The disadvantages of the systems should also be noted:

Environment – Heterologously expressed protein is not in the native environment (especially in the cell membranes of *E. coli*) and therefore may exhibit abnormal catalytic activity.

Specificity – Over-expression of enzymes can lead to a loss of substrate specificity and thus gives misleading profiles.

18.4.3 Choice of expression systems

The expression systems commonly used within industrial research can be divided into four main groups, determined by the host cell type. These are bacterial-based, yeast-based, insect cell-based and mammalian cell-based systems. The selection of the optimum cell system for the expression of drug-metabolising enzymes depends on a variety of factors. Some considerations for the expression of P450s are listed below and summarised in Table 18.1.

Mammalian P450s are membrane bound to either the SER or the mitochondrial inner membrane and require phospholipids to function normally. The NH_2-terminus of the protein contains a signal recognition/insertion sequence which both targets and anchors the protein to the appropriate membrane. This sequence does not play any further role in the catalytic activity of the enzyme, as the enzyme is still functional if the region has been deleted.

The cytochrome P450 enzyme requires a source of reducing agents and in the SER this is provided by NADPH-cytochrome P450 reductase (and in some cases cytochrome b_5). In the mitochondria, this is replaced by a two-component system consisting of adrenodoxin and NADPH-adrenodoxin reductase. A purified enzyme can be reconstituted to its active form *in vitro* by the addition of NADPH-cytochrome P450 reductase and phospholipids. The species from which the reductase is isolated is not crucial and heterologously expressed recombinant reductase has been successfully used in various reconstitution experiments.

Cytochrome P450 contains a non-covalently bound haem molecule and the expression system must be able to produce and insert the haem into the nascent enzyme if functional expression is to be achieved. There is therefore a requirement to supplement the culture with a suitable haem source such as D-amino levulinic acid or hemin Cl.

Table 18.1 *A comparison of expression systems and their suitability for P450 expression*

	Expression system			
Properties	**Mammalian**	**Insect**	**Yeast**	**Bacteria**
Vector system	Vaccinia	Baculovirus	Plasmid	Plasmid
Ease of culture	++	++	+++	+++
Expression levels (Hlms = 100%)	25%	200%	75%	300%
Haem incorporation	++	++	++	+++
Microsomal membranes	✓	✓	✓	5
Endogenous reductase	P450 reductase	P450 reductase	P450 reductase	Puteroredo xin
Endogenous P450s	+++	++	++	+

Cytochrome P450 is a globular protein and the host cell must have the ability to fold the protein correctly if a functional enzyme is to be produced.

Expression in bacteria

Bacterial expression

Bacteria, especially *E. coli*, are a good system for the expression of foreign proteins as, like yeast, it is well understood genetically and can be manipulated to suit the specific requirements. The cells can also be grown to high densities with ease. However, the bacteria have significant structural differences from the eukaryotic cells. There is no SER or NADPH-P450 reductase although a bacterial version is present and has been shown to have some activity with heterologous P450s.

Surprisingly, work with *E. coli* has shown that these differences are not insurmountable and several groups have reported the expression of functional P450s in such a system (see Table 18.2).

Cell types

E. coli

The work horses of bacterial expression are the variants of *E. coli* that have been developed for molecular biology. The principal strains used JM109 and DH5a which are both commercially available from most and can be used for general cloning work and expression. Another *E. coli*-derived cell line is BL21(DE3) which is specifically designed for use with the T7 promotor system. The majority of bacterial expression listed in Table 18.2 utilises these strains.

Salmonella typhimurium

This is the strain used in the Ames assay for mutagenic compounds and their metabolites. Traditionally compounds are incubated with rat S9 fraction and the resulting metabolites tested for their abilities to revert *S. typhimurium* mutants back to wild type. By transforming these mutants with a recombinant P450 it is possible to re-create the assay without the need for S9. This approach has been used to express human CYP1A2 in T1538.

Bacterial expression protocols

Protocols for the expression of P450s in bacteria are reviewed by Barnes (1996) and are based on the methods devised by Gillam *et al.* (1993).

Expression in yeast

Yeast expression

Yeast systems have the advantage of well-characterised genetics and ease of growth in large volumes. There are also endogenous reductase systems and SER membranes with which the expressed proteins can associate. This system has been used successfully to produce a wide range of P450s (see *Methods in Enzymology*, **206**, pp. 132–133) including human CYP2C9, 2C10 and 3A4. The catalytic rates of the expressed enzymes for specific probe substrates are comparable to those in human liver microsomes (Masimirembwa *et al.*, 1999).

Cell types

Saccharomyces cerevisiae

This is the most common strain of yeast used for the expression of P450s and other enzymes. There have been some reports of poor haem incorporation but these are in a minority.

It is possible to make stable yeast clones where multiple copies of the human cDNAs are incorporated into the yeast genome. Co-expression of OR and cytochrome b_5 is also stably incorporated to give functional expression systems.

Pichia pastoralis

A new system utilising *P. pastoralis* has recently been developed by invitrogen and claims to give higher yields than existing systems although this has yet to be tried for P450 expression.

Yeast expression protocols

Yeast expression protocols are described by Masimirembwa *et al.* (1999). The heterologous P450s are inserted into the yeast ER and therefore standard microsomal preparation techniques may be employed for their recovery once the cell wall is broken. This can be achieved by the addition of a yeast lytic enzyme (e.g. zymolase).

Expression in baculovirus

Insect cell expression systems

The baculovirus expression system is a highly effective system for the large-scale production of recombinant proteins in insect cells. The major attraction of baculovirus as an expression vector system was originally the virus-encoded polyhedrin and *p10* genes.

These genes produce large amounts of polyhedrin and *p10* proteins in virus-infected insect cells in the later stages of the virus replication cycle. The polyhedrin protein, controlled by the *polh* promoter, is required in the normal infection cycle to package virus particles within occlusion bodies or polyhedra, which protect the virus particles in the environment between susceptible hosts.

The function of the *p10* protein is not clear as yet but it is thought to be involved in polyhedra formation and is controlled by the *p10* promoter. Polyhedrin and *p10* are not required to maintain an infection in cultured cells *in vitro*. The polyhedrin

TABLE 18.2 *Expression of human drug metabolising enzymes in different host cells*

Enzyme	Bacteria	Yeast	Baculovirus	Mammalian COS cells, CHO, V79, HepG2/ Vaccinia	β-Lymphoblastoid
CYP1A1	Guo *et al.*, 1994	Eugster *et al.*, 1990	Buters *et al.*, 1995	McManus *et al.*, 1990	Crespi *et al.*, 1993
CYP1A2	Fisher *et al.*, 1992	Eugster and Sengstag, 1993	Christopherson *et al.*, 1995	Aoyama *et al.*, 1989a; McManus *et al.*, 1990	Crespi *et al.*, 1990a
CYP1B1	Shimada *et al.*, 1998	Fujita *et al.*, 2001	Crespi and Miller, 1999		Crespi *et al.*, 1997
CYP2A6	Kushida *et al.*, 2000	Lessard *et al.*, 1997	Grogan *et al.*, 1995	Yamano *et al.*, 1989a; Miles *et al.*, 1990	Crespi *et al.*, 1991
CYP2B6	Gervot *et al.*, 1999	Gervot *et al.*, 1999	Roy *et al.*, 1999	Yamano *et al.*, 1989b	Chang *et al.*, 1993
CYP2C8	Richardson *et al.*, 1995	Srivastava *et al.*, 1991	Zeldin *et al.*, 1995	Veronese *et al.*, 1993; Rettie *et al.*, 1994	Crespi *et al.*, 1993
CYP2C9	Sandhu *et al.*, 1993	Yasumori *et al.*, 1989	Grogan *et al.*, 1995	Veronese *et al.*, 1993; Rettie *et al.*, 1994	Crespi *et al.*, 1993
CYP2C18	Richardson *et al.*, 1995	Goldstein *et al.*, 1994	Crespi and Miller, 1999	Furuya *et al.*, 1991	
CYP2C19	Richardson *et al.*, 1995	Goldstein *et al.*, 1994	Christopherson *et al.*, 1995		Crespi and Miller, 1999
CYP2D6	Gillam *et al.*, 1995a	Ellis *et al.*, 1992	Christopherson *et al.*, 1995	Tyndale *et al.*, 1991	Penman *et al.*, 1993

CYP2E1	Gillam *et al.*, 1994		Patten and Koch, 1995	Patten *et al.*, 1992; Tassaneeyakul *et al.*, 1993	Crespi *et al.*, 1990b
CYP3A4	Gillam *et al.*, 1993	Renaud *et al.*, 1990	Lee *et al.*, 1995	Aoyama *et al.*, 1989b; Ball *et al.*, 1992	Crespi *et al.*, 1991
CYP3A5	Gillam *et al.*, 1995b	Fujita *et al.*, 2001	Crespi and Miller, 1999	Aoyama *et al.*, 1989b; Ball *et al.*, 1992	
CYP4A11	Palmer *et al.*, 1993		Imaoka *et al.*, 1993	Imaoka *et al.*, 1993	Crespi and Miller, 1999
UDPGT	Ouzzine *et al.*, 1994		Sheen *et al.*, 1998	Ouzzine *et al.*, 1999; Forsman *et al.*, 2000	
SULT	Guengerich *et al.*, 1996		Falany *et al.*, 2000		
FMO	Cashman *et al.*, 1997	Itoh *et al.*, 1993	Haining *et al.*, 1997		
MAO	Lu *et al.*, 1996	Miller and Edmondson, 1999	Rebrin *et al.*, 2001		
NAT	Delomenie *et al.*, 1997			Blum *et al.*, 1990; Yanagawa *et al.*, 1994	
GST	Thier *et al.*, 1995	Cho *et al.*, 2001			

and *p10* genes can be replaced with foreign gene sequences and thus express recombinant protein from the polyhedrin (*polh*) and *p10* (*p10*) promoters.

The insect cell-baculovirus expression system provides a eukaryotic environment that is generally conducive to the proper folding, disulphide bond formation, oligomerisation and/or other post-translation modifications required for the biological activity of some eukaryotic proteins. These modifications are performed using insect cell-derived sugars and are therefore near-authentic versions of the original proteins.

The baculovirus insect cell system has been used for the expression of several P450 enzymes (see Table 18.2) and is the method of choice for the generation of high-activity microsomes (Crespi and Miller, 1999).

Insect host cell types

Insect cell lines can be obtained from commercial suppliers or from the American type culture collection (Rockville, MD).

Spodoptera frugiperda

S. frugiperda is the fall army worm and the most common insect cell donor and is found as the *SF9* and *SF21* cell lines. These cells are used to grow, maintain and titre baculovirus stocks and can be used for enzyme expression.

Tricoplusia ni

T. ni is the cabbage looper worm and its cells are smaller and more adaptable to fermentation as they can be grown to higher density than SF9 cells (Lee *et al.*, 1995).

Drosophilla melanogaster

Drosophilla has been the basis of genetic studies for decades and is therefore well understood. This has lead to the development of stably transfected (transgenic) *Drosophilla* cells. The advantage of these cells is that they do not need a virus system for expression and are therefore easier to maintain. This has been proposed as a possible *in vivo* model for various isoforms but it would be more difficult to extract pure enzymes due to the multicellular nature and size of the insect (Jowett *et al.*, 1991).

Baculovirus expression protocols

The handling of insect cells requires cell culture facilities and good aseptic technique, and the cultures are prone to fungal and bacterial infections. The heterologous P450s are inserted into the ER membranes of the insect cells and therefore standard microsomal preparation techniques may be employed for their recovery. The insect cells are robust and can be cultured in large volume sparged fermenters designed for bacterial production. This has allowed cultures up to 50 L to be fermented, harvested and 2 g of microsomal protein isolated from a single batch.

Protocols for generation and maintenance of baculovirus stocks, and the expression and scale up of insect cell can be found in Hood *et al.* (1998).

Expression in mammalian cells

Mammalian expression systems

Mammalian cell systems most closely resemble the *in vivo* environment of the enzyme and as such are potentially the most likely to produce the protein in its functional state.

The main disadvantage is the cells have endogenous P450s which may interfere with the purification of the enzyme and give a background activity in microsomal catalytic studies. The cells may also show low expression of the P450s and poor haem incorporation. Therefore, scale up for isolation of protein can be both costly and difficult to engineer (Crespi and Miller, 1999).

Cell types and vectors

COS cells

These cells are derived from an African green monkey kidney cell line (CV-1) that has been immortalised with SV40 viral DNA. This cell line produces the SV40 T antigen which allows plasmids containing the SV40 origin to replicate and express in this cell line. The most common vector used is the pCMV system which contains the promotor from the cytomegalovirus (Clark and Waterman, 1991).

HepG2

These cells are derived from a human hepatoma and are well characterised in the literature. They can be transformed using a plasmid system, but the main utilisation has been for vaccinia virus-mediated expression.

These cells are lysed during the expression process and can therefore only be used for membrane preparations. There is also a risk inherent in the infective nature of the virus that requires special containment to prevent operator exposure.

V79/CHO

These cells are derived from lung fibroblasts and ovaries of the Chinese hamster, respectively. The expression is driven by an SV40-containing plasmid which can result in a stable expression of the enzyme of choice. The non-lytic nature of this system allows the use of whole cells for toxicology and bioreactor experiments.

NIH 3T3

This is another fibroblast-derived cell line that can be transformed using the vaccinia virus system.

β-Lymphoblastoid

The AHH-1 human β-lymphoblastoid cell line has been transformed using epstein barr virus (EBV)-based vectors. This system has been used to express single and multiple P450s and was the basis of the first commercially available recombinant microsomes (Crespi *et al.*, 1993).

Caco-2/MDCK

Epithelial cell monolayers are now routinely being used as models of intestinal permeability for drug candidates, and common cell lines are MDCK, Caco-2 and LLC-PK. In native intestinal cells, high levels of CYP3A4 are expressed and act as a metabolic barrier, but the cell models lack such an expression level. Using the vector systems developed for CYP3A4 expression β-lymphoblastoid cells, Crespi *et al.* (2000) have developed cell lines that are metabolically closer to the endogenous gut epithelia.

Expression protocols

The culture conditions vary with the vector:cell line combinations, and protocols can be obtained from the references cited above. Cells can be used as intact bioreactors or to be processed to microsomal membranes for use in metabolism studies.

Care must be taken to minimise the risk of contamination, both from the environment into the cell culture and, in the cases of the virally transformed cells, from the cell culture to the operator.

Applications of expressed enzymes

Drug metabolism and enzyme inhibition studies

The principal uses of recombinant enzymes are the determination of route of metabolism and the assessment of the inhibitory potential of candidate drugs. Both areas are reviewed extensively in the literature (Crespi and Miller, 1999; Masimirembwa *et al.*, 1999). Care must be taken to ensure that the recombinant enzyme selected has the appropriate kinetic parameters (Clarke, 1998) and that it is compatible with the *in vitro* system in which it is studied.

Bioreactors

Bioreactors are growing cultures of cells expressing endogenous or heterologous enzymes that can be used to metabolise drug compounds to their metabolites. The advantages of bioreactors over conventional incubations are as follows.

Because the cells are growing, the culture can be sustained for longer periods of time and therefore a higher yield of metabolites can be obtained. This is especially useful if the rate of metabolite formation is slow.

Cultures can be scaled up to allow the extraction of enough low-abundance metabolite for structural determination (NMR, MS).

Bioreactors can also perform reactions that are difficult to reproduce by synthetic chemistry and are therefore invaluable for the production of authentic metabolite standards and drug products. The most common recombinant bioreactor systems are based on whole, baculovirus-infected insect cells and primary hepatocytes from various species. The drive for hepatocyte bioreactor is the result of research into artificial livers.

Site-directed mutagenesis (SDM)

The development of expression systems that can produce functional P450 protein from a cDNA has allowed the manipulation of the proteins by site-directed mutagenesis. This is a process where the sequence of the cDNA is deliberately altered to change the protein structure of the encoded enzyme. This technique has had three main applications in the field of drug metabolism.

Correction of cloning artefacts

During the late 1980s there was a race to isolate, sequence and publish the gene sequences for P450 enzymes. In the rush to publish, mistakes were made and retractions printed. Some of these mistakes were due to cloning errors which were subsequently corrected by SDM.

A significant example of such a mix up concerned the cDNA for human CYP2D6 where two forms existed, differing by a valine to methionine change at amino acid residue 374. While the enzymes appeared to have the same catalytic activity, studies with the probe substrate metoprolol and comparison to a human liver bank showed that the 374 met form was the correct one and that the 374 val form was probably a cloning artefact (Ellis *et al.*, 1996). The validated gene sequences are now available on the bioinformatics databases and a list of accession numbers is periodically updated (Nelson *et al.*, 1996).

Modelling of enzyme active sites

The ability to change individual residues has allowed extensive modelling of the active site of enzymes. This has led to a greater understanding of the interaction between enzymes and substrates, allowing rational drug design.

Producing soluble for crystallisation studies

In order to obtain good crystals, the protein must be reasonably soluble in a pure form, a problem for mammalian P450s which tend to form insoluble precipitates when removed from the membrane environment.

Recently, this problem has been overcome by a combination of removing the membrane anchor region and mutation surface residues to make them more polar. Using this approach Cosme and Johnson (2000) have managed to produce crystals for the rabbit CYP2C5, the first mammalian P450 to be studied in this way.

Immobilised P450s for biosensors

One application of expressed enzymes is that of biosensors, where an enzyme is immobilised to a chip and activity determined electronically. The complex membrane requirements of drug-metabolising enzymes (especially P450s) have hindered progress in this area as a lipid membrane is difficult to build onto a chip.

A novel solution has been proposed by Sligar and his group (Bayburt *et al.*, 1998) where the membrane is enclosed by a border of the HDL protein apolipoprotein A1. This form 'Nanodiscs' of membrane ranging from 7 to 19 nm in diameter into which P450 and reductase molecules can be inserted. These nanodiscs then provide a means of attaching the enzymes to the surface of a chip.

Transgenic organisms

The development of transgenic technologies has allowed the study of gene function in the whole organism (animal or plant). Such studies have taken the form of gene addition (transgenics), gene deletions (knockouts), gene substitutions (knockins) or nuclear transfer (cloning). The methodology and application of these methods to DMPK is discussed below.

Gene additions: transgenics

Gene additions enable the study of the protein in a whole organism. This can take the form of the over-expression of an endogenous protein or insertion of a gene from another species into a host organism to study the effect against the endogenous background. Such approaches have been used to study the effects of human P450 (Imaoka *et al.*, 2001) in mice. Human P450s expressed in plants have been used in bio-remuneration and detoxification.

Transgenics are produced by the method of *pro-nuclear injection*. Fertilised eggs are removed from the donor animal and the pro-nucleus is injected with a vector containing the gene of interest. The egg is implanted into a surrogate mother and the transgene integrates randomly into the host genome. The resulting off-spring will express the foreign gene in a site-dependent manner and not necessarily at a level proportional to the number of copies integrated into the genome.

Gene deletions: knockouts

The ultimate way to inhibit an enzyme is to delete its expression from the test organism. This can be done by utilising transgenic knockout techniques. This method has been widely used to study the function of enzymes, nuclear hormone receptors and transport proteins (Nebert and Duffy, 1997).

The method of choice for knockouts utilises embryonic stem cells. The gene for the enzyme to be knocked out is identified in an embryonic stem cell line. Using homologous recombination the gene is disrupted (usually by the insertion of a selectable marker), and the modified stem cells are injected into an embryonic host. The embryos are then allowed to mature into adult animals and the knockout is assessed. Using selective breeding, a line of animals can be produced with both of the genomic copies of the gene deleted. These animals can then be used in routine *in vivo* and *in vitro* experiments to determine the effect of the knockout. This technique is currently confined to mice due to the difficulty of culturing embryonic stem cells from other organisms, although true rat ES cells may be available soon.

Gene substitution: knockins

Knockins use the same methodology as knockouts but instead of deleting the target gene, it is replaced with a new gene. This new gene may be a mutated version of the target gene, allowing the study of a polymorphism in an animal model. Another application is to replace the host gene with one from another species which has allowed the 'humanisation' of mice where the effects of the human gene can then be studied in a mouse model (Xie *et al.*, 2000).

Nuclear transfer

The field of nuclear transfer or 'cloning' is new and under the media spotlight. After the arrival of Dolly the Sheep, Gene the Calf, Copy Cat and cloned mice in Hawaii, the media and scientific press are full of the ethical and practical issues surrounding this technology. The application of cloning to DMPK will develop, once the ethical barriers have been resolved.

18.5 *Induction or suppression?*

18.5.1 Background

Drug-metabolising enzymes can be modulated by the action of compounds on nuclear receptors. This can lead to significant drug–drug interactions where the metabolism of one drug is affected by the co-administration of a second. These changes can be detected at various stages of the protein expression. Increases in protein amounts can be detected by Western blotting, ELISA and proteomic techniques.

Increases in the mRNA levels (translational regulation) can be detected by Northern blotting, RT-PCR, Riboprobes, RNA protection assays, differential gene expression and Northern ELISA techniques.

Finally regulation at a transcriptional level can be detected with the use of reporter gene constructs.

The majority of these techniques can be performed with commercially available kits, as per the manufacturer's protocols.

18.5.2 Determination of changes in protein levels

Western blotting

Western blotting is a method of identifying a specific protein that has been separated on an acrylamide gel, transferred to a nylon membrane and then detected using a specific antibody. This antibody is then detected with a second antibody, labelled with radioactivity or an enzyme that can be detected with a coloured substrate.

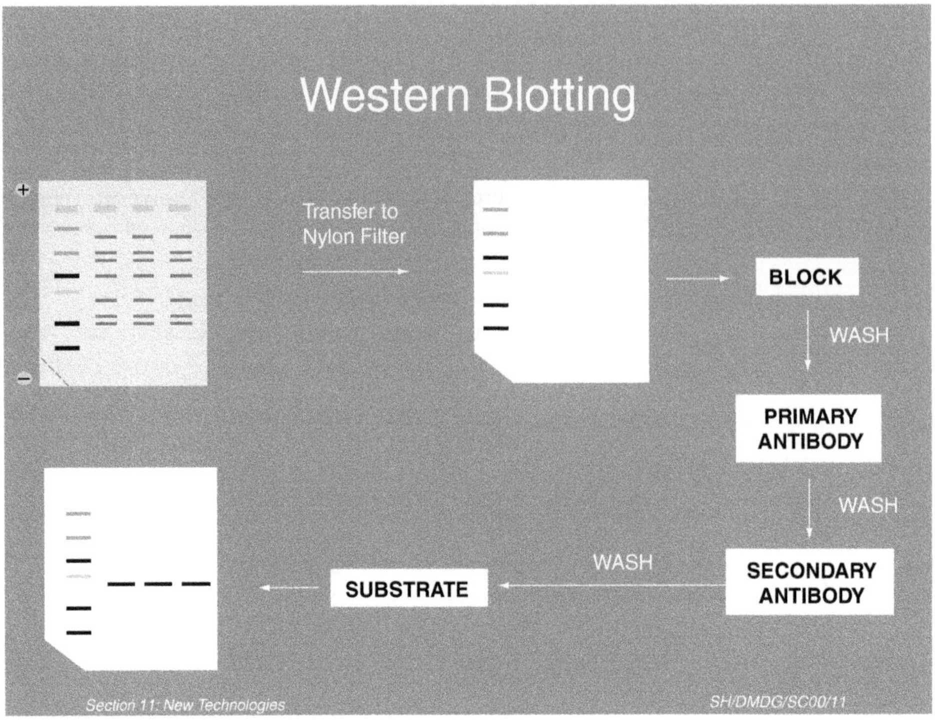

FIGURE 18.4 *Western blotting.*

As the amount of antibody binding to the membrane is proportional to the amount of specific protein, this method can be semi-quantitative, providing that a suitable analysis system is utilised to determine the band intensities (densitometer or image analyser). This process is illustrated in Figure 18.4.

Enzyme-linked immunosorbent assay (ELISA)

ELISA is a variation of the Western blot where the protein to be determined is immobilised to the surface of a microtitre well and then detected by the addition of an antibody specific to the protein of interest. A second, enzyme-labelled, antibody is then used to detect the first. Using a range of substrates which give coloured or chemiluminescent products, the concentration of the protein can be determined to some accuracy.

Due to the 96-well microtitre format of this assay it is possible to run several samples and a standard curve simultaneously. Using automated plate washers and readers, it is possible to get accurate readings of specific protein abundance. This will give numerical data on the induction of enzymes at a protein level.

For more details see 'Immunoassay: A Practical Guide', B. Law (ed.) (1996), ISBN 0–7484–0560–7.

Proteomics

Proteomics is a technique that combines gel electrophoresis and MS analysis to identify changes in the levels of expression of all the proteins in a given biological sample (Yoshida *et al.*, 2001). This technique is currently being used to 'fingerprint' the expression changes in cells following exposure to toxic compounds in the hope that a few 'key' proteins can be identified as markers of toxicity.

Proteins are separated from a biological matrix by two-dimensional gel electrophoresis. The proteins are first separated by their net charge using isoelectric focussing on an immobilised pH gradient (IPG) strip. The strip is then placed in contact with a polyacrylamide gel and the proteins are then separated by molecular weight using standard PAGE methods. The resulting spots of protein can then be sampled, analysed by TOF MS and identified against a database of known protein structures. By comparing gels from control and induced cells, it is possible to determine the changes in protein expression profiles.

18.5.3 Determination of changes in mRNA levels

Polymerase chain reaction (PCR)

The polymerase chain reaction (PCR) has become a core technique for molecular biologists and has allowed the development of several assays applicable to drug metabolism. PCR allows the logarithmic amplification of a specific double-stranded sequence of DNA from a background of other genes, proteins and cell debris.

The reaction is divided into three stages (see Figure 18.5):

Denaturation – The two strands in the target DNA are separated by heating the reaction mixture to >95 °C.

Annealing – Oligonucleotide primers bind to the ends of the template DNA. These primers are designed to bind specifically to these sequences.

Elongation – The polymerase enzyme makes a copy of each strand using the primers as a starting point until the target sequence has been duplicated. The cycle then repeats with the newly copied versions of the target DNA acting as template for the next cycle. As each cycle doubles the number of double-stranded template, the product increases exponentially. Reactions are run for a minimum of 25 cycles which results in 2^{24} copies of each original template molecule.

This technique has been made possible by the discovery of thermostable polymerases that can withstand the repeated heating and cooling during the cycling of the reaction. The reactions themselves are run in precision-controlled heating blocks which can change temperature quickly and accurately and can be

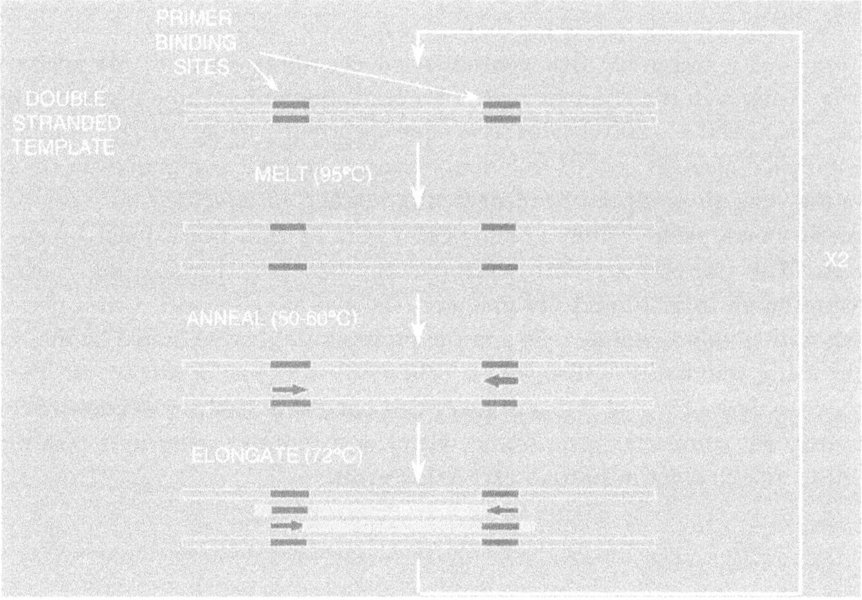

FIGURE 18.5 *The PCR amplification process.*

programmed for complex cycle profiles. For extensive methods, see PCR Protocols: Methods in Molecular Biology, 15 (1993), B. White (ed.).

RT-PCR

As described previously, PCR requires double-stranded DNA to act as a template for the amplification reaction and since mRNA is single stranded, it is therefore not suitable for direct amplification by PCR. This problem can be overcome by the use of a reverse-transcriptase enzyme which synthesises the complementary strand to the mRNA, thus creating a double-stranded template for the PCR reaction.

This reaction has been optimised in a series of kits, and single polymerases have been discovered that will perform the RT and PCR steps, thus making it a one-tube reaction.

Such a technique can be used to detect very low levels of a specific mRNA from a tissue sample or cell culture. This technique has been used successfully in the evaluation of gene therapy products.

Quantitative RT-PCR

The use of RT-PCR to determine changes in mRNA levels is becoming widespread within drug metabolism and toxicology. The advantage of the technique is that only a small amount of starting material (tissue or cell culture) is required to provide the template for the reaction. This allows a higher throughput to be achieved in induction studies (Morris and Davila, 1996). In most methods, the changes in the amount of mRNA are normalised against a control mRNA, whose expression level remains constant. These controls are usually the mRNA for 'housekeeping' genes such as glyceraldehyde phosphate dehydrogenase (GAPDH) or b-actin. It should be noted that the levels of expression of these proteins may vary on xenobiotic challenge and must be closely monitored.

The original method of analysis for the RT-PCR products was to run them on a gel and determine the staining intensity by desitometry on image analysis. This approach was limited by the poor linearity of the stain intensity over a concentration range. Also, because the concentration of the products increases sigmoidaly, linearity is lost at higher concentrations.

To overcome these problems, real-time measurement of product formation was developed utilising fluorescent dyes to monitor the progress of the reaction. Two approaches have been utilised.

Incorporation of intercollating dyes – Fluorescent dyes such as ethidium bromide and *sybr green* only bind to double-stranded DNA and can therefore be used to follow the production of the double-stranded products in a PCR reaction. This approach has been used in the development of the LightCycler system by Roche Molecular Biochemicals.

Use of dye-labelled primers – An alternative approach, called *Taqman*, has been developed by applied biosystems and utilises a dye-labelled primer which hybridises within the PCR product. One end of the primer is labelled with a fluorescent dye and the other with a second dye which acts as a quencher. In its native state, the light emitted from the first dye is absorbed by the second one, thus giving no signal. During the PCR reaction the primer is degraded by the polymerase and the reporter dye then dissociates from the quenching and is free to fluoresce.

Because both these techniques allow for real-time measurement of PCR product formation, the rate of formation can be estimated from the linear part of the curve (Figure 18.6). This leads to a more accurate determination of original copy number and therefore mRNA induction. By comparing against a standard curve, it is possible to calculate the amount of starting target mRNA in each sample.

Riboprobes

Riboprobes are short lengths (150–300 bp) of single-stranded RNA used as specific probes for an mRNA of interest. The sequence of the cDNA of interest is examined by computer to identify areas that are specific to that gene. Care must be taken in selecting a region that has a sequence unique to the gene of interest. Such a region is usually found in the 3′ non-coding region (3′-NCR) where the homology between genes is low.

This region is then cloned (usually by PCR) into a vector whose multiple cloning site is flanked by the promoters for RNA polymerase (most commercial vectors have

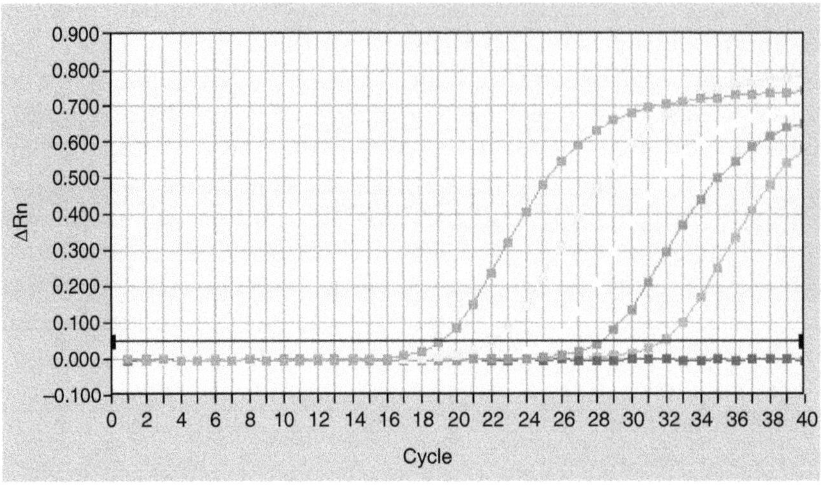

FIGURE 18.6 *A typical standard curve plot from a Taqman run showing the threshold line from which the cycle number is calculated.*

this configuration). Utilising an *in vitro* transcription kit, it is possible to produce the riboprobe in both the sense and anti-sense strands. Incorporation of labelled nucleotides in the polymerisation mix allows the production of labelled riboprobes. These probes can then be hybridised to the target mRNA and thus used to detect the presence of the mRNA in a sample (Rae *et al.*, 2001).

Riboprobes may be used to determine mRNA concentration (see below) or used in *in situ* hybridisation to locate the expression of the mRNA within a tissue of interest. The latter approach has been used extensively to map the regulation of gene expression in developmental biology.

RNase protection assay

The RNase protection assay is another method of quantifying the levels of a specific mRNA extracted from a tissue (see Figure 18.7).

A riboprobe is designed to a short region of the target mRNA and is labelled (usually with a ^{32}P dCTP). Total mRNA is extracted from the tissue and the probe is added and allowed to hybridise to the target message. The mRNA is then treated with RNAse, which selectively degrades single-stranded RNA. The mRNA/probe hybrid is double stranded and is therefore not degraded in this digest. The digestion products are run on an SDS-PAGE gel, imaged by autoradiography and the amount of probe/mRNA hybrid is quantified against known standard. This allows a semi-quantitative determination of the concentration of the target mRNA in the tissue of interest (Rae *et al.*, 2001). This technique requires the generation of highly labelled probes and non-radioactive versions of this method have been developed to reduce the amount of radioactivity utilised.

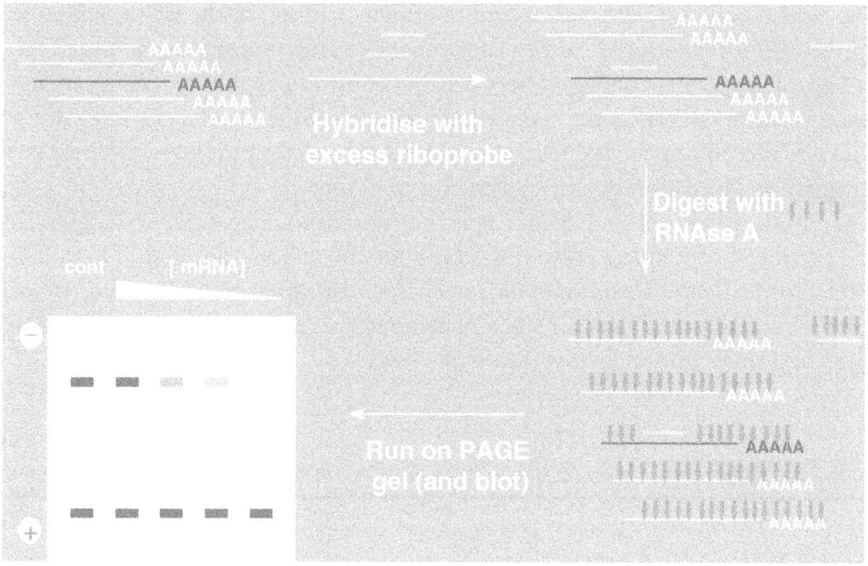

FIGURE 18.7 *The RNase protection assay.*

Northern ELISA

Northern ELISA is a technique under development from Bohringer Manheim which combines riboprobes and ELISA to give a more quantifiable readout. It is currently experimental and little data exists on its utility for drug metabolism studies.

Differential gene expression (DGE)

Differential gene expression is a hybridisation technique that allows the comparison of the mRNA levels in a specific tissue from different individuals or from different tissues in the same individual. This enables the study of the modulation of mRNA in induced or diseased animals. The developing technologies of radioactive and non-radioactive imaging coupled with powerful image analysis software have enabled thousands of genes to be studied in a single experiment. If the number of genes of interest is small it is possible to simplify this procedure to a 96-well format. Efforts are also underway to reduce the scale even more and by incorporation of microchip technology, develop a 'metabolism' and 'tox chip'.

The following example is for the study of genes regulated by an inducing agent. A representative cDNA library for the tissue of interest (e.g. liver) is gridded out in duplicate onto two nylon membranes. The livers from control and induced animals are removed and mRNA isolated. The mRNA is converted to cDNA and radiolabelled or fluorescently labelled nucleotides incorporated in the process.

The labelled cDNA from the control liver is hybridised to the first membrane and the cDNA from the induced liver to the other one. The intensity of the signal on each of the gridded spots is compared between the control and induced samples, and the imaging software identifies the spots where there is a difference in the intensity of the signal. The identity of the induced gene can then be determined by referring back to the original gridded library and sequencing the clone.

If the study is only interested in a specific subset of genes, smaller 'focused' arrays can be produced containing only the cDNAs for the genes of interest. This allows for simpler and quicker analysis and lends itself for adaptation to a microchip format. A popular version of this is the Clonetech Atlas array that covers many drug-metabolising enzymes and transcription factors (Rae *et al.*, 2001).

18.5.4 Determination of changes in gene transcription

Reporter gene assays

Reporter systems allow the study of gene regulation at a transcriptional level. The promoter of the gene to be studied is cloned in front of the cDNA for a protein, usually an enzyme, whose activity can be easily determined. The promoter/reporter construct can then be introduced to a cell line or hepatocyte and used as a testy for the induction of the target gene. Compounds that would normally modulate the target gene will now have the same effect on the reporter gene and therefore such modulation can be determined (Figure 18.8). Common reporter genes include chloramphenecol acetyl transferase (CAT), secreted placental alkaline phosphatase (SPAP), luciferase and green fluorescent protein (GFP).

For a reporter system to be representative of the true *in vivo* regulation of the gene the complete promoter/enhancer region must be mapped and cloned. This is not a trivial

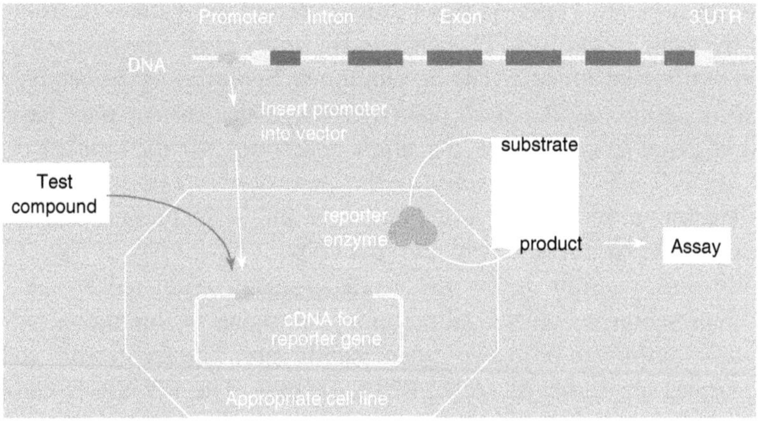

FIGURE 18.8 *Basis of reporter gene assay.*

task as many genes are controlled by several regulatory elements, some of which may be found at a significant distance from the promoter region. To date, therefore, reporter systems have been confined to a few enzymes (CYP1A, 2B, 3A and 4A). The use of these reporter genes to study enzyme induction is reviewed by Masimirembwa *et al.* (2001).

18.6 *Population genetics and polymorphisms*

18.6.1 Introduction to polymorphisms

The phrase 'no two people are the same' has been confirmed by the Human Genome Sequencing project where the structure and regulation of human genes are being determined. During this project inter-individual differences in the gene sequences, called as single nucleotide polymorphisms (SniPs for short), have been identified and used to map the chromosomes on which they occur. By comparing the distribution of these SNPs with known disease states, it is becoming possible to find connections and possible causes of these problems.

Genetic polymorphisms in drug-metabolising enzymes and endogenous targets have been shown to affect both the efficacy and safety of a variety of prescription medicines. As the nucleic acid sequence of the human genome is determined, our understanding of the importance of genetic polymorphisms on the pharmacokinetics and pharmacodynamics of a drug is increasing. This knowledge has lead to the development of simple genotyping tests that can help predict the disposition and/or efficacy of a drug prior to administration. Genotyping technology will impact the drug development process in the following ways:

1 Enable one to predict and understand the pharmacokinetic and pharmacodynamic variability due to polymorphic drug-metabolising enzymes, receptors and other molecular targets.
2 Used in disease diagnosis to confirm that the disease-causing mutation is present in patient being treated; the relevance of polymorphisms in drug-metabolising enzymes is reviewed by Nebert.

18.6.2 Polymorphisms and microheterogeneity

It is important to note that not all phenotypic differences seen in the metabolism of xenobiotics are due to genetic polymorphisms. Inter-individual variation due to expression levels of the same 'wild type' gene can lead to significant differences in the rates of metabolism for probe drugs. Such variation is described as microheterogeneity and are less easy to assay for.

18.6.3 Polymorphisms in drug-metabolising enzymes

Modern genetic analysis is continually expanding the list of known polymorphism in drug-metabolising enzymes. Some of these mutations result in coding changes while others are located in the regulatory regions of the gene and cause differences in basal expression levels and inducibility. The most common polymorphic forms are:

CYP2C19

The polymorphisms of CYP2C19 and their detection are discussed in Goldstein and de Morais (1994).

CYP2D6

The polymorphisms of CYP2D6 and their detection are discussed in Sachse *et al.* (1997).

CYP2C9

The polymorphisms of CYP2C9 and their detection are discussed in Stubbins *et al.* (1996).

CYP2E1

The polymorphisms of CYP2E1 and their detection are discussed in Powell *et al.* (1998).

18.6.4 Detection of polymorphisms

Sequencing

Once an SNP has been identified, work is done to determine the frequency of this polymorphism in a given population. This is usually done by obtaining genomic DNA from hundreds of individuals and re-sequencing the part of the genomic DNA containing the mutation. If the donors are part of a clinical trial panel or from a liver bank it may be possible to determine if the SNP is associated with a specific phenotypic change.

Once the SNP has been identified, it is possible to detect it with a variety of analytical techniques and thus build a polymorphism screen. These techniques include restriction fragment length polymorphism (RFLP) analysis, amplification refractory mutation system (ARMS), single-strand conformation polymorphism (SSCP) and the use of gene chips.

RFLP

RFLP analysis was the first technique developed to identify SNPs. It relies on the SNP creating or removing a restriction enzyme site and is therefore not applicable for all polymorphisms. A fragment spanning the SNP is amplified by PCR and then digested with the appropriate enzyme. The digests are run on an agarose or polyacrylamide gel, and if an SNP is present in one or both of the alleles a differential banding pattern will be observed. This technique is widely used in the identification of the multiple CYP2D6 alleles (Daly *et al.*, 1998).

ARMS

The ARMS is a PCR-based method which allows the detection of SNPs directly from the genomic DNA. For a PCR reaction to be successful, the 3′-end of the primer must be exactly the same as the target sequence. A mismatch in this position will lead to a failure of the polymerase to elongate the new strand and no product will be formed.

Two primers are made which match the DNA sequence immediately adjacent to the SNP site with the last base of the primer complementary to the wild type or the mutant sequence. If the target DNA contains the SNP of interest, a PCR product will be obtained from the mutant primer but not the wild type. If there is no polymorphism present then the pattern will be reversed. This technique has been used successfully to identify polymorphisms in CYP2C9 (Stubbins *et al.*, 1996).

SSCP

SSCP relies on the physical properties of the PCR-amplified fragments. The rate of migration of the single-stranded fragment through a polyacrylamide gel is determined by its sequence, and by comparing the banding patterns under different gel conditions it is possible to identify polymorphic variants. SSCP has been used to identify polymorphisms in CYP2C9 (Stubbins *et al.*, 1996).

Gene chips

Gene chips rely on determining the sequence of the target DNA by hybridisation to fluorescently labelled oligonucleotides. The oligonucleotides are designed to bind the DNA around the site of the SNP and can detect mismatches caused by polymorphisms. As it is possible to look for multiple SNP from a single DNA sample spotted onto a chip, this method may offer a considerable increase in throughput and the possibility of automated genotyping from a single drop of blood.

18.7 References

Aoyama, T., Gonzalez, F.J. and Gelboin, H.V. (1989a) Human cDNA-expressed cytochrome P450 IA2: mutagen activation and substrate specificity. *Mol. Carcinog.* 2(4), 192–198.

Aoyama, T., Yamano, S., Waxman, D.J., Lapenson, D.P., Meyer, U.A., Fischer, V., Tyndale, R., Inaba, T., Kalow, W. and Gelboin, H.V. (1989b) Cytochrome P-450 hPCN3, a novel cytochrome P-450 IIIA gene product that is differentially expressed in adult human liver. cDNA and deduced amino acid sequence and distinct specificities of cDNA-expressed hPCN1 and hPCN3 for the metabolism of steroid hormones and cyclosporine. *J. Biol. Chem.* 264(18), 10388–10395.

Ball, S.E., Maurer, G., Zollinger, M., Ladona, M. and Vickers, A.E. (1992) Characterisation of the cytochrome P-450 gene family responsible for the N-dealkylation of the ergot alkaloid CQA 206–291 in humans. *Drug Metab. Dispos.* 20(1), 56–63.

Barnes, H.J. (1996) Maximising expression of eukaryotic cytochrome P450s in *E. coli*. *Methods Enzymol.* 272, 3–14.

Bayburt, T.H., Carlson, J.W. and Sligar, S.G. (1998) Reconstitution and imaging of a membrane protein in a nanometer-size phospholipid bilayer. *J. Struct. Biol.* **123**, 337–344.

Blum, M., Grant, D.M., McBride, W., Heim, M. and Meyer, U.A. (1990) Human arylamine *N*-acetyltransferase genes: isolation, chromosomal localization, and functional expression. *DNA Cell Biol.* 9(3), 193–203.

Buters, J.T., Shou, M., Hardwich, J.P., Korzekwa, K.R. and Gonzalez, F.J. (1995) cDNA-directed expression of human cytochrome P450 CYP1A1 using baculovirus. *Drug. Met. Dispos.* 23(7), 696–701.

Cashman, J.R., Bi, Y.A., Lin, J., Youil, R., Knight, M., Forrest, S. and Treacy, E. (1997) Human flavin-containing monooxygenase form 3: cDNA expression of the enzymes containing amino acid substitutions observed in individuals with trimethylaminuria. *Chemical Res. Toxicol.* 10(8), 837–841.

Chang, T.K., Teixeira, J., Gil, G. and Waxman, D.J. (1993) The lithocholic acid 6 beta-hydroxylase cytochrome P-450, CYP 3A10, is an active catalyst of steroid-hormone 6 beta-hydroxylation. *Biochem. J.* 15 April; **291**(Pt 2), 429–433.

Cho, S.G., Lee, Y.H., Park, H.S., Ryoo, K., Kang, K.W., Park, J., Eom, S.J., Kim, M.J., Chang, T.S., Choi, S.Y., Shim, J., Kim, Y., Dong, M.S., Lee, M.J., Kim, S.G., Ichijo, H. and Choi, E.J. (2001) Glutathione *S*-transferase mu modulates the stress-activated signals by suppressing apoptosis signal-regulating kinase 1. *J. Biol. Chem.* **276**(16), 12749–12755.

Christopherson, R.I., Williams, N.K., Schoettle, S.L., Szabados, E., Hambley, T.W. and Manthey, M.K. (1995) Inhibitors of dihydro-orotase, amidophosphoribosyltransferase and IMP cyclohydrolase as potential drugs. *Biochem. Soc. Trans.* November; 23(4), 888–893.

Clarke, S.E. (1998) *In vitro* assessment of human cytochrome P450. *Xenobiotica* 28(12), 1167–1202.

Clarke, B.J. and Waterman, M.R. (1991) Heterologous expression of mammalian P450 in COS cells. *Methods Enzymol.* **206**, 100–108.

Cosme and Johnson (2000) Engineering microsomal cytochrome P450 2C5 to be a soluble, monomeric enzyme. Mutations that alter aggregation, phospholipid dependence of catalysis, and membrane binding. *J. Biol. Chem.* 28 January; **275**(4), 2545–2553.

Crespi, C.L. and Miller, V.P. (1999) The use of heterologously expressed drug metabolizing enzymes – state of the art and prospects for the future. *Pharmacol. Ther.* **84**, 121–131.

Crespi, C.L., Langenbach, R. and Penman, B.W. (1990a) The development of a panel of human cell lines expressing specific human cytochrome P450 cDNAs. *Prog. Clin. Biol. Res.* **340B**, 97–106.

Crespi, C.L., Steimel, D.T., Aoyama, T., Gelboin, H.V. and Gonzalez, F.J. (1990b) Stable expression of human cytochrome P450IA2 cDNA in a human lymphoblastoid cell line: role of the enzyme in the metabolic activation of aflatoxin B1. *Mol. Carcinog.* 3(1), 5–8.

Crespi, C.L., Gonzalez, F.J., Steimel, D.T., Turner, T.R., Gelboin, H.V., Penman, B.W. and Langenbach, R. (1991) A metabolically competent human cell line expressing five cDNAs encoding procarcinogen-activating enzymes: application to mutagenicity testing. *Chem. Res. Toxicol.* 4(5), 566–572.

Crespi, C.L., Langenbach, R. and Penman, B.W. (1993) Human cell lines, derived from AHH-1 TK + /− human lymphoblasts, genetically engineered for expression of cytochromes P450. *Toxicol.* **82**(1–3), 89–104.

Crespi, C.L., Penman, B.W., Steimel, D.T., Smith, T., Yang, C.S. and Sutter, T.R. (1997) Development of a human lymphoblastoid cell line constitutively expressing human CYP1B1 cDNA: substrate specificity with model substrates and promutagens. *Mutagenesis* 12(2), 83–89.

Crespi, C.L., Fox, L., Stocker, P., Hu, M. and Steimel, D.T. (2000) Analysis of drug transport and metabolism in cell monolayer systems that have been modified by cytochrome P4503A4 cDNA-expression. *Eur. J. Pharm. Sci.* 12(1), 63–68.

Daly, A.K., Monkman, S.C., Smart, J., Steward, A. and Cholerton, S. (1998) Analysis of cytochrome P450 polymorphisms. *Methods Mol. Biol.* **107**, 405–422.

Delomenie, C., Goodfellow, G.H., Krishnamoorthy, R., Grant, D.M. and Dupret, J.M. (1997) Study of the role of the highly conserved residues Arg9 and Arg64 in the catalytic function of human *N*-acetyltransferases NAT1 and NAT2 by site-directed mutagenesis. *Biochem. J.* 323 (Pt 1), 207–215.

Ellis, S.W., Ching, M.S., Watson, P.F., Henderson, C.J., Simula, A.P., Lennard, M.S., Tucker, G.T. and Woods, H.F. (1992) Catalytic activities of human debrisoquine 4-hydroxylase cytochrome P450 (CYP2D6) expressed in yeast. *Biochem. Pharmacol.* 44(4), 617–620.

Ellis, S.W., Rowland, K., Ackland, M.J., Rekka, E., Simula, A.P., Lennard, M.S., Wolf, C.R. and Tucker, G.T. (1996) Influence of amino acid residue 374 of cytochrome P-450 2D6 (CYP2D6) on the regio- and enantio-selective metabolism of metoprolol. *Biochem. J.* 316(Pt 2), 647–654.

Eugster, H.P. and Sengstag, C. (1993) *Saccharomyces cerevisiae*: an alternative source for human microsomal liver enzymes and its use in drug interaction studies. *Toxicol.* **82**(1–3), 61–73.

Eugster, H.P., Sengstag, C., Meyer, U.A., Hinnen, A. and Wurgler, F.E. (1990) Constitutive and inducible expression of human cytochrome P450IA1 in yeast Saccharomyces cerevisiae: an alternative enzyme source for in vitro studies. *Biochem. Biophys. Res. Commun.* 30 October; 172(2), 737–744.

Falany, C.N., Xie, X., Wang, J., Ferrer, J. and Falany, J.L. (2000) Molecular cloning and expression of novel sulphotransferase-like cDNAs from human and rat brain. *Biochem. J.* 346(3), 857–864.

Fischer, C.W., Caudle, D.L., Martin-Wixtrom, C., Quattrochi, L.C., Tuckey, R.H., Waterman, M.R. and Estabrook, R.W. (1992) High level expression of functional P450 1A2 in *E. coli*. *FASEB J.* 6, 759–764.

Forsman, T., Lautala, P., Lundstrom, K., Monastyrskaia, K., Ouzzine, M., Burchell, B., Taskinen, J. and Ulmanen, I. (2000) Production of human UDP-glucuronosyltransferases 1A6 and 1A9 using the semliki forest virus expression system. *Life Sci.* 67(20), 2473–2484.

Fujita, K.K., Nakayama, K., Yamazaki, Y., Tsuruma, K., Yamada, M., Nohmi, T. and Kamataki, T. (2001) Construction of *Salmonella typhimurium* YG7108 strains, each coexpressing a form of human cytochrome P450 with NADPH-cytochrome P450 reductase. *Environ. Mol. Mutagen.* **38**(4), 329–338.

Furuya, H., Meyer, U.A., Gelboin, H.V. and Gonzalez, F.J. (1991) Polymerase chain reaction-directed identification, cloning, and quantification of human CYP2C18 mRNA. *Mol. Pharmacol.* **40**(3), 375–382.

Gervot, L., Rochat, B., Gautier, J.C., Bohnenstengel, F., Kroemer, H., de Berardinis, V., Martin, H., Beaune, P. and de Waziers, I. (1999) Human CYP2B6: expression, inducibility and catalytic activities. *Pharmacogenetics* 9(3), 295–306.

Gillam, E.M., Baba, T., Kim, B.R., Ohmori, S. and Guengerich, F.P. (1993) Expression of modified human cytochrome P450 3A4 in *Escherichia coli* and purification and reconstitution of the enzyme. *Arch. Biochem. Biophys.* **305**(1), 123–131.

Gillam, E.M., Guo, Z. and Guengerich, F.P. (1994) Expression of modified human cytochrome P450 2E1 in *Escherichia coli*, purification, and spectral and catalytic properties. *Arch. Biochem. Biophys.* 312(1), 59–66.

Gillam, E.M., Guo, Z., Martin, M.V., Jenkins, C.M. and Guengerich, F.P. (1995a) Expression of cytochrome P450 2D6 in *Escherichia coli*, purification, and spectral and catalytic characterization. *Arch. Biochem. Biophys.* **319**(2), 540–550.

Gillam, E.M., Guo, Z., Ueng, Y.F., Yamazaki, H., Cock, I., Reilly, P.E., Hooper, W.D. and Guengerich, F.P. (1995b) Expression of cytochrome P450 3A5 in *Escherichia coli*: effects of 5′ modification, purification, spectral characterization, reconstitution conditions, and catalytic activities. *Arch. Biochem. Biophys.* 317(2), 374–384.

Goldstein, J.A. and de Morais, S.M. (1994) Biochemistry and molecular biology of the human CYP2C subfamily. *Pharmacogenetics* 4(6), 285–299.

Goldstein, J.A., Faletto, M.B., Romkes-Sparks, M., Sullivan, T., Kitareewan, S., Raucy, J.L., Lasker, J.M. and Ghanayem, B.I. (1994) Evidence that CYP2C19 is the major (S)-mephenytoin 4′-hydroxylase in humans. *Biochem.* **33**(7), 1743–1752.

Grogan, J., Shou, M., Andrusiak, E.A., Tamura, S., Buters, J.T., Gonzalez, F.J. and Korezekwa, K. (1995) Cytochrome P4502A1, 2E1 and 2C9 cDNA-expression by insect cells and partial purification using hydrophobic chromatography. *Biochem. Pharmacol.* **50**(9), 1509–1515.

Guengerich, F.P., Gillam, E.M. and Shimada, T. (1996) New applications of bacterial systems to problems in toxicology. *Critical Rev. Toxicol.* **26**(5), 551–583.

Guo, Z., Gillam, E.M., Ohmori, S., Tukey, R.H. and Guengerich, F.P. (1994) Expression of modified human cytochrome P450 1A1 in Escherichia coli: effects of 5′ substitution, stabilization, purification, spectral characterization, and catalytic properties. *Arch. Biochem. Biophys.* 1 August; 312(2), 436–446.

Haining, R.L., Hunter, A.P., Sadeque, A.J., Philpot, R.M. and Rettie, A.E. (1997) Baculovirus-mediated expression and purification of human FMO3: catalytic, immunochemical, and structural characterization. *Drug Metab. Dispos.* 25(7), 790–797.

Hood, S.R., Shah, G. and Jones, P. (1998) Expression of cytochromes P450 in a baculovirus system. *Methods Mol. Biol.* **107**, 203–218.

Imaoka, S., Hayashi, K., Hiroi, T., Yabusaki, Y., Kamataki, T. and Funae, Y. (2001) A transgenic mouse expressing human CYP4B1 in the liver. *Biochem. Biophys. Res. Commun.* 15 June; 284(3), 757–762.

Imaoka, S., Ogawa, H., Kimura, S. and Gonzalez, F.J. (1993) Complete cDNA sequence and cDNA-directed expression of CYP4A11, a fatty acid omega-hydroxylase expressed in human kidney. *DNA Cell Biol.* 12(10), 893–899.

Itoh, K., Kimura, T., Yokoi, T., Itoh, S. and Kamataki, T. (1993) Rat liver flavin-containing monooxygenase (FMO): cDNA cloning and expression in yeast. *Biochim. Biophys. Acta* 1173(2), 165–171.

Jowett, T., Wajidi, M.F., Oxtoy, E. and Wolf, C.R. (1991) Mamalian genes expressed in *Drosophila*. A transgenic model for the study of chemical mutagenesis and metabolism. *EMBO J.* **10**, 1075–1081.

Kushida, H., Fujita, K., Suzuki, A., Yamada, M., Nohmi, T. and Kamataki, T. (2000) Development of a salmonella tester strain sensitive to promutagenic *N*-nitrosamines: expression of recombinant CYP2A6 and human NADPH-cytochrome P450 reductase in *S. typhimurium* YG7108. *Mutat. Res.* 471(1–2), 135–143.

Lee, C.A., Kadwell, S.H., Kost, T.A. and Serabjit-Singh, C.J. (1995) CYP3A4 expressed in insect cells infected with a recombinant baculovirus containing both CYP3A4 and human NADPH-cytochrome P450 reductase is catalytically similar to human liver microsomal CYP3A4. *Arch. Biochem. Biophys.* **319**(1), 157–167.

Lessard, E., Fortin, A., Belanger, P.M., Beaune, P., Hamelin, B.A. and Turgeon, J. (1997) Role of CYP2D6 in the N-hydroxylation of procainamide. (Journal Article) *Pharmacogenetics* October; 7(5), 381–390.

Lu, G., Unge, T., Owera-Atepo, J.B., Shih, J.C., Ekblom, J. and Oreland, L. (1996) Characterization and partial purification of human monoamine oxidase-B expressed in *Escherichia coli. Protein Expr. Purif.* 7(3), 315–322.

Masimirembwa, C.M., Otter, C., Berg, M., Jonsson, M., Leidvik, B., Jonsson, E., Johansson, T., Backman, A., Edlund, A. and Andersson, T.B. (1999) Heterologous expression and kinetic characterization of human cytochromes P-450: validation of a pharmaceutical tool for drug metabolism research. *Drug Metab. Dispos.* October; 27(10), 1117–1122.

Masimirembwa, C.M., Thompson, R. and Andersson, T.B. (2001) *In vitro* high throughput screening of compounds for favorable metabolic properties in drug discovery. *Comb. Chem. High Throughput Screen.* 4(3), 245–263.

McManus, M.E., Burgess, W.M., Veronese, M.E., Huggett, A., Quattrochi, L.C. and Tukey, R.H. (1990) Metabolism of 2-acetylaminofluorene and benzo(a)pyrene and activation of food-derived heterocyclic amine mutagens by human cytochromes P-450. *Cancer Res.* **50**(11), 3367–3376.

Miles, J.S., McLaren, A.W., Forrester, L.M., Glancey, M.J., Lang, M.A. and Wolf, C.R. (1990) Identification of the human liver cytochrome P-450 responsible for coumarin 7-hydroxylase activity. *Biochem. J.* 267(2), 365–371.

Miller, J.R. and Edmondson, D.E. (1999) Influence of flavin analogue structure on the catalytic activities and flavinylation reactions of recombinant human liver monoamine oxidases A and B. *J. Biol. Chem.* 274(33), 23515–23525.

Morris, D.L. and Davila, J.C. (1996) Analysis of rat cytochrome P450 isoenzyme expression using semi-quantitative reverse transcriptase-polymerase chain reaction (RT-PCR). *Biochem. Pharmacol.* 52(5), 781–792.

Nebert, D.W. and Duffy, J.J. (1997) How knockout mouse lines will be used to study the role of drug-metabolising enzymes and their receptors during reproduction and development, and in environmental toxicity, cancer, and oxidative stress. *Biochem. Pharmacol.* 53(3), 249–254.

Nelson, D.R., Koymans, L., Kamataki, T., Stegeman, J.J., Feyereisen, R., Waxman, D.J., Waterman, M.R., Gotoh, O., Coon, M.J., Estabrook, R.W., Gunsalus, I.C. and Nebert, D.W. (1996) P450 superfamily: update on new sequences, gene mapping, accession numbers and nomenclature. *Pharmacogenetics* 6(1), 1–42.

Ouzzine, M., Fournel-Gigleux, S., Pillot, T., Burchell, B., Siest, G. and Magdalou, J. (1994) Expression of the human UDP-glucuronosyltransferase UGT1*6 in *Escherichia coli*. Influence of bacterial signal peptides on the production and localization of the recombinant protein. *FEBS Lett.* 339(1–2), 195–199.

Ouzzine, M., Magdalou, J., Burchell, B. and Fournel-Gigleux, S. (1999) Expression of a functionally active human hepatic UDP-glucuronosyltransferase (UGT1A6) lacking the *N*-terminal signal sequence in the endoplasmic reticulum. *FEBS Lett.* 454(3), 187–191.

Palmer, C.N.A., Richardson, T.H., Griffin, K.J., Hsu, M.-H., Muerhoff, A.S., Clark, J.E. and Johnson, E.F. (1993) Characterisation of a cDNA encoding a human kidney, cytochrome P450 4A fatty acid w-hydroxylase and the cognate enzyme expressed in *Escherichia coli Biochim. Biophys. Acta* 1172(1–2), 161–167.

Patten, C.J. and Koch, P. (1995) Baculovirus expression of human P450 2E1 and cytochrome b_5. *Arch. Biochem. Biophys.* 238(1), 143–150.

Patten, C.J., Ishizaki, H., Aoyama, T., Lee, M., Ning, S.M., Huang, W., Gonzalez, F.J. and Yang, C.S. (1992) Catalytic properties of the human cytochrome P450 2E1 produced by cDNA expression in mammalian cells. *Arch. Biochem. Biophys.* 299(1), 163–171.

Penman, B.W., Reece, J., Smith, T., Yang, C.S., Gelboin, H.V., Gonzalez, F.J. and Crespi, C.L. (1993) Characterization of a human cell line expressing high levels of cDNA-derived CYP2D6. *Pharmacogenetics* 3(1), 28–39.

Powell, H., Kitteringham, N.R., Pirmohamed, M., Smith, D.A. and Park, B.K. (1998) Expression of cytochrome P4502E1 in human liver: assessment by mRNA, genotype and phenotype. *Pharmacogenetics* October; 8(5), 411–421.

Rae, J.M., Johnson, M.D., Lippman, M.E. and Flockhart, D.A. (2001) Rifampin is a selective, pleiotropic inducer of drug metabolism genes in human hepatocytes: studies with cDNA and oligonucleotide expression arrays. (Journal Article) *J. Pharmacol. Exp. Ther.* 299(3), 849–857.

Rebrin, I., Geha, R.M., Chen, K. and Shih, J.C. (2001) Effects of carboxyl-terminal truncations on the activity and solubility of human monoamine oxidase B. *J. Biol. Chem.* 276(31), 29499–29506.

Renaud, J.P., Cullin, C., Pompon, D., Beaune, P. and Mansuy, D. (1990) Expression of human liver cytochrome P450 IIIA4 in yeast. A functional model for the hepatic enzyme. *Eur. J. Biochem.* 194(3), 889–896.

Rettie, A.E., Wienkers, L.C., Gonzalez, F.J., Trager, W.F. and Korzekwa, K.R. (1994) Impaired (S)-warfarin metabolism catalysed by the R144C allelic variant of CYP2C9. *Pharmacogenetics* 4(1), 39–42.

Richardson, T.H., Jung, F., Griffin, K.J., Wester, M., Raucy, J.L., Kemper, B., Bornheim, L.M., Hassett, C., Omiecinski, C.J. and Johnson, E.F. (1995) A universal approach to the expression of human and rabbit cytochrome P450s of the 2C subfamily in *Escherichia coli*. *Arch. Biochem. Biophys.* 323(1), 87–96.

Roy, P., Yu, L.J., Crespi, C.L. and Waxman, D.J. (1999) Development of a substrate-activity based approach to identify the major human liver P-450 catalysts of cyclophosphamide and ifosfamide activation based on cDNA-expressed activities and liver microsomal P-450 profiles. *Drug Metab. Dispos.* 27(6), 655–666.

Sachse, C., Brockmoller, J., Bauer, S. and Roots, I. (1997) Cytochrome P450 2D6 variants in a Caucasian population: allele frequencies and phenotypic. *Am. J. Hum. Gen.* February; 60(2), 284–295.

Sandhu, P., Baba, T. and Guengerich, F.P. (1993) Expression of modified cytochrome P450 2C10 (2C9) in *Escherichia coli*, purification, and reconstitution of catalytic activity. *Arch. Biochem. Biophys.* 306(2), 443–450.

Sheen, Y.Y., Owens, I.S., Kim, S.S. and Kim, J.E. (1998) UDPGT cDNA expression and UDPGT1 in human liver. *J. Toxicol. Sci.* 23 (Suppl 2), 136–139.

Shimada, T., Wunsch, R.M., Hanna, I.H., Sutter, T.R., Guengerich, F.P. and Gillam, E.M. (1998) Recombinant human cytochrome P450 1B1 expression in *Escherichia coli*. *Arch. Biochem. Biophys.* 357(1), 111–120.

Srivastava, P.K., Yun, C.H., Beaune, P.H., Ged, C. and Guengerich, F.P. (1991) Separation of human liver microsomal tolbutamide hydroxylase and (*S*)-mephenytoin 4′-hydroxylase cytochrome P-450 enzymes. *Mol. Pharmacol.* 40(1), 69–79.

Stubbins, M.J., Harries, L.W., Smith, G., Tarbit, M.H. and Wolf, C.R. (1996) Genetic analysis of the human cytochrome P450 CYP2C9 locus. *Pharmacogenetics* 6(5), 429–439.

Tassaneeyakul, W., Veronese, M.E., Birkett, D.J., Gonzalez, F.J. and Miners, J.O. (1993) Validation of 4-nitrophenol as an *in vitro* substrate probe for human liver CYP2E1 using cDNA expression and microsomal kinetic techniques. *Biochem. Pharmacol.* 46(11), 1975–1981.

Thier, R., Muller, M., Taylor, J.B., Pemble, S.E., Ketterer, B. and Guengerich, F.P. (1995) Enhancement of bacterial mutagenicity of bifunctional alkylating agents by expression of mammalian glutathione *S*-transferase. *Chem. Res. Toxicol.* 8(3), 465–472.

Tyndale, R., Aoyama, T., Broly, F., Matsunaga, T., Inaba, T., Kalow, W., Gelboin, H.V., Meyer, U.A. and Gonzalez, F.J. (1991) Identification of a new variant CYP2D6 allele lacking the codon encoding Lys-281: possible association with the poor metabolizer phenotype. *Pharmacogenetics* 1(1), 26–32.

Veronese, M.E., Doecke, C.J., Mackenzie, P.I., McManus, M.E., Miners, J.O., Rees, D.L., Gasser, R., Meyer, U.A. and Birkett, D.J. (1993) Site-directed mutation studies of human liver cytochrome P-450 isoenzymes in the CYP2C subfamily. *Biochem. J.* 289(2), 533–538.

Xie, W., Barwick, J.L., Downes, M., Blumberg, B., Simon, C.M., Nelson, M.C., Neuschwander-Tetri, B.A., Brunt, E.M., Guzelian, P.S. and Evans, R.M. (2000) Humanized xenobiotic response in mice expressing nuclear receptor SXR. *Nat.* 406(6794), 435–439.

Yamano, S., Nhamburo, P.T., Aoyama, T., Meyer, U.A., Inaba, T., Kalow, W., Gelboin, H.V., McBride, O.W. and Gonzalez, F.J. (1989a) cDNA cloning and sequence and cDNA-directed expression of human P450 IIB1: identification of a normal and two variant cDNAs derived from the CYP2B locus on chromosome 19 and differential expression of the IIB mRNAs in human liver. *Biochem.* 28(18), 7340–7348.

Yamano, S., Nagata, K., Yamazoe, Y., Kato, R., Gelboin, H.V. and Gonzalez, F.J. (1989b) cDNA and deduced amino acid sequences of human P450 IIA3 (CYP2A3). *Nucleic Acids Res.* 17(12), 4888.

Yanagawa, Y., Sawada, M., Deguchi, T., Gonzalez, F.J. and Kamataki, T. (1994) Stable expression of human CYP1A2 and *N*-acetyltransferases in Chinese hamster CHL cells: mutagenic activation of 2-amino-3-methylimidazo[4,5-f]quinoline and 2-amino-3,8-dimethylimidazo [4,5-f]quinoxaline. *Cancer Res.* 54(13), 3422–3427.

Yasumori, T., Murayama, N., Yamazoe, Y., Abe, A., Nogi, Y., Fukasawa, T. and Kato, R. (1989) Expression of a human P-450IIC gene in yeast cells using galactose-inducible expression system. *Mol. Pharmacol.* 35(4), 443–449.

Yoshida, M., Loo, J.A. and Lepleya, R.A. (2001) Proteomics as a tool in the pharmaceutical drug design process. *Curr. Pharm. Des.* March; 7(4), 291–310.
Zeldin, D.C., DuBois, R.N., Falck, J.R. and Capdevila, J.H. (1995) Molecular cloning, expression and characterisation of an endogenous human cytochrome P450 arachadonic acid epoxygenase isoform. *Arch. Biochem. Biophys.* 232(1), 76–86.

18.8 *Bibliography*

There are several good introductions to this subject. I have listed them in order of complexity (and weight!).

Stryer, L. (1995) Biochemistry, 4th edn, USA, ISBN 0–7167–2009–4.
Alberts, B. *et al.* (1994) Molecular biology of the cell, 3rd edn, USA, Garland publishing, ISBN 0–8153–1620–8.
Lewin, B., Genes, V. (1994) UK, Oxford University Press, ISBN0–19–854288–7.
Sambrook, J. (1989) Molecular cloning: A laboratory manual, 2nd edn, USA, Cold Spring Harbor Laboratory Press, ISBN0–87969–309–6.

CHAPTER 19

The role of drug metabolism and pharmacokinetics in drug discovery: past, present and future

Mike Tarbit

19.1 *Introduction*

It is tempting to begin this chapter with the view that the role of drug metabolism and pharmacokinetics (DMPK) in the processes of lead optimisation in drug discovery is now well established. After all, the drug metabolism departments in several of the major pharmaceutical R&D companies have been moving progressively further into a supporting role for drug discovery over the past twenty years or so, as realisation has dawned that inappropriate kinetics has been a major reason for high attrition rates in the costly process of candidate development (Lin and Lu, 1997). The value assessment of this evolution has been fed by a few case histories of highly successful optimisation processes, where some companies synthesised compounds with a very effective balance of potency, safety and pharmacokinetics (Beresford *et al.*, 1988; Richardson *et al.*, 1990). It is salutary to note that in each case these drugs made near blockbuster impact on the market place and represented difficult targets for their competitors. Thus there is now clear evidence that a drug with the correct balance of potency and kinetics will be a highly effective medicine.

So why the hesitancy in declaring that this is now an established, efficient, process of the norm, rather than the exception? The problem is one of the slow pace of integration of DMPK into the overall process of drug discovery at a sufficiently early stage. There are still some major companies where DMPK support for drug discovery is non-existent, or patchy and inconsistent. This often correlates with a significant polarisation between the more flexible, non-regulatory 'research' elements of the company, and the somewhat conservative good laboratory practice, traditional 'development' departments. Resource maps in the drug metabolism departments in these companies tend to favour the latter activities, with little realisation of the value of committing effort in optimising compounds prior to candidate selection. Even those major companies where a significant investment of resource has been made in discovery support, there is often a serial process in place, whereby project chemists optimise on potency first, then attempt to 'fix' kinetics on their most potent molecules through a cyclical or iterative process. This usually occurs in the absence of a realisation that in many cases potency can be titrated against good kinetic characteristics and lead to a very effective drug. In the ideal world, recognised by some of the more enlightened companies, the process of optimising potency, safety and kinetics should be carried out more in parallel, in an integrated fashion, and should occur as early in the process of identifying lead molecules as analytical methods allow. Project teams should include DMPK scientists at their genesis, and such scientists should provide their knowledge and wisdom from first principles of lead optimisation. The later this process is left, the more costly and time-consuming it becomes to correct any deficient properties in a molecular series. Proof that insufficient kinetic input is still occurring in major league companies is all too plain when compounds are withdrawn soon after marketing for kinetic reasons (Honig *et al.*, 1993; Griffin, 1998) at a cost of multiple millions.

As if this was not enough, the recent revolutionary changes in chemistry technology now enable project chemists to produce libraries of hundreds to millions of combinatorial analogues in project life-cycles (Berman and Howard, 2000). Coupled with the incredible rates at which these compounds can now be screened against their target receptor or enzyme, this has all but swamped the ability of DMPK groups to provide kinetic and metabolic information of any value to lead optimisation groups. Thus even in the enlightened companies mentioned above, which may have significant resources committed to discovery support, the DMPK processes have, once more, become a major choke point in sifting out compounds with the correct balance. Some companies are responding to this challenge by attempting to emulate the screening revolution, and bring high-throughput screening into DMPK (Rodrigues, 1997; Tarbit and Berman, 1998; Eddershaw and Dickins, 1999; Eddershaw *et al.*, 2000). It is early in the evolution of this technology, but the pace of application will undoubtedly speed up with increasing need and with development of new methods, some of which may be borrowed from partners in biological high-throughput screening.

It is against this complex, but rapidly changing, background that this chapter will attempt to highlight the key principles and parameters of DMPK input into lead optimisation and provide some insight into likely future developments.

19.2 *The first principle: potency versus efficacy*

Most discovery projects base their primary screening of compounds on *in vitro* assays. This is logical. It isolates the primary target from complicating factors that may influence a compound's behaviour *in vivo*, enabling them to get to structure–activity relationships in the most direct manner. It also has a major practical advantage in that it enables the very high-throughput rates mentioned above; rates which would prove impossible to achieve *in vivo*. However, it is important to realise that the conditions of these assays bear little resemblance to conditions likely to be experienced *in vivo*. Thus in these *in vitro* tests, the compound remains in contact with the target throughout the period of the test; the drug concentration is usually constant; there is generally no metabolism of the compound, and thus no generation of metabolites; and there is little or no protein present to bind the drug and reduce the availability of the 'active' concentration. This can be described as a 'static' test. Conditions are entirely different when compounds are administered *in vivo*, and there is much more dynamic interplay between the physiological processes in the body and the physicochemical properties of the molecule. Thus the compound needs to be delivered in a medium that will render it soluble at the site of absorption in the gastrointestinal tract, and it needs to possess suitable physicochemical properties to cross the intestinal mucosa, just to gain access to the systemic circulation. Even when absorbed, the compound has to bypass the liver, the body's main organ of metabolism and defence against environmental xenobiotic challenge; exposure to metabolism on this 'first pass' may remove part, or all, of the fraction of drug absorbed (Figure 19.1). Once present in the systemic circulation the drug may bind avidly to proteins in both plasma and tissues, resulting in a significant reduction in the availability of effective drug. In some cases, the tissue distribution of the drug may be such that it does not even reach the organ containing the target receptor (Figure 19.2). Finally, the body will attempt to clear the drug from the systemic circulation by metabolism and/or renal clearance; thus the concentration may decrease rapidly with time, resulting in insufficient exposure of the target to the compound. Under these conditions, the relative potency of a compound in a project favoured *in vitro* assay can be completely negated by its pharmacokinetic profile *in vivo*. For similar reasons, a compound that has a less promising *in vitro* potency may perform admirably against its more promising

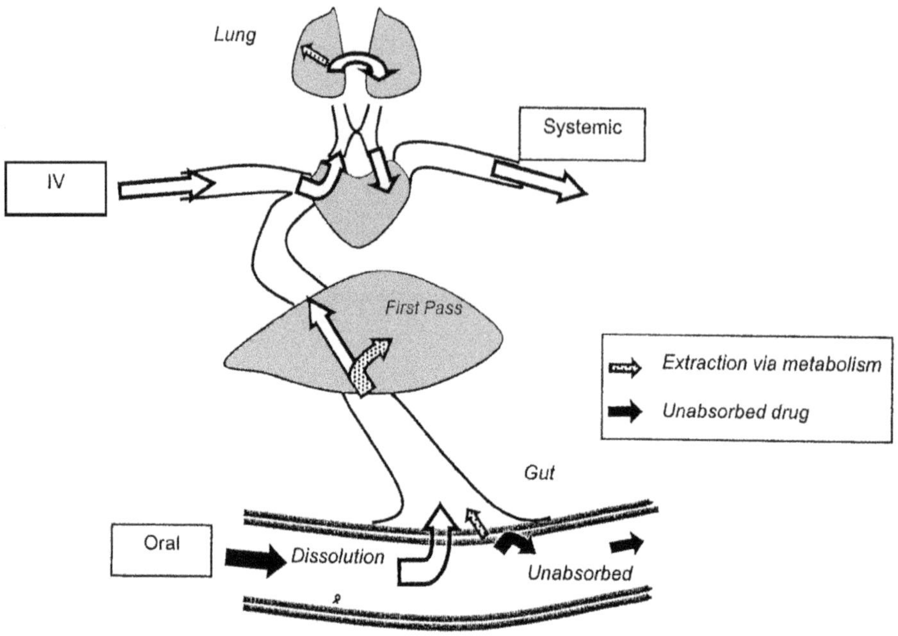

FIGURE 19.1 *'First pass' may remove part, or all, of the fraction of drug absorbed.*

potent analogue cousins, if it has a more suitable kinetic profile. Thus, for example, a compound with a relatively poor potency, but with complete oral bioavailability will show better *in vivo* efficacy than a compound with a 50-fold more potency, but less than one per cent systemic availability.

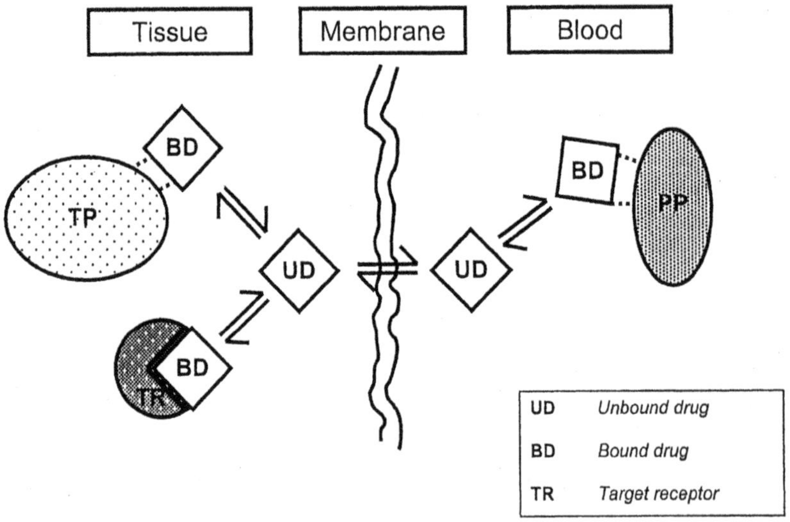

FIGURE 19.2 *Effect of binding on drug pharmacology.*

One corollary of these factors is that pharmacokinetics is a major explanatory factor for the so-called '*in vitro–in vivo* correlation failures' that often result in bemused looks on the faces of project scientists when their most potent lead fails to work at all in the secondary *in vivo* animal disease models. It goes without saying, therefore, that *in vitro* potency should never be the sole basis of selecting candidates. As mentioned previously, the ideal drug will be one that has been designed with a view to gaining the best balance possible between inherent potency and a suitable kinetic profile to translate that potency into appropriate efficacy.

19.3 *Which are the key kinetic parameters to measure?*

Pharmacokinetics is essentially a mathematical science, and can evolve into fairly complex and tortuous equations in the hands of the serious practitioner. Indeed 'whole body' physiological simulations are frequently attempted by aficionados in their efforts to predict total patterns of behaviour from knowledge of a compound's structure and properties. Fortunately for the lead optimisation process, the key parameters that need to be assessed when making decisions on the appropriateness of a kinetic profile are fairly simple to calculate, yet refined enough to make suitably narrow distinctions between structural analogues within a project series.

19.4 *Assessment of absorption and systemic availability*

Not surprisingly, given that most clinically used drugs are administered orally, absorption tends to attract the initial attention of projects in establishing their preferred product profile. In addition, most project tests, or animal models, *in vivo* tend to involve oral administration, to avoid the necessity of complex parenteral formulation, and to enable administration of reasonably high dose-levels. Thus this is usually the first 'alarm' call on kinetics for a project, when apparent efficacy in these models apparently fails to translate from *in vitro* potency. From the more recent perspective, the production of combinatorial libraries has evolved from chemical reactions based broadly on peptide principles. Although chemistries are developing quickly in more 'drug-like' directions, these libraries tend to present collections of compounds with high molecular weights and polar properties. Absorption has, therefore, proved to be a major kinetic barrier to the generation of drug candidates from combinatorial libraries.

Assessments of systemic absorption are complicated by the fact that there are a number of processes affecting the systemic bioavailability of an orally administered drug. Two of the major factors are permeation of the drug across the intestinal mucosa, i.e. absorption *per se*, and the extent to which the liver can then extract and metabolise the drug on its first pass through the portal system. The latter process is a well-developed homeostatic mechanism for protecting the systemic circulation from xenobiotic challenge; consequently drugs need to be somewhat resistant to metabolic attack to achieve significant systemic levels.

The overall systemic availability of a drug is classically determined by ratio of systemic exposure, measured as area under the plasma concentration time curve (Figure 19.3), after sequential intravenous and oral administrations of a compound. However, this measure has inherent basic assumptions which need to be considered when evaluating results and comparing compounds. Thus the calculation assumes that:

(a) all of the drug administered via the intravenous route is delivered to the systemic circulation; and
(b) that the resultant systemic exposure (*AUC*) represents the theoretical maximum which would be seen if 100 per cent of a corresponding oral dose was absorbed into the system. This is based on the premises that the intravenous dose will reach the arterial system without pre-systemic modification, and that once drug has successfully survived any problems of oral absorption and hepatic first pass, and reached the arterial system, then any subsequent systemic clearance will be independent of delivery route. This is generally the case, although in rare cases pulmonary first pass (see Figure 19.1), which occurs after intravenous administration, may have some impact on this.

Somewhat more contentious in calculating bioavailability, and often the cause of misinterpretation of results, is the necessary assumption that systemic clearance of the drug remains the same after either dose-route. This assumption is often invalid. Systemic clearance of drugs via metabolic routes can be saturated if the concentration of the drug reaching the enzymes exceeds their capacity to function under first order processes. This is relatively rare following intravenous routes of administration, as the drug is distributed to the tissues via the arterial system before it reaches the liver at resultant low concentrations. However, very high concentrations of drug are usually present in the portal vein following oral administration and absorption, which may lead to saturation of the hepatic metabolic enzymes, and thus reduced systemic clearance. The degree of any saturation will also be affected by the total dose administered, consequently relationships are likely to be non-linear and unpredictable (Figure 19.4). Formulation difficulties, which are common in the discovery

$$F = \frac{AUC_{po}}{AUC_{iv}} \times \frac{D\text{–}L_{iv}}{D\text{–}L_{po}}$$

Note. $$Cl_p = \frac{AUC_{iv}}{D\text{–}L_{iv}}$$

FIGURE 19.3 *Bioavailability and clearance.*

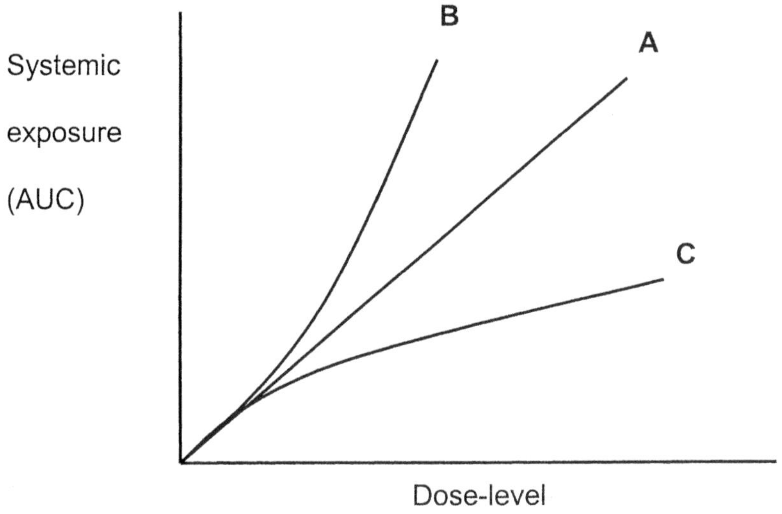

FIGURE 19.4 *Non-linear kinetics caused by saturation of clearance.*

phases of drug development, often result in administration of much lower dose-levels for the intravenous phase of these studies than the oral phase, pre-disposing the study to the complications outlined. Evidence of any degree of saturation – apparent bioavailabilities that exceed 100 per cent, for example – invalidates straightforward calculations of oral systemic availability and means that any conclusions should be drawn with caution. In the case of the apparent super bioavailability cited, for example, the unwary will draw the conclusions that bioavailabilities that exceed 100 per cent are *actually* 100 per cent, or 'total'. They are not. The data cannot lead to any conclusion about the fraction of the oral dose absorbed, in the case of saturation, without further and more complicated experimentation.

Judging a compound's oral systemic bioavailability provides valuable information on its potential for use as an oral agent. However, it is not a wholly effective means of dissecting out the nature of any problem and addressing it. As discussed above, there are two key processes that have a major impact on the final systemic availability of a drug, mucosal permeation and hepatic first pass, and chemistry approaches to optimising molecules for each of these processes may be very different. Measuring the absolute degree of absorption of a drug across the intestinal mucosa is not a simple exercise *in vivo*. Models exist which examine the rate of disappearance of drug from the lumen of a cannulated loop of gut into, presumably, the portal blood supply, or, measure the rate and extent of appearance of drug in the portal vein after direct administration into the gut. Neither models are convenient, or high throughput, enough to examine large numbers of compounds on a routine basis, and both are prone to error and complicating factors.

How do we get to the judgement of which factors contribute most to a compound's overall availability *in vivo* then? The straightforward approach in discovery project support is to forget about absorption, initially, and concentrate on measuring the intrinsic systemic clearance of the drug. This can be done readily after an intravenous, or parenteral, dose (see Chapter 7 on kinetics). Reasonable conclusions can then be drawn about the likely fate of any subsequently orally administered dose. Thus if intrinsic systemic clearance of a compound is high and metabolic, equating with liver blood flow for example, then the likelihood of any orally administered drug escaping first pass extraction by the liver and achieving systemic levels is low, even if the compound was completely absorbed across the intestinal mucosa. The conclusion here would be that absorption is patently not the primary project issue with compounds exhibiting these properties, and clearance issues must be solved first (Figure 19.5). If systemic clearance is moderate, however, say 50 per cent of liver blood flow, then one would expect such a drug to show systemic exposure equal to, or greater than, half that of the intravenous dose if it was completely orally absorbed, in keeping with some first pass extraction of a fraction of the oral dose. If oral systemic exposure is much lower than half of the intravenous value, then it is reasonable to conclude that the difference must be due to poor absorption. Obviously this can be affected by any saturation of first pass, so care in interpretation is needed if apparent exposure after oral administration is much higher than would have been predicted by consideration of systemic clearance versus hepatic blood flow. Finally, if systemic clearance is low after intravenous administration, say less than 10 per cent of liver blood flow, then it is likely that any first pass metabolism of such a compound would be negligible. Thus any marked reduction in oral *AUC* versus the corresponding intravenous value, would clearly indicate that absorption, per se, was a problem.

These guidelines are not infallible, and factors such as renal or non-hepatic metabolic clearance and active transport of drugs can complicate their use. Some

<u>High Clearance Drug</u>

Cl_m after iv dose = ~ 40 ml/min/kg

LBF in dog = ~ 40 ml/min/kg

Thus liver can eliminate all drug in portal flow

If "f" is low, could be due to fpm or absorption

<u>Low Clearance Drug</u>

Cl_m after iv dose = ~ 4 ml/min/kg

LBF in dog = ~ 40 ml/min/kg

Thus impact of fpm = ~10%; i.e. predicted "f" = ~90

If actual "f" is low, probably due to absorption

FIGURE 19.5 *High and low clearance.*

mitigation of these complications can be planned ahead. Thus, for example, urine should always be collected in support kinetic studies, and levels of excretion of unchanged drug determined. This provides improved confidence in determining what fraction of the dose is metabolised, and enables an appropriate correction of the impact of any potential first pass on calculations of theoretical fraction absorbed. In fact, within limitations mentioned above about saturation of first pass metabolism, comparisons of the fraction of unchanged drug excreted in urine after corresponding intravenous and oral doses can be used to estimate systemic availability in a non-invasive manner.

Despite these limitations, this clearance-based approach has the advantage of being a simple yet reasonable basis for making decisions about the relatively large number of molecules likely to be encountered in a lead optimisation programme, without the necessity for using complex and error-prone *in vitro*, or surgically prepared animal models.

19.5 *Cell-based models of absorption*

Given the significant difficulties of measuring absolute absorption values *in vivo*, many workers have tried to develop predictive *in vitro* models over the past 30 years since the early work of Borchardt (Hildalgo *et al.*, 1989). These have generally been based on immortalised intestinal cell-lines such as various clones of the human Caco2 line (Artursson *et al.*, 1996; Rubas *et al.*, 1996). These cell lines have some major advantages: they are undoubtedly cheap and have relatively high throughput, thus large numbers of compounds can be examined in relatively short time (Taylor *et al.*, 1996); they 'isolate mechanism', in the sense that they have fewer complicating factors than would be encountered *in vivo*, thereby allowing greater chance of understanding structure–activity relationships between permeation and molecular properties; and the conditions of the test can be carefully controlled. However, there are major drawbacks in their use, which should lead the wary to interpret data from such studies with caution. Thus, as with all immortal and cultured cells, their phenotypic characteristics are not the same as the mucosal cells *in vivo*, nor do they present the full range of differentiated cells likely to be encountered by drugs crossing the intestinal barrier. In addition, despite the best efforts of many workers to modify media and environmental factors, the conditions of cell-based assays are not those present in the gut. There is little of the dynamic changes that occur in gut transit, blood flow, membrane properties, pH, dissolution rates, etc. Under these conditions, it is usually a step too far to interpret the behaviour of drugs in cell-based assays as indicative of the extent of absorption *in vivo*. Where these assays can add value to project support is in judging and comparing the permeation properties of a series of molecules, in the belief that such intrinsic properties as rate of permeation and overall extent, taken in conjunction with other properties such as the aqueous solubility of the drugs, will give useful information on the potential of the drug to be absorbed.

In general, and not unexpectedly, these studies have shown that increased lipophilicity tends to promote improved permeation across the mucosal cells via the so-called transcellular route, whilst small polar molecules may percolate, generally more slowly, through the polar channels in the mucosal layer via the so-called paracellular route. A general conclusion is thus that the more lipophilic a molecule is, the more likely it is to be rapidly absorbed across the mucosa after oral administration. As with most kinetic optimisation strategies, however, a balance is needed between increasing the lipophilicity of molecules to aid their absorption, and taking this too far, so that it markedly decreases their solubility at the site of absorption, essentially becoming self-defeating. As outlined below, increasing lipophilicity can also have the effect of promoting first pass metabolic clearance. The recent development of a rules-based method for defining an appropriate balance of physicochemical properties for absorption has gained wide usage among medicinal chemists, and demonstrates the value of predictive methods in discovery chemistry (Lipinski *et al.*, 1997).

19.6 *The importance of clearance*

The considerations above highlight the significance of clearance as a primary parameter in the pharmacokinetic optimisation of drugs. Project teams that develop the ability to titrate their potency structure–activity relationships with the appropriate chemical strategies to build low systemic clearance into the molecules have a high probability of achieving successful candidates and marketed medicines. There are three major physiological routes of systemic clearance, viz. biliary, metabolic and renal, and it is instructive to understand the basic mechanisms, when targeting molecular modifications to defeat them. In essence, biliary and renal clearances represent the major routes of systemic elimination of unwanted chemicals. Both are based on aqueous media. Consequently xenobiotic molecules cannot be excreted from the systemic circulation unless they are polar enough to partition into body water, which is the source of urine or bile. (NB. The corollary to this is that any administered drugs that are polar enough to partition into body water are likely to be rapidly eliminated from the body, hence, for example, the high renal clearance and relatively short systemic exposure of polar antibiotics.) The various processes of endobiotic and xenobiotic biotransformation which comprise metabolic clearance (see Chapter 13) have, therefore, evolved to transform any lipophilic molecules into polar 'metabolites', which will subsequently favour their partition into the aqueous media and excretion. Thus the 'drug-metabolising enzymes' generally increase the overall polarity of molecules, either by direct oxidative attack in areas of high electron density (e.g. cytochromes P-450), or by conjugating molecules with highly polar moieties such as glucuronic acid, sulphate or amino-acids (e.g. glucuronyl transferases). This interplay between metabolic processes and renal clearance has significant consequences for drug optimisation. Many of the therapeutic targets for projects comprise either receptors or enzymes that sit in lipophilic cell membranes. Understandably, this means that compound potency tends to increase with lipophilicity, as this tends to drive the molecules into the receptor environment. Unfortunately, the metabolising enzymes have evolved to conserve cellular homeostasis, and consequently they also sit in the membranes. Thus strategies aimed at increasing potency tend also to increase the prospect of rapid metabolic clearance of compounds to more polar, and thus less potent, metabolites.

So what are the approaches that DMPK support groups can offer projects to aid the evolution of a balance between potency and clearance in lead optimisation? As mentioned above, the primary pieces of information relate to a quantification of overall systemic clearance, and a determination of which fraction is metabolic versus renal. This is readily achievable by collecting urine over the course of a kinetic study and determining the fraction of dose excreted unchanged. By definition, renal clearance is then equal to the same fraction of total clearance. Metabolic clearance (Figure 19.6) is assumed to represent the difference. Biliary clearance is normally discounted, as bile flow is low, although active transport into bile can undermine this assumption with certain classes of compounds. If metabolic clearance of the test molecule is high, then chemical optimisation needs to be directed towards decreasing the metabolic opportunities on the molecule. This is greatly aided by

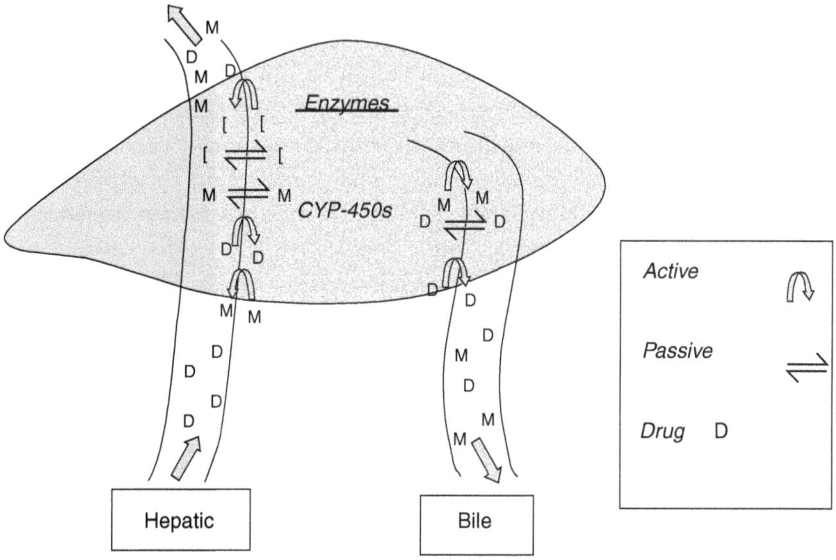

FIGURE 19.6 *Metabolic clearance.*

any identification of metabolites of the test compound, as this provides target sites for blocking substitutions. However, comprehensive identification of metabolites in discovery support is hindered by a lack of radiolabelled drugs (not practical, given the number of molecules examined), and a lack of knowledge of the overall routes of elimination of metabolites. Urine, collected as above, should always be examined by spectroscopy techniques in these circumstances, preferably versus a control sample from the same animal, to identify any possible molecular ions indicative of metabolites. However, in general, the identification of potential sites of metabolism depends upon paper, or in silico prediction, or on *in vitro* experiments with enzyme preparations. Consideration of the previous paragraph indicates that the simplest way of decreasing metabolic attack is to increase the overall polarity of the molecule, thereby reducing its access to the lipophilic membranes containing the metabolising enzymes. However, most project chemists are wary of taking this route, for fear of losing potency.

If renal clearance of the molecule is high and represents the major route of elimination, then any improvement in duration of exposure should be targeted by increasing the lipophilicity of follow-up molecules. The basis of this strategy is that renal filtrate concentrates in the kidney tubule, due to the reabsorption of some of the water. This alters the concentration of solutes and can drive their reabsorption across the tubular epithelium, with consequent greater systemic exposure. Thus increasing lipophilicity of renally cleared compounds will promote their reabsorption. Naturally, this cannot be carried too far, as it may lead to a vicious circle between metabolic clearance and renal clearance. However, it is possible to design molecules that are sufficiently polar to avoid significant involvement in metabolic clearance, yet which have sufficient lipophilicity to undergo significant renal tubular reabsorption (Humphrey *et al.*, 1985). The binding of drugs to plasma proteins is another key factor that modulates renal clearance, as only the unbound drug can be filtered in the glomerulus. Thus drugs which have similar polarities, but markedly different protein-binding coefficients, will demonstrate very different renal clearances. The corollary to this is that it may seem that one approach to reducing renal clearance would be to increase protein binding of follow-on drugs. The drawback to this approach is that we have relatively little knowledge of which molecular characteristics affect protein binding other than the ubiquitous lipophilicity, and, as described above, that approach is common to promoting renal reabsorption anyway. More fundamental is the fact that any marked increase in protein binding may have a significant impact on efficacy, as it is generally considered to be the free drug that is pharmacologically active.

Overall, projects will spend much of their optimisation effort in balancing the potency of molecules with modifications that lead to low or moderate systemic clearance. Molecules that have been designed to be relatively resistant to metabolic attack, and which are lipophilic enough to avoid rapid renal clearance, stand a very high chance of providing efficacy as systemic medicines, even if other kinetic parameters are not optimal.

19.7 *Distribution and protein binding*

Major frustrations can occur in lead optimisation when projects, having spent significant time cycling through numerous iterations of synthesis and testing to optimise potency and clearance, arrive at compounds that appear to be potent *in vitro*, and which possess the desired low clearance *in vivo*, yet still do not work in animal models of efficacy. There are a number of potential causes for this, including the oft over-looked fact that animal models are not always a true reflection of the *in vitro* test, i.e. the pharmacology is incorrect. However, the more probable cause of lack of efficacy in these circumstances is the pattern of tissue distribution of the drug, and more specifically, its binding to plasma and tissue proteins. As mentioned above, the tests of *in vitro* potency usually relate to free drug concentrations in the test wells in a screening campaign. There may be some complicating factors, such as the presence of cell membranes and proteins, but these are usually in low abundance relative to the acting drug concentration, and thus do not exert much influence on the effect seen, which is invariably taken to relate directly to the concentration added. In a sense 'all hell breaks loose' *in vivo*. There are relatively massive amounts of different proteins in the body, which can bind the drug to a greater or lesser extent. In addition, protein mixtures differ between blood/plasma and the tissues it bathes. Consequently, some drugs may be differentially distributed between plasma and tissues on the basis of these protein differences (Figure 19.2). Thus another major discriminatory factor between drugs needs to be faced: the extent to which they bind to proteins. Binding is usually expressed in percentage terms, which describes the fraction of the concentration of drug in plasma that is bound to the plasma proteins. It is commonly accepted that the unbound fraction of drug is the active concentration in pharmacological (and toxicological) terms. It is also the unbound, un-ionised drug concentration that is in diffusion equilibrium throughout the body. Any apparent differences in tissue concentrations relate to the differences in tissue-specific protein binding and in tissue pH, which may cause ionic trapping of drugs. It is vital to understand the fundamental impact this has on apparent efficacy *in vivo*. Take the example of two drugs that are equipotent in *in vitro* tests, and which demonstrate the same concentration in plasma, but which have protein binding values of 99 and 10 per cent, respectively. In the *in vivo* animal models, the former drug will appear to be around 90 times less effective than the latter in dose-level terms (Table 19.1). Differences in protein binding may not be as apparent as the example cited, yet still have a significant effect on the interpretation of efficacy. Thus two equipotent drugs which have protein-binding values of 99 and 99.9 per cent may not appear to be that different on first examination, until it is realised that the free drug concentrations actually differ 10-fold (Table 19.2). Thus it is apparent that protein-binding differences can mask the true potency of molecules *in vivo*.

One major drawback in understanding the impact of protein binding in project support campaigns is the major difficulty in measuring it accurately enough to

TABLE 19.1 *A comparison of the effect of protein binding on the effective dose of two equipotent drugs*

	Drug A	**Drug B**
Potency (ng/ml)	50	500
Vd (l/kg)	0.6	0.6
PPB (%)	99	10
Plasma conc. (ng/ml)	5000	555
Effective d/l (mg/kg)	3.0	0.33

TABLE 19.2 *The importance of minor differences in protein binding on free drug concentrations*

	Drug A	**Drug B**
Potency (ng/ml)	50	50
Vd (l/kg)	0.6	6.0
PPB (%)	99.0	99.9
Plasma conc. (ng/ml)	5000	5000
Effective d/l (mg/kg)	3.0	30

interpret the pharmacokinetic studies. Accurate assessments of protein binding normally require the use of expensive radiolabelled drug, as methods typically use dialysis to equilibrium followed by measurement of free drug concentration. These free drug concentrations are typically very low, especially with lipophilic drugs, where binding is usually high. Thus given the large numbers of molecules emerging in discovery projects, and the impracticalities of radiolabelling them, protein binding is usually confined to the determination of 'rough estimates', denoting whether protein binding is high, medium or low. This is often good enough, however, to focus attention on the fact that protein binding may be having a major impact on efficacy, and whether novel compounds are improving in their efficacy or not.

19.8 *Half-life and duration of action*

One of the principles of lead optimisations studies in DMPK is to fit the pharmacokinetic profile of the compound to its therapeutic purpose. For example, there is little point in spending many months building in metabolic stability to molecules that are targeted to the liver after an oral dose, or are designed for topical effects in lungs. Indeed, in such circumstances systemic metabolic *lability* may be the key kinetic target of the project. It is important, therefore, to give continuing consideration to the impact that a particular kinetic profile, often defined in animal models, will have on the duration of action of a drug, and its consequent therapeutic utility in man. In most disease strategies a 'once a day oral dose' represents an ideal regimen for the therapeutic market place. Given that about 90 per cent of a dose is eliminated within three plasma half-lives of a compound (see Chapter 7), this would suggest that a half-life of about 7–10 hours in man would be ideal to achieve this. This can be written into the product profile of a project as an optimisation target. However, there are several important considerations when aiming at this target. It is important to realise, for example, taking into account species-scaling factors (see Chapter 7), that this 'ideal' half-life in man will be shorter in dog, and much shorter in rat. Thus, for example, a half-life of about 3–4 hours in rat is likely to translate to the ideal profile in man. On the converse, compounds that demonstrate half-lives in double figure in the animal test species may be progressed into candidate selection without a realisation that the half-life in man may be extremely long and wholly inappropriate for efficacy. Compounds which have half-lives in man much in excess of 10–12 hours will show systemic accumulation on daily dosing, as all of the previous day's dose will not be eliminated before a new dose. In extreme cases this can be a serious drawback to both efficacy and adverse event potential. A compound demonstrating a half-life more than 24 hours in man will take longer than four days to reach dosing equilibrium, thus effective treatment may be significantly delayed. The drug will also accumulate in the systemic circulation, to an extent driven by the half-life, and will take longer than that period to be cleared from the system. Thus any adverse events in individual patients may be prolonged.

Plasma half-life is not the only mediator of duration of action. In fact the primary factor of duration will be the relative affinity of the compound for its receptor or enzyme target. In some circumstances compounds may show very high affinity for a receptor yet be eliminated from the systemic circulation rapidly. Compounds of this profile are often described as 'magic bullets', since they achieve efficacy, but limit potentially therapeutic index risking systemic exposure. In these cases, there may be no clearly apparent relationship between plasma half-life (PK) and duration of action (PD). How does a project build lead optimisation strategies when this occurs? These PK–PD relationships can be dissected out from animal data, using so-called 'effect compartment' models (see Chapter 8). However, this exercise depends on good quality data for both PK and PD and thus can be relatively low throughput. The pragmatic course is still to optimise kinetic profile, and half-life, to the 'once a day' regimen mentioned above. An appropriately long half-life guarantees efficacy at the target site; whatever the affinity (on/off rate) of the compound there will always be drug present, due to the half-life.

19.9 *Modifying structures to block metabolism*

Much of the above kinetic profile of project compounds emerges from *in vivo* pharmacokinetic studies carried out in experimental animals and is often a read out of empirical changes made within a series of molecules. Such experiments are low throughput, costly, in that a significant amount of drug has to be synthesised, and time-consuming. A consequence of this is that *in vivo* pharmacokinetic studies are usually focused around compounds that a project team has vested a significant interest in; as discussed earlier, this is often based on *in vitro* potency values as a first principle. It is therefore difficult to be systematic about the assessment of structure–activity surrounding metabolic stability within a project's chemical series *in vivo.* Even with the modern development of cassette dosing of heterologous mixtures of compounds *in vivo* (Berman *et al.*, 1997; Olah *et al.*, 1997; McLoughlin *et al.*, 1997; Frick *et al.*, 1998), which has provided marked increase in the throughput of *in vivo* kinetic studies, the testing of any hypotheses for increasing the stability of project molecules is highly constrained. An added complication of this situation is that tracing the metabolic fate of molecules, and assessing which sites are prone to metabolic attack, is all but impossible *in vivo* unless radiolabelled drug is being used, or significant clearance of the metabolites occurs into the urine. Unfortunately in the absence of excretion balance data, the experimenter will not know whether a particular metabolite identified in the urine is a major route or a minor one. Notwithstanding that caveat, urine should always be taken during *in vivo* experimentation and examined for any metabolic evidence.

The traditional solution to the constraints of *in vivo* throughput has been to invoke *in vitro* studies examining the metabolic fate of compounds using a range of vectors from recombinant enzyme preparations, through liver microsomes, up to whole cells and liver slices (Parkinson, 1996; Carlile *et al.*, 1997; Lave *et al.*, 1997; Eddershaw and Dickins, 1999). This approach has the major advantage of control of the metabolic environment and knowledge of how much compound has been added, and how much remains, over a given period of time. The methodology has also provided a higher throughput than *in vivo* studies, albeit, up until the last four to five years, still not of sufficient capacity to examine the libraries of compounds being produced from modern combinatorial and parallel chemistry methods (Rodrigues, 1997; Tarbit and Berman, 1998). Such *in vitro* studies can provide valuable information about rates and sites of metabolism in a series of molecules, and are particularly good at selecting out compounds that would have poor resistance to metabolic attack *in vivo*. They have two main drawbacks, however, which limit their usefulness: (a) they are generally short-term incubations over an hour or so, and (b) the differences in morphology and physiological conditions between the test tube and the liver mean that projecting any findings *in vitro* to an *in vivo* kinetic outcome is highly risky. In practical terms this means that these approaches are often used as a selection filter prior to *in vivo* studies. Thus compounds that exhibit significant instability over that period can be selected out, as they would be unlikely to show metabolic stability *in vivo.* It is also probable that significant amounts of metabolite will be formed in these circumstances, thereby providing some information on sites of metabolic vulnerability. The drawback, however, is that compounds that are stable over the short incubation period will not guarantee appropriate systemic clearances *in vivo* and will provide little information to guide improvements.

Methods and protocols for *in vitro* studies are now changing rapidly, and with the application of robotics and modern hyphenated techniques involving liquid chromatography, tandem mass spectrometry and NMR, very high-throughput *in vitro* studies, often achieving 1,000 compounds per week, are now possible (Eddershaw and Dickins, 1999; Ekins *et al.*, 2000). It now becomes feasible to take a large diverse set of molecules within a chemical series and examine both their relative stability and, in many cases, their metabolites, leading to information on their vulnerable points of metabolism. The metabolism practitioner can therefore plan low cost, high throughput, experiments that do not need to be focused on potency per se, and which, for example, can examine the impact of structural and physicochemical properties within a series on metabolic stability. As mentioned below, this enhanced capacity has also resulted in a major opportunity for understanding the rules governing metabolism, which begin to suggest the possibility of drug design in the future (Selick *et al.*, 2002).

19.10 *What do we do about inhibitors and inducers?*

In many respects, the drug-metabolising enzymes and drug transporters, which are the main active components contributing to a kinetic profile, are exactly analogous to the enzyme or receptor targets that the compounds are aimed at. They can be inhibited, down regulated, blocked, or induced by administered compounds, dietary or environmental chemicals. In many cases, they have specifically evolved to incorporate adaptive mechanisms that allow the organism to respond to external chemical challenge, or to regulate potent endogenous signalling lipids and steroids. Some classes of enzymes, in particular the cytochromes P-450, show a high degree of overlap in their structural features between those which may be legitimate project targets for therapeutic intervention, e.g. aromatase, thromboxane synthase, cycloxygenase, etc. and those involved in metabolising drugs. In addition to this overlap, heterocycles are a common moiety used in medicinal chemistry, and molecules incorporating a lone pair nitrogen in a heterocycle are potential ligands for the haem domain of cytochrome P-450. It is not surprising, therefore, that projects will often encounter molecules that interact with the broad P-450 catalytic and regulatory mechanisms, thereby altering the expression levels of metabolising enzymes, or inhibiting their activity. Judging the impact of any compounds as inhibitors or inducers of metabolising enzymes needs a combined consideration of the relative selectivity of the compound for its specific target versus the degree of induction and the importance of the therapeutic indication.

In the case of induction, the primary concern is that potent inducers will markedly increase the metabolic clearance of either the drug itself (auto-induction) or of co-administered compounds. The former carries implications for both toxicity testing of the drug (lack of safety cover) and clinical use (decreasing or total loss of efficacy), the latter for clinical and marketing consequences (e.g. increased clearance of oral contraceptives or epilepsy drugs). However, there are mitigating circumstances. Most compounds tend to be fairly weak inducers, and their effects are often associated with the high dose-levels administered in the animal safety tests. The low, therapeutic, dose-levels used in man are often the 'saving grace' of compounds that show clear evidence of induction in rat and dog. In addition, the planned therapeutic use for the drug is a strong context for any evidence of induction with a molecule. Thus, for example, compounds designed for acute or sub-acute administration are not likely to be robbed of their efficacy by virtue of any potential to induce enzymes chronically, even though repeat dose toxicity tests may be complicated by induction seen in the test species. Similarly, compounds that represent the only, or most effective, treatments for life-threatening conditions will still find substantial therapeutic utility in the presence of some induction. It is worth bearing in mind that some of the leading drugs on the market place, including omeprazole (Diaz *et al.*, 1990) and the azole antifungal drugs (Suzuki *et al.*, 2000), show clear evidence of induction in animals and humans without a serious impact on their therapeutic use or marketability.

Inhibition of drug-metabolising enzymes can present more serious complications to the therapeutic use of a drug. There are now a number of well-documented cases where the inhibitory effects of a drug on the clearance of co-administered therapeutic agents have led to serious consequences for patients (Honig *et al.*, 1993; Griffin, 1998; Fung *et al.*, 2001). There is an increasing body of knowledge about which clinically used drugs are metabolised by which particular pathways. Drug metabolism departments are also increasingly armed with tools which can determine the effects of compounds on specific enzymes. Thus, although not wholly prescriptive to any extent as yet, early knowledge of the inhibitory potency of a compound against human enzymes, and which specific pathways are affected, does allow project decision-making to be conducted with some forward knowledge of the potential consequences for therapeutic use or market risk.

So how should projects react when they encounter compounds which show significant induction or inhibition potential? The short answer is with caution. Neither is inherently a reason for terminating interest in a compound sine die, but they may represent a major factor for consideration, among others, when making choices between particular series of compounds, or when deciding which factors to optimise alongside potency. Potential vulnerability on the market place from competitor compounds that may lack any induction or inhibition potential means that they should be avoided if there is a choice.

19.11 *What does the ideal drug look like?*

The obvious answer, from the kinetic viewpoint, is one that has the ideal pharmacokinetic profile for its intended therapeutic use. Assuming a systemic treatment, such a compound might be one that is completely absorbed after oral dosing and undergoes no first pass metabolism, so that the whole dose is available; displays no protein binding, so that all of the drug in the body is in the pharmacologically active form; has a tissue distribution that is limited to total body water, thus keeping the concentrations relatively high, and favours the site of action; and has a half-life that delivers a once-a-day regimen. Such drugs have been designed successfully and have made major impact on therapeutic use in their class (Beresford *et al.*, 1988; Richardson *et al.*, 1990). An additional ideal characteristic would be the 'magic bullet' profile mentioned above; in other words a drug that doped up the target with a high affinity ligand, but was then rapidly eliminated from the rest of the body's systemic circulation, thereby leaving the efficacy without any potential 'non-specific' drug effect complications. Unfortunately 'magic bullets' are extremely difficult to design, given our great lack of knowledge about the relationship between physicochemical properties of compounds and their pharmacokinetic behaviour *in vivo*. It is not surprising, therefore that project support teams tend to be conservative and attempt to build in systemic efficacy by reducing systemic clearance and promoting duration of action via longer half-lives.

The need to optimise on reduced systemic clearance always presents a challenge to project chemists. They have developed a strong cultural background in optimising on potency against the targets, and this obviously is of prime importance. However, the recent perceived need to optimise compounds for kinetic features has added significant complication and can lead to chemical strategies that appear contradictory. Thus, for example, the fastest way towards the 'ideal profile' mentioned above would be by introducing greater polarity into molecules. This would reduce metabolic clearance, promote low volume of distribution, low protein binding and maintain high concentrations of effective drug. The problem is, however, that this runs counter-intuitive to the fact that increasing potency is usually driven by increasing lipophilicity in molecules, the latter promoting increased metabolism, high protein binding and extensive tissue distribution. This situation leads to the need for the metabolic blocking strategies mentioned above and results in the drive to obtain molecules with the best balance of properties. Good kinetic properties are not generally wholly exclusive of good pharmacophores in molecules, but they can take significant time to get into balance.

19.12 *The future*

The role of pharmacokinetic support in drug discovery has expanded exponentially over the past 20 years, and very few large pharmaceutical companies would attempt a programme of drug discovery now without some DMPK input. However, the recent revolutionary changes in combinatorial chemistry methods and the burgeoning high-throughput screening capacity, mentioned above, mean that DMPK optimisation can now represent a significant bottleneck in the discovery process. Realisation of this, and the growing awareness of the value of gaining DMPK and toxicity information at the earliest, and cheapest, phases of drug development, is driving an innovatory wave into drug metabolism departments. We are now entering a phase where the conversion of the relatively low-throughput methods of kinetic and metabolic profiling is being replaced by 'industrialised' screening methods, based on *in vitro* tools that isolate mechanism, whether it be metabolism, permeation or drug transport. The linkage of the high volumes of information derived from these screens with similarly high volumes of physicochemical property determinations, is also opening up the prospect of rules-based modelling and prediction of kinetic outcomes (Lipinski *et al.*, 1997; Selick *et al.*, 2002). It is now possible to see that the future of DMPK input to lead optimisation will not comprise empirical and observational kinetic studies, but will increasingly be driven by informatics and data mining approaches which will lead to predictive models of kinetic outcome in man. The development and refinement of these models will then enable the 'golden age' of drug design, wherein compounds can be designed and virtually screened for kinetic properties *in silico*, before they are even synthesised.

Genetics is another area where revolutionary developments have had a major impact on the pharmaceutical industry, and, again, the DMPK departments cannot stand apart from these changes. The whole basis of the genetics revolution is predicated on the concept of 'right medicine to the right patient at the right time', whereby the patients' individual genotype sets the success criteria for a medicine whose therapeutic target has been clearly defined by genetic analysis. The extra complication in this somewhat ideal scenario is the fact that polymorphism and genetic variability exist in the drug-metabolising enzymes and other factors that underpin a pharmacokinetic profile in a particular patient. Thus 'right medicine to the right patient' needs to encompass a clear understanding of the impact that the 'kinetic genotype' of the patient will have on efficacy. The accelerating drive to bring full disclosure of a compound's properties to the earliest phases of drug discovery, generating so-called 'molecules with a CV', is now also developing with genetics, which is increasingly being seen as the start of the discovery process. The impact on this for DMPK groups, is that they will need to develop higher throughput tools to determine not only metabolic turnover of compounds but also which specific enzymes are involved in those pathways, and whether or not those pathways are polymorphic in one or more of the human ethnic groups. Again, this information will be available to projects that are likely to generate multiple hits and leads, and will enable informed choices to be made on full information, rather than having to put compounds into development to find out the information serially and at significant cost in time and resource.

Overall, the trend for the future is one of a need for increasing amounts of information at earlier phases of the discovery process (Beresford *et al.*, 2002). This is driving a need for increased innovation in automation and informatics, which in turn will enable availability of much more predictive knowledge in DMPK. The implications of this are that companies will need to invest more resources into the discovery support phase, possibly at the expense of the more traditional development phases. However, the compensation will be that the latter groups will need to spend less time 'uncovering' properties of the candidate molecules, as these will already have been determined in early discovery.

19.13 *Summary*

The role of DMPK input in drug discovery has been growing progressively over the past 20 years. Its value has been clearly established such that the leading pharmaceutical companies all now incorporate kinetic input, via sizeable dedicated groups, into the optimisation programmes within projects. The major target of these groups is to obtain the best balance of properties in a molecule that will convert the *in vitro* potency of the compound to an *in vivo* efficacy. Translation failures usually relate to poor absorption and metabolic stability, and these generally comprise the major elements of optimisation, although tissue distribution and protein binding can have fundamental impact. The conduct of optimisation studies has been 'traditional', using protocols that would be recognisable to scientists operating in development mode some 20 years ago. This seems set to change rapidly, as the realisation grows that DMPK and toxicology optimisation represent significant bottlenecks in the modern process. However, these needs also provide great opportunity for DMPK scientists in that they will allow the industry to move from a descriptive, observational mode, born out of a need to provide prescriptive information to regulators, to a more predictive, influencing mode. The latter will increasingly be based on models and simulations that are derived from the high-throughput possibilities of modern DMPK screening. In addition to the change in the traditional methods, new opportunities for these groups are arriving from the recent rapid developments and industrial interest in genetics and surrogates. It is clear, therefore, that the realm of DMPK support for discovery is entering a new era, and the successful companies will be those that harness this rapidly and effectively to drive better drug design.

19.14 *References*

Artursson, P., Palm, K. and Luthman, K. (1996) Caco-2 monolayers in experimental and theoretical predictions of drug transport. *Adv. Drug Deliv. Rev.* 22, 67–84.

Beresford, A.P., McGibney, D., Humphrey, M.J., Macrae, P.V. and Stopher, D.A. (1988) Metabolism and kinetics of amlodipine in man. *Xenobiotica* 19, 245–254.

Beresford, A.P., Selick, H.E. and Tarbit, M.H. (2002) The emerging importance of predictive ADME simulation in drug discovery. *Drug Discov. Today* 7(2), 109–116.

Berman, J., Halm, K., Adkison, K. and Shaffer, J. (1997) Simultaneous pharmacokinetic screening of a mixture of compounds in the dog using API LC/MS/MS analysis for increased throughput. *J. Med. Chem.* 40, 827–829.

Berman, J. and Howard, R.J. (2000) Combinatorial drug discovery: concepts. In: *Combinatorial Chemistry and Molecular Diversity in Drug Discovery*, Gordon, E. and Kerwin, J. (eds) London, Wiley.

Carlile, D.J., Zomorodi, K. and Houston, J.B. (1997) Scaling factors to relate drug metabolic clearance in hepatic microsomes, isolated hepatocytes, and the intact liver – studies with induced livers involving diazepam. *Drug Metab. Dispos.* 25, 903–911.

Diaz, D., Fabre, I., Daujat, M., Saint Aubert, B., Bories, P., Michel, H. and Maurel, P. (1990) Omeprazole is an aryl hydrocarbon-like inducer of human hepatic cytochrome P450. *Gastroenterol.* 99, 737–747.

Eddershaw, P.J., Beresford, A.P. and Bayliss, M.K. (2000) ADME/PK as part of a rational approach to drug discovery. *Drug Discov. Today* 4, 409–414.

Eddershaw, P.J. and Dickins, M. (1999) Advances in in vitro drug metabolism screening. *Pharm. Sci. Technol. Today* 2, 13–19.

Ekins, S., Ring, B.J., Grace, J., McRobie-Belle, D.J. and Wrighton, S.A. (2000) Present and future in vitro approaches for drug metabolism. *J. Pharmacol. Toxicol. Methods* 44, 313–324.

Fung, M., Thornton, A., Mybeck, K., Wu, J.H., Hornbuckle, K. and Muniz, E. (2001) Evaluation of the characteristics of safety withdrawal of prescription drugs from worldwide pharmaceutical markets – 1960 to 1999. *Drug Inf. J.* 35, 293–317.

Frick, L.W., Adkison, K.K., Wells-Knecht, K.J., Woollard, P. and Higton, D.M. (1998) Cassette dosing: rapid in vivo assessment of pharmacokinetics. *Pharm. Technol. Today* 1, 12–19.

Griffin, J.P. (1998) The withdrawal of mibefradil (Posicor). *Adverse Drug React. Toxicol. Rev.* 17, 59–60.

Hidalgo, I.J., Raub, T.J. and Borchardt, R.T. (1989) Characterization of the human colon carcinoma cell line (Caco-2) as a model system for intestinal epithelial permeability. *Gastroenterol.* 96, 736–749.

Honig, P.K., Wortham, D.C., Zamani, K., Conner, D.P., Mullin, J.C. and Cantelina, L.R. (1993) Terfenadine-ketoconazole interaction. Pharmacokinetic and electrocardiographic consequences. *JAMA* 269, 1513–1518.

Humphrey, M.J., Jevons, S. and Tarbit, M.H. (1985) Pharmacokinetic evaluation of UK-49,858, a metabolically stable triazole antifungal drug, in animals and humans. *Antimicrob. Agents Chemother.* 28, 648–653.

Lave, T., Dupin, S., Schmitt, C., Valles, B., Ubeaud, G., Chou, R.C., Jaeck, D. and Coassolo, P. (1997) The use of human hepatocytes to select compounds based on their expected hepatic extraction ratios in humans. *Pharm. Res.* 14, 152–155.

Lin, J.-L. and Lu. A.Y.H. (1997) Role of pharmacokinetics and metabolism in drug discovery and development. *Pharm. Rev.* 49, 403–449.

Lipinski, C.A., Lombardo, F., Dominy, B.W. and Feeney, P.J. (1997) Experimental and computational approaches to estimate solubility and permeability in drug discovery and development settings. *Adv. Drug Deliv. Rev.* 23, 3–25.

McLoughlin, D.A., Olah, T.V. and Gilbert, J.D. (1997) A direct technique for the simultaneous determination of 10 drug candidates in plasma by liquid chromatography atmospheric pressure chemical ionization mass spectrometry interfaced to a Prospekt solid-phase extraction system. *J. Pharm. Biomed. Anal.* 15, 1893–1901.

Olah, T.V., McLoughlin, D.A. and Gilbert, J.D. (1997) The simultaneous determination of mixtures of drug candidates by liquid chromatography/atmospheric pressure chemical ionization mass spectrometry as an in vivo drug screening procedure. *Rapid Commun. Mass Spectrom.* 11, 17–23.

Parkinson, A. (1996) An overview of current cytochrome P-450 technology for assessing the safety and efficacy of new materials. *Toxicol. Pathol.* 24, 45–57.

Richardson, K., Cooper, K., Marriott, M.S., Tarbit, M.H., Troke, P.F. and Whittle, P.J. (1990) Discovery of fluconazole, a novel antifungal agent. Reviews of infectious diseases. 12 (Suppl 3), S267–S271.

Rodrigues, A.D. (1997) Preclinical drug metabolism in the age of high-throughput screening: an industrial perspective. *Pharm. Res.* 14, 1504–1510.

Rubas, W., Cromwell, M.E.M., Mrsny, R.J., Ingle, G. and Elias, K.A. (1996) An integrated method to determine epithelial transport and bioactivity of oral drug candidates in vitro. *Pharm. Res.* 13, 23–26.

Selick, H.E., Beresford, A.P. and Tarbit, M.H. (2002) The emerging importance of predictive ADME simulation in drug discovery. *Drug Discov. Today* 15 January; 7(2), 109–116.

Suzuki, S., Kurata, N., Nishimura, Y., Yasuhara, H. and Satoh, T. (2000) Effects of imidazole antimycotics on the liver microsomal cytochrome P450 isoforms in rats: comparison of in vitro and ex vivo studies. *Eur. J. Drug Metab. Pharmacokinet.* 25, 121–126.

Tarbit, M.H. and Berman, J. (1998) High-throughput approaches for evaluating absorption, distribution, metabolism and excretion properties of lead compounds. *Curr. Opin. Chem. Biol.* 2, 411–416.

Taylor, E.W., Gibbons, J.A., Braeckman, R.A. (1996) Screening of chemical mixtures from combinatorial libraries in the Caco-2 model of intestinal absorption. *Pharm. Res.* 13, S-242.

Index

For Product Safety Concerns and Information please contact our EU representative GPSR@taylorandfrancis.com
Taylor & Francis Verlag GmbH, Kaufingerstraße 24, 80331 München, Germany

www.ingramcontent.com/pod-product-compliance
Ingram Content Group UK Ltd.
Pitfield, Milton Keynes, MK11 3LW, UK
UKHW031042080625
459435UK00013B/559

* 9 7 8 0 3 6 7 3 9 4 4 2 4 *